RN Nursing Care of Children
Review Module Edition 9.0

P9-CNI-745

CONTRIBUTORS

Sheryl Sommer, PhD, RN, CNE
VP Nursing Education & Strategy

Janean Johnson, MSN, RN
Nursing Education Strategist

Karin Roberts, PhD, MSN, RN, CNE
Nursing Education Coordinator

Sharon R. Redding, EdD, RN, CNE
Nursing Education Specialist and Content Project Coordinator

Lois Churchill, MN, RN
Nursing Education Specialist

Carrie B. Elkins, DHSc, MSN, BC
Nursing Education Specialist

Pamela Roland, MSN, RN
Nursing Education Specialist

EDITORIAL AND PUBLISHING

Derek Prater
Spring Lenox
Michelle Renner
Mandy Tallmadge
Kelly Von Lunen

CONSULTANTS

Claire M. Creamer, PhD(c), RN, CPNP-PC
Judy Drumm, DNS, RN, CPN
Christi Glesmann, MSN, RN-BC

Intellectual Property Notice

Important Notice to the Reader

User's Guide

Welcome to the Assessment Technologies Institute® RN Nursing Care of Children Review Module Edition 9.0. The mission of ATI's Content Mastery Series® review modules is to provide user-friendly compendiums of nursing knowledge that will:

- Help you locate important information quickly.

- Assist in your learning efforts.

- Provide exercises for applying your nursing knowledge.

- Facilitate your entry into the nursing profession as a newly licensed RN.

Organization

This review module is organized into units covering the foundations of nursing care of children, nursing care of children with systems disorders, and nursing care of children with special needs. Chapters within these units conform to one of four organizing principles for presenting the content:

- Nursing concepts

- Growth and development

- Procedures

- Systems disorders

Nursing concepts chapters begin with an overview describing the central concept and its relevance to nursing. Subordinate themes are covered in outline form to demonstrate relationships and present the information in a clear, succinct manner.

Procedures chapters include an overview describing the procedure(s) covered in the chapter. These chapters will provide you with nursing knowledge relevant to each procedure, including indications, interpretations of findings, nursing actions, and complications.

Systems disorders chapters include an overview describing the disorder(s) and/or disease process. These chapters may provide information on health promotion and disease prevention before addressing assessments, including risk factors, subjective data, and objective data. Next, you will focus on patient-centered care, including nursing care, medications, teamwork and collaboration, therapeutic procedures, surgical interventions, and care after discharge. Finally, you will find complications related to the disorder, along with nursing actions in response to those complications.

Application Exercises

Questions are provided at the end of each chapter so you can practice applying your knowledge. The Application Exercises include NCLEX-style questions, such as multiple-choice and multiple-select items, and questions that ask you to apply your knowledge in other formats, such as by using an ATI Active Learning Template. After the Application Exercises, an answer key is provided, along with rationales for the answers.

NCLEX® Connections

To prepare for the NCLEX-RN, it is important for you to understand how the content in this review module is connected to the NCLEX-RN test plan. You can find information on the detailed test plan at the National Council of State Boards of Nursing's Web site: https://www.ncsbn.org/. When reviewing content in this review module, regularly ask yourself, "How does this content fit into the test plan, and what types of questions related to this content should I expect?"

To help you in this process, we've included NCLEX Connections at the beginning of each unit and with each question in the Application Exercises Answer Keys. The NCLEX Connections at the beginning of each unit will point out areas of the detailed test plan that relate to the content within the section or unit. The NCLEX Connections attached to the Application Exercises Answer Keys will demonstrate how each exercise fits within the detailed content outline.

These NCLEX Connections will help you understand how the detailed content outline is organized, starting with major client needs categories and subcategories and followed by related content areas and tasks. The major client needs categories are:

- Safe and Effective Care Environment
  - Management of Care
  - Safety and Infection Control
- Health Promotion and Maintenance
- Psychosocial Integrity
- Physiological Integrity
  - Basic Care and Comfort
  - Pharmacological and Parenteral Therapies
  - Reduction of Risk Potential
  - Physiological Adaptation

An NCLEX Connection might, for example, alert you that content within a unit is related to:

- Physiological Adaptation
  - Alterations in Body Systems
    - Identify clinical manifestations and incubation periods of infectious diseases.

QSEN Competencies

As you use the review modules, you will note the integration of the Quality and Safety Education for Nurses (QSEN) competencies throughout the chapters. These competencies are integral components of the curriculum of many nursing programs in the United States and prepare you to provide safe, high-quality care as a newly licensed RN. Icons appear to draw your attention to the six QSEN competencies:

- Safety: The minimization of risk factors that could cause injury or harm while promoting quality care and maintaining a secure environment for clients, self, and others.

- Patient-Centered Care: The provision of caring and compassionate, culturally sensitive care that addresses clients' physiological, psychological, sociological, spiritual, and cultural needs, preferences, and values.

- Evidence-Based Practice: The use of current knowledge from research and other credible sources, on which to base clinical judgment and client care.

- Informatics: The use of information technology as a communication and information-gathering tool that supports clinical decision-making and scientifically based nursing practice.

- Quality Improvement: Care related and organizational processes that involve the development and implementation of a plan to improve health care services and better meet clients' needs.

- Teamwork and Collaboration: The delivery of client care in partnership with multidisciplinary members of the health care team to achieve continuity of care and positive client outcomes.

Icons

Icons are used throughout the review module to draw your attention to particular areas. Keep an eye out for these icons:

  This icon is used for NCLEX connections.

  This icon is used for content related to safety and is a QSEN competency. When you see this icon, take note of safety concerns or steps that nurses can take to ensure client safety and a safe environment.

  This icon is a QSEN competency that indicates the importance of a holistic approach to providing care.

  This icon, a QSEN competency, points out the integration of research into clinical practice.

  This icon is a QSEN competency and highlights the use of information technology to support nursing practice.

  This icon is used to focus on the QSEN competency of integrating planning processes to meet clients' needs.

  This icon highlights the QSEN competency of care delivery using an interprofessional approach.

M This icon indicates that a media supplement, such as a graphic, animation, or video, is available. If you have an electronic copy of the review module, this icon will appear alongside clickable links to media supplements. If you have a hardcopy version of the review module, visit www.atitesting.com for details on how to access these features.

Feedback

ATI welcomes feedback regarding this review module. Please provide comments to: comments@atitesting.com.

TABLE OF CONTENTS

UNIT 1   Foundations of Nursing Care of Children

SECTION: PERSPECTIVES OF NURSING CARE OF CHILDREN

> Family-Centered Nursing Care
> Physical Assessment Findings
> Health Promotion of Infants (1 Month to 1 Year)
> Health Promotion of Toddlers (1 to 3 Years)
> Health Promotion of Preschoolers (3 to 6 Years)
> Health Promotion of School-Age Children (6 to 12 Years)
> Health Promotion of Adolescents (12 to 20 Years)

NCLEX® CONNECTIONS

When reviewing the chapters in this unit, keep in mind the relevant sections of the NCLEX® outline, in particular:

Client Needs: Safety and Infection Control	Client Needs: Health Promotion and Maintenance	Client Needs: Pharmacological and Parenteral Therapies

> Relevant topics/tasks include:
» Accident/Injury Prevention
  > Identify and facilitate correct use of infant and child car seats.
	> Relevant topics/tasks include:
	» Aging Process
	  > Provide care and education for the newborn less than 1 month old through the infant or toddler client through 2 years.
	» Developmental Stages and Transitions
	  > Provide education to clients/staff members about expected age-related changes and age-specific growth and development.
	» Techniques of Physical Assessment
	  > Choose physical assessment equipment and techniques appropriate for the client.
		> Relevant topics/tasks include:
		» Medication Administration
		  > Review pertinent data prior to medication administration (e.g., contraindications, lab results, allergies, potential interactions).

chapter 1

CHAPTER 1   Family-Centered Nursing Care

Overview

- Families are groups that should remain constant in children's lives.
- Family is defined as what an individual considers it to be.
- Families often include individuals with a biological, marital, or adoptive relationship, but in the absence of these characteristics, families also consist of individuals who have a strong emotional bond and commitment to one another.
- Due to the expanding concepts of family, the term household is sometimes used.
- Positive family relationships are characterized by parent-child interactions that show mutual warmth and respect.
- Family-centered nursing care includes the following:
  - Agreed-upon partnerships between families of children, nurses, and providers, in which the families and children benefit.
  - Respecting cultural diversity, and incorporating cultural views in the plan of care.
  - Understanding growth and developmental needs of children and their families.
  - Treating children and their families as clients.
  - Working with all types of families.
  - Collaborating with families regarding hospitalization, home, and community resources.
  - Allowing families to serve as experts regarding their children's health conditions, usual behaviors in different situations, and routine needs.
- Promoting family-centered care
  - Nurses should perform comprehensive family assessments to identify strengths and weaknesses.
    - Characteristics of healthy families
      - Members communicate well and listen to each other.
      - There is affirmation and support for all members.
      - Members teach respect for others.
      - There is a sense of trust.
      - Members play and share humor together.
      - Members interact with one another.
      - There is a shared sense of responsibility.
      - There are traditions and rituals.
      - Members seek help for their problems.
  - Nurses should pay close attention when family members state that a child "isn't acting right" or has other concerns.
  - Children's opinions should be considered when providing care.

Family Theories

THEORY	DESCRIPTION
Family systems	› The family is viewed as a whole system, instead of the individual members. › A change to one member affects the entire system. › The system can both initiate and react to change. › Too much and too little change can lead to dysfunction.
Family stress	› Describes stress as inevitable. › Stressors can be expected or unexpected. › Explains the reaction of a family to stressful events. › Offers guidance for adapting to stress.
Developmental	› Views families as a small group that interacts with the larger social system. › Emphasizes similarities and consistencies in how families develop and change. › Uses Duvall's family life cycle stages to describe the changes a family goes through over time. › How the family functions in one stage has a direct effect on how the family will function in the next stage.

Family Composition

TYPE	MEMBERS
Traditional nuclear family	› Married couple and their biologic children (only full brothers and sisters)
Nuclear family	› Two parents and their children (biologic, adoptive, step, foster)
Single-parent family	› One parent and one or more children
Blended family (also called reconstituted)	› At least one stepparent, stepsibling, or half-sibling
Extended family	› At least one parent, one child, and other individuals either related or not
Gay/lesbian family	› Two members of the same sex who have children and a legal or common-law tie
Foster family	› A child or children who have been placed in an approved living environment away from the family of origin – usually with one or two parents
Binuclear family	› Parents who have terminated spousal roles but continue their parenting roles
Communal family	› Individuals who share common ownership of property and goods and exchange services without monetary consideration

- Changes that occur with the birth (or adoption) of the first child
  - Parents' sense of self as they transition to the new parental role
  - Division of labor and roles within the relationships of couples
  - Relationships with grandparents
  - Work relationships
  - Increased financial responsibilities and possible loss of income
  - Necessary sleep habit changes

Parenting Styles

TYPE	DESCRIPTION	EXAMPLE
Dictatorial or authoritarian	› Parents try to control the child's behaviors and attitudes through unquestioned rules and expectations.	› The child is never allowed to watch television on school nights.
Permissive	› Parents exert little or no control over the child's behaviors, and consult the child when making decisions.	› The child assists with deciding whether or not he will watch television.
Democratic or authoritative	› Parents direct the child's behavior by setting rules and explaining the reason for each rule setting. › Parents negatively reinforce deviations from the rules.	› The child can watch television for 1 hr on school nights after completing all of his homework and chores. › The privilege is taken away but later reinstated based on new guidelines.
Passive	› Parents are uninvolved, indifferent, and emotionally removed.	› The child may watch television whenever he wants.

- Positive parental influences
  - Parents have good mental health.
  - Structure and routine is maintained in the household.
  - Parents engage in activities with the child.
  - There is communication that validates the child's feelings.

  - The child is monitored for safety with special consideration for her developmental needs.
- Guidelines for promoting acceptable behavior in children
  - Set clear and realistic limits and expectations based on the developmental level of the child.
  - Validate the child's feelings, and offer sympathetic explanations.
  - Provide role modeling and reinforcement for appropriate behavior.
  - Focus on the child's behavior when disciplining the child.

Family Assessment

- History – Medical history for parents, siblings, and grandparents
- Structure – Family members (mother, father, son)
- Developmental tasks – Tasks a family works on as the child grows (parents with a school-age child helping her to develop peer relations)
- Family characteristics – Cultural, religious, and economic influences on behavior, attitudes, and actions
- Family stressors – Expected (birth of a child) and unexpected (illness of a child, divorce, disability, or death of a family member) events that cause stress
- Environment – Availability of and family interactions with community resources
- Family support systems – Availability of extended family, work and peer relationships, as well as social systems and community resources to assist the family in meeting needs or adapting to a stressor

APPLICATION EXERCISES

1. A nurse manager on a pediatric floor is preparing an education program on working with families for a group of newly hired nurses. Which of the following should the nurse include when discussing the developmental theory?

    A. Describes that stress is inevitable

    B. Emphasizes that change with one member affects the entire family

    C. Provides guidance to assist families adapting to stress

    D. Defines consistencies in how families change

2. A nurse is assisting a group of parents of adolescents to develop skills that will improve communication within the family. The nurse hears one parent state, "My son knows he better do what I say." Which of the following parenting styles is the parent exhibiting?

    A. Authoritarian

    B. Permissive

    C. Authoritative

    D. Passive

3. A nurse is performing family assessment. Which of the following should the nurse include? (Select all that apply.)

    _____ A. Medical history

    _____ B. Parents' education level

    _____ C. Child's physical growth

    _____ D. Support systems

    _____ E. Stressors

4. A nurse is providing anticipatory guidance to the mother of a toddler. The nurse learns that the household includes the mother, toddler, an older brother, and a grandmother. Use the ATI Active Learning Template: Basic Concept to complete this item to include the following:

    A. Related Content: Describe the composition of this family.

    B. Underlying Principles:
        • Two methods the parent can use to positively influence the child
        • Two ways the parent can promote acceptable behavior in the child

    C. Nursing Interventions: Two additional family assessments the nurse should perform

APPLICATION EXERCISES KEY

1.   A. INCORRECT: The family stress theory describes that stress is inevitable.

     B. INCORRECT: The family systems theory emphasizes that change with one member affects the entire family.

     C. INCORRECT: The family stress theory provides guidance to assist families adapting to stress.

     D. **CORRECT:** The nurse should include that the developmental theory defines consistencies in how families change.

     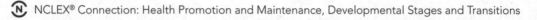 NCLEX® Connection: Health Promotion and Maintenance, Developmental Stages and Transitions

2.   A. **CORRECT:** This parent is exhibiting an authoritarian parenting style. Using this style, the parent controls the adolescent's behaviors and attitudes through unquestioned rules and expectations.

     B. INCORRECT: This parent is not exhibiting a permissive parenting style. Using this style, the parent exerts little or no control over the adolescent's behaviors, and consults the adolescent when making decisions.

     C. INCORRECT: This parent is not exhibiting an authoritative parenting style. Using this style, the parent directs the adolescent's behavior by setting rules and explaining the reason for each rule setting.

     D. INCORRECT: This parent is not exhibiting a passive parenting style. Using this style, the parent is uninvolved, indifferent, and emotionally removed.

     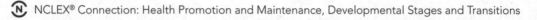 NCLEX® Connection: Health Promotion and Maintenance, Developmental Stages and Transitions

3.   A. **CORRECT:** The nurse should include a medical history on the parents, siblings, and grandparents when performing a family assessment.

     B. **CORRECT:** The nurse should include the family structure, which includes family members, family size, roles/position within the family, and occupation and education of family members, when performing a family assessment.

     C. INCORRECT: The nurse should include the child's physical growth when performing an individual assessment on the child.

     D. **CORRECT:** The nurse should include support systems to determine the availability of extended family, work and peer relationships, and social systems and community resources to assist the family in meeting needs when performing a family assessment.

     E. **CORRECT:** The nurse should include stressors, both expected and unexpected, when performing a family assessment.

     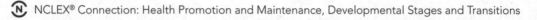 NCLEX® Connection: Health Promotion and Maintenance, Health Promotion/Disease Prevention

4. *Using the ATI Active Learning Template: Basic Concept*

   A. Related Content

   - Family composition: This is an extended family, which includes at least one parent, one or more children, and other individuals who are either related or not related.

   B. Underlying Principles

   - Positive parental influences

     ○ Have good mental health.

     ○ Maintain structure and routine in the household.

     ○ Engage in activities with the child.

     ○ Validate the child's feelings when communicating.

     ○ Monitor for safety concerns with special consideration for the child's developmental needs.

   - Promoting acceptable behavior

     ○ Validate the child's feelings, and offer sympathetic explanations.

     ○ Provide role modeling and reinforcement for acceptable behavior.

     ○ Set clear and realistic limits and expectations based on the child's developmental level.

     ○ Focus on the behavior when implementing discipline.

   C. Nursing Interventions

   - Family assessments

     ○ Medical history on parents, siblings, and grandparents

     ○ Family structure for roles/position within the family, as well as occupation and education of family members

     ○ Developmental tasks a family works on as the child grows

     ○ Family characteristics, such as cultural, religious, and economic influences on behavior, attitudes, and actions

     ○ Family stressors, such as expected (birth of a child) and unexpected (illness of a child, divorce, disability or death of a family member) events that cause stress

     ○ Availability of and family interactions with community resources

     ○ Family support systems, such as availability of extended family, work and peer relationships, as well as social systems and community resources to assist the family in meeting needs or adapting to a stressor

   Ⓝ NCLEX® Connection: Health Promotion and Maintenance, Aging Process

chapter **2**

Overview

- Perform examinations in nonthreatening environments.
- Take time to play and develop rapport prior to beginning an examination.
- Alter exams to accommodate developmental needs.
- Observe for behaviors such as interacting with nurse, making eye contact, permitting physical touch, and willingly sitting on the examination table to determine the child's readiness to cooperate.
- If the child is uncooperative, assess reasons, be firm and direct about expected behavior, complete the assessment quickly, and use a calm voice.
- Involve children and family members in examinations.
- Praise children for cooperation during exams.

Nursing Considerations

- Keep the room warm and well lit.
- Keep medical equipment out of sight.
- Provide privacy. Determine whether older school-age children and adolescents prefer a caregiver to remain during examination.
- Explain each step of the examination to the child.
  - Use age-appropriate language.
  - Demonstrate what will happen using dolls, puppets, or paper drawings.
  - Allow child manipulate and handle equipment.
  - Encourage child to use equipment on others.
- Examine the child in a secure, comfortable position. For example, a toddler may sit on a parent's lap if desired.
- Proceed to examine the child in an organized sequence when possible.
- Encourage the child and/or family to ask questions during physical exams.

Expected Vital Signs

- Temperature

AGE	RECOMMENDED ROUTES	EXPECTED LEVEL
3 months	› Axillary › Rectal (if exact measurement necessary)	37.5° C (99.5° F)
6 months		37.5° C (99.5° F)
1 year		37.7° C (99.9° F)
3 years	› Axillary › Tympanic › Oral (if child cooperative) › Rectal (if exact measurement necessary)	37.2° C (99.0° F)
5 years		37.0° C (98.6° F)
7 years	› Oral › Axillary › Tympanic › Oral	36.8° C (98.2° F)
9 years		36.7° C (98.1° F)
11 years		36.7° C (98.1° F)
13 years		36.6° C (97.9° F)

- Pulse Rate
  - Newborn – 80 to 180/min (depending on activity)
  - 1 week to 3 months – 80 to 220/min (depending on activity)
  - 3 months to 2 years – 70 to 150/min (depending on activity)
  - 2 to 10 years – 60 to 110/min (depending on activity)
  - 10 years and older – 50 to 90/min (depending on activity)
- Respirations
  - Newborn to 1 year – 30 to 35/min
  - 1 to 2 years – 25 to 30/min
  - 2 to 6 years – 21 to 25/min
  - 6 to 12 years – 19 to 21/min
  - 12 years and older – 16 to 19/min

- Blood Pressure
  - Age, height, and gender all influence blood pressure readings. Readings should be compared with standard measurements (National High Blood Pressure Education Program Working Group on High Blood Pressure in Children and Adolescents).
  - Infants – 65 to 80 mm Hg systolic and 40 to 50 mm Hg diastolic
  - The following chart provides examples of expected ranges of blood pressure by age and gender.

	GIRLS		BOYS	
	Systolic (mm Hg)	Diastolic (mm Hg)	Systolic (mm Hg)	Diastolic (mm Hg)
1 year	83 to 114	38 to 67	80 to 114	34 to 66
3 years	86 to 117	47 to 76	86 to 120	44 to 75
6 years	91 to 122	54 to 83	91 to 125	53 to 84
10 years	98 to 129	59 to 88	97 to 130	58 to 90
16 years	108 to 138	64 to 93	111 to 145	63 to 94

Expected Physical Assessment Findings

- General Appearance
  - Appears undistressed
  - Appears clean and well-kept
  - Muscle tone
    - Erect head posture is expected in infants after 4 months of age.
  - Has no body odors
  - Makes eye contact when addressed (except infants)
  - Follows simple commands as age appropriate
  - Uses speech, language, and motor skills spontaneously
  - Growth – Growth can be evaluated using weight, height, body mass index (BMI), and head circumference. Growth charts are tools that can be used to assess the overall health of a child. To see growth charts by age and gender, visit the website for the Centers for Disease Control and Prevention (http://www.cdc.gov).
- Skin, Hair, and Nails
  - Skin
    - Variations in skin color are expected based on race and ethnicity.
    - Temperature should be warm or slightly cool to the touch.
    - Skin turgor exhibits brisk elasticity with adequate hydration.
    - Skin texture should be smooth and slightly dry, not oily.
    - Lesions are not expected findings.
    - Skin folds should be symmetric.

- ○ Hair and Scalp
  - Hair should be evenly distributed, smooth, and strong.
    - □ Manifestations of nutritional deficiencies include hair that is stringy, dull, brittle, and dry.
    - □ Hair loss or balding spots on infants may indicate he is spending too much time in the same position.
  - Assess children approaching adolescence for the presence of secondary hair growth.
  - Scalp should be clean and absent from any scaliness, infestations, and trauma.
- ○ Nails
  - Pink over the nail bed and white at the tips
  - Smooth and firm (but slightly flexible in infants)
  - No clubbing
- • Lymph nodes should be nonpalpable. Lymph nodes that are small, palpable, nontender, and mobile may be an expected finding in children.
- • Head and Neck
  - ○ Head
    - The shape of the head should be symmetric.
    - Fontanels should be flat. The posterior fontanel usually closes between 6 and 8 weeks of age, and the anterior fontanel usually closes between 12 and 18 months of age.
  - ○ Face
    - Symmetric appearance and movement
    - Proportional features
  - ○ Neck
    - Short in infants
    - No palpable masses
    - Midline trachea
    - Full range of motion present whether assessed actively or passively
- • Eyes
  - ○ Visual acuity – May be difficult to assess in children younger than 3 years of age
    - Visual acuity in infants can be assessed by holding an object in front of the eyes and checking to see whether the infant is able to fix on the object and follow it.
    - Use the tumbling E or HOTV test to check visual acuity of children who are unable to read letters and numbers.
    - Older children should be tested using a Snellen chart or symbol chart.
  - ○ Color vision should be assessed using the Ishihara color test or the Hardy-Rand-Rittler test. The child should be able to correctly identify shapes, symbols, or numbers.

- Peripheral visual fields should be
    - Upward 50°
    - Downward 70°
    - Nasally 60°
    - Temporally 90°
- Extraocular movements may not be symmetric in newborns.
    - Corneal light reflex should be symmetric.
    - Cover/uncover test should demonstrate equal movement of the eyes.
    - Six cardinal fields of gaze should demonstrate no nystagmus.
- Eyebrows should be symmetric and evenly distributed from the inner to the outer canthus.
- Eyelids should close completely and open to allow the lower border and most of the upper portion of the iris to be seen.
- Eyelashes should curve outward and be evenly distributed with no inflammation around any of the hair follicles.
- Conjunctiva
    - Palpebral is pink.
    - Bulbar is transparent.
- Lacrimal apparatus is without excessive tearing, redness, or discharge.
- Sclera should be white.
- Corneas should be clear.
- Pupils should be
    - Round
    - Equal in size
    - Reactive to light
    - Accommodating
- Irises should be round with the permanent color manifesting around 6 to 12 months of age.
- Internal Exam
    - Red reflex should be present in infants.
    - Arteries, veins, optic discs, and maculas may be visualized in older children and adolescents.
- Ears
    - Alignment
        - The top of the auricles should meet in an imaginary horizontal line that extends from the outer canthus of the eye.
    - External Ear
        - The external ear should be free of lesions and nontender.
        - The ear canal should be free of foreign bodies or discharge.
        - Cerumen is an expected finding.

- ○ Internal Ear
  - In infants and toddlers, pull the pinna down and back to visualize the tympanic membrane.
  - In children older than 3 years of age, pull the pinna up and back to visualize.
  - The ear canal should be pink with fine hairs.
  - The tympanic membrane should be pearly pink, or gray.
  - The light reflex should be visible.
  - Umbo (tip of the malleolus) and manubrium (long process or handle) are the bony landmarks that should be visible.
- ○ Hearing
  - Newborns should have intact acoustic blink reflexes to sudden sounds.
  - Infants should turn toward sounds.
  - Older children can be screened by whispering a word from behind to see whether they can identify the word.
- Nose
  - ○ The position should be midline.
  - ○ Patency should be present for each nostril without excessive flaring.
  - ○ Internal structures
    - The septum is midline and intact.
    - The mucosa is deep pink and moist with no discharge.
  - ○ Smell can be assessed in older children.
- Mouth and Throat
  - ○ Lips
    - Darker pigmented than facial skin
    - Smooth, soft, moist, and symmetric
  - ○ Gums
    - Coral pink
    - Tight against the teeth
  - ○ Mucous membranes
    - Without lesions
    - Moist, pink, smooth, and glistening
  - ○ Tongue
    - Infants may have white coatings on their tongues from milk that can be easily removed. Oral candidiasis coating is not easily removed.
    - Children and adolescents should have pink, symmetric tongues that they are able to move beyond their lips.
  - ○ Teeth
    - Infants should have six to eight teeth by 1 year of age.
    - Children and adolescents should have teeth that are white and smooth, and begin replacing the 20 deciduous teeth with 32 permanent teeth.

- ○ Hard and soft palates – Intact, firm, and concave
- ○ Uvula – Intact and moves with vocalization
- ○ Tonsils
  - ▪ Infants – May not be able to visualize
  - ▪ Children – Barely visible to prominent, same color as surrounding mucosa, deep crevices that hold food particles
- ○ Speech
  - ▪ Infants – Strong cry
  - ▪ Children and adolescents – Clear and articulate
- Thorax and Lungs
  - ○ Chest shape
    - ▪ Infants – Shape is almost circular with anteroposterior diameter equaling the transverse or lateral diameter.
    - ▪ Children and adolescents – The transverse diameter to anteroposterior diameter changes to 2:1.
  - ○ Ribs and sternum – More soft and flexible in infants; symmetric and smooth, with no protrusions or bulges
  - ○ Movement – Symmetric, no retractions
    - ▪ Infants – Irregular rhythms are common.
    - ▪ Children younger than 7 – More abdominal movement is seen during respirations.
  - ○ Breath sounds
    - ▪ Inspiration is longer and louder than expiration
    - ▪ Vesicular, or soft, swishing sounds, are heard over most of the lungs
  - ○ Breasts
    - ▪ Newborns – Breasts may be enlarged during the first few days.
    - ▪ Children and adolescents – Nipples and areolas are darker pigmented and symmetric.
      - ▫ Females – Breasts typically develop between 10 to 14 years of age. The breasts should appear asymmetric, have no masses, and be palpable.
      - ▫ Males may develop gynecomastia, which is unilateral or bilateral breast enlargement that occurs during puberty.
- Circulatory System
  - ○ Heart sounds – S_1 and S_2 heart sounds should be clear and crisp. S_1 is louder at the apex of the heart. S_2 is louder near the base of the heart. Sinus arrhythmias that are associated with respirations are common. Physiologic splitting of S_2 and S_3 heart sounds are expected findings in some children.
  - ○ Pulses
    - ▪ Infants – Brachial, temporal, and femoral pulses should be palpable, full, and localized.
    - ▪ Children and adolescents – Pulse locations and expected findings are the same as those in adults.

- Abdomen – Without tenderness, no guarding. Peristaltic waves may be visible in thinner children.
  - Shape – Symmetric and without protrusions around the umbilicus
    - Infants and toddlers have rounded abdomens.
    - Children and adolescents should have flat abdomens.
  - Bowel sounds should be heard every 5 to 30 seconds.
- Genitalia
  - Male
    - Hair distribution is diamond shaped after puberty in adolescent males. No pubic hair is noted in infants and small children.
    - Penis
      - Penis should appear straight.
      - Urethral meatus should be at the tip of the penis.
      - Foreskin may not be retractable in infants and small children.
      - Enlargement of the penis occurs during adolescence.
      - The penis may look abnormally small in males who are obese because of skin folds partially covering the base.
    - Scrotum
      - The scrotum hangs separately from the penis.
      - The skin on the scrotum has a rugated appearance and is loose.
      - The left testicle hangs slighter lower than the right.
      - The inguinal canal should be absent of swelling.
      - During puberty, the testes and scrotum enlarge with darker scrotal skin.
  - Female
    - Hair distribution over the mons pubis should be documented in terms of amount and location during puberty. Hair should appear in an inverted triangle. No pubic hair should be noted in infants or small children.
    - Labia – Symmetric, without lesions, moist on the inner aspects
    - Clitoris – Small, without bruising or edema
    - Urethral meatus – Slit-like in appearance with no discharge
    - Vaginal orifice – The hymen may be absent, or it may completely or partially cover the vaginal opening prior to sexual intercourse.
  - Anus – Surrounding skin should be intact with sphincter tightening noted if the anus is touched. Routine rectal exams are not done with the pediatric population.
- Musculoskeletal System
  - Length, position, and size are symmetric.
  - Joints – Stable and symmetric with full range of motion and no crepitus or redness

- Spine
    - Infants – Spines should be without dimples or tufts of hair. They should be midline with an overall C-shaped lateral curve.
    - Toddlers appear squat with short legs and protuberant abdomens.
    - Preschoolers appear more erect than toddlers.
    - Children should develop the cervical, thoracic, and lumbar curvatures like that of adults.
    - Adolescents should remain midline (no scoliosis noted).
- Gait
    - Toddlers and young children – A bowlegged or knock-knee appearance is a common finding. Feet should face forward while walking.
    - Older children and adolescents – A steady gait should be noted with even wear on the soles of shoes.
- Neurologic System
    - Infant Reflexes

REFLEX	EXPECTED FINDING	EXPECTED AGE
Sucking and rooting reflexes	› Elicited by stroking an infant's cheek or the edge of an infant's mouth » The infant turns her head toward the side that is touched and starts to suck.	Birth to 4 months
Palmar grasp	› Elicited by placing an object in an infant's palm » The infant grasps the object.	Birth to 3 months
Plantar grasp	› Elicited by touching the sole of an infant's foot » The infant's toes curl downward.	Birth to 8 months
Moro reflex	› Elicited by allowing the head and trunk of an infant in a semi-sitting position to fall backward to an angle of at least 30° » The infant's arms and legs symmetrically extend, then abduct while fingers spread to form C shape.	Birth to 4 months
Startle reflex	› Elicited by clapping hands or by a loud noise. » The newborn will abduct arms at the elbows, and the hands will remain clenched.	Birth to 4 months
Tonic neck reflex (fencer position)	› Elicited by turning an infant's head to one side » The infant extends the arm and leg on that side and flexes the arm and leg on the opposite side.	Birth to 3 to 4 months
Babinski reflex	› Elicited by stroking the outer edge of the sole of an infant's foot up toward the toes » The infant's toes fan upward and out.	Birth to 1 year
Stepping	› Elicited by holding an infant upright with his feet touching a flat surface » The infant makes stepping movements.	Birth to 4 weeks

○ Cranial Nerves

CRANIAL NERVE	EXPECTED FINDINGS INFANTS	EXPECTED FINDINGS CHILDREN/ADOLESCENTS
I Olfactory	› Difficult to test	› Identifies smells through each nostril individually
II Optic	› Looks at face and tracks with eyes	› Has intact visual acuity, peripheral vision, and color vision
III Oculomotor	› Blinks in response to light › Has pupils that are reactive to light	› Has no nystagmus and PERRLA is intact
IV Trochlear	› Looks at face and tracks with eyes	› Has the ability to look down and in with eyes
V Trigeminal	› Has rooting and sucking reflexes	› Is able to clench teeth together › Detects touch on face with eyes closed
VI Abducens	› Looks at face and tracks with eyes	› Is able to see laterally with eyes
VII Facial	› Has symmetric facial movements	› Has the ability to differentiate between salty and sweet on tongue › Has symmetric facial movements
VIII Acoustic	› Tracks a sound › Blinks in response to a loud noise	› Does not experience vertigo › Has intact hearing
IX Glossopharyngeal	› Has an intact gag reflex	› Has an intact gag reflex › Is able to taste sour sensations on back of tongue
X Vagus	› Has no difficulties swallowing	› Speech clear, no difficulties swallowing › Uvula is midline
XI Spinal Accessory	› Moves shoulders symmetrically	› Has equal strength of shoulder shrug against examiner's hands
XII Hypoglossal	› Has no difficulties swallowing › Opens mouth when nares are occluded	› Has a tongue that is midline › Is able to move tongue in all directions with equal strength against tongue blade resistance

○ Deep tendon reflexes should demonstrate the following:
  ▪ Partial flexion of the lower arm at the biceps tendon
  ▪ Partial extension of the lower arm at the triceps tendon
  ▪ Partial extension of the lower leg at the patellar tendon
  ▪ Plantar flexion of the foot at the Achilles tendon
○ Cerebellar function (children and adolescents)
  ▪ Finger to nose test – Rapid coordinated movements
  ▪ Heel to shin test – Able to run the heel of one foot down the shin of the other leg while standing
  ▪ Romberg test – Able to stand with slight swaying while eyes are closed
○ Language, cognition, and fine and gross motor development can be screened using a standardized tool such as the Denver Developmental Screening Test – Revised (Denver II). A combination of data collected from psychosocial and medical histories and a physical examination is used to determine need and make a referral for further evaluation.

APPLICATION EXERCISES

1. A nurse is preparing to assess a preschool-age child. Which of the following is an appropriate action by the nurse to prepare the child?

    A. Allow the child to role-play using miniature equipment.

    B. Use medical terminology to describe what will happen.

    C. Separate the child from her parent during the examination.

    D. Keep medical equipment visible to the child.

2. A nurse is checking the vital signs of a 3-year-old child during a well-child visit. Which of the following findings should the nurse report to the provider?

    A. Temperature 37.2° C (99.0° F)

    B. Pulse 106/min

    C. Respirations 30/min

    D. Blood pressure 88/54 mm Hg

3. A nurse is assessing a child's ears. Which of the following is an expected finding?

    A. Light reflex is located at the 2 o'clock position.

    B. Tympanic membrane is red in color.

    C. Bony landmarks are not visible.

    D. Cerumen is present bilaterally.

4. A nurse is assessing a 6-month-old infant. Which of the following reflexes should the infant exhibit?

    A. Moro

    B. Plantar grasp

    C. Stepping

    D. Tonic neck

5. A nurse is performing a neurological assessment on an adolescent. Which of the following is an appropriate reaction by the adolescent when the nurse checks the trigeminal cranial nerve? (Select all that apply.)

_____ A. Clenching teeth together tightly

_____ B. Recognizing sour tastes on the back of the tongue

_____ C. Identifying smells through each nostril

_____ D. Detecting facial touches with eyes closed

_____ E. Looking down and in with the eyes

6. A nurse is preparing to examine a preschool-age child. Use the ATI Active Learning Template: Basic Concept to complete this item to include the following:

A. Underlying Principles: Two behaviors that indicate the child is ready to cooperate.

B. Nursing Interventions:

- Two actions to take if child is uncooperative.

- Three actions to promote the child's comfort during the examination.

APPLICATION EXERCISES KEY

1. A. **CORRECT:** The nurse should allow the child to role-play, or manipulate, actual or miniature equipment to reduce the anxiety and fear related to the examination.

    B. INCORRECT: The nurse should use neutral words and avoid overestimating the child's understanding of words when describing what will happen.

    C. INCORRECT: The nurse should encourage parental presence during the examination.

    D. INCORRECT: The nurse should keep medical equipment out of sight unless showing or using it on the child.

    ⓝ NCLEX® Connection: Health Promotion and Maintenance, Aging Process

2. A. INCORRECT: A temperature of 37.2° C (99.0° F) is within the expected reference range for a 3-year-old child and should not be reported to the provider.

    B. INCORRECT: A pulse of 106/min is within the expected reference range for a 3-year-old child and should not be reported to the provider.

    C. **CORRECT:** Respirations of 30/min is above the expected reference range for a 3-year-old child and should be reported to the provider.

    D. INCORRECT: A blood pressure of 90/52 mm Hg is within the expected reference range for a 3-year-old child and should not be reported to the provider.

    ⓝ NCLEX® Connection: Management of Care, Collaboration with Interdisciplinary Team

3. A. INCORRECT: The light reflex should be located around the 5 or 7 o'clock position.

    B. INCORRECT: The tympanic membrane should be a pearly pink, gray color.

    C. INCORRECT: Bony landmarks should be visible.

    D. **CORRECT:** The presence of cerumen bilaterally is an expected finding.

    ⓝ NCLEX® Connection: Reduction of Risk Potential, Potential for Alterations in Body Systems

4.   A. INCORRECT: The moro reflex is exhibited by infants from birth to the age of 4 months.

    B. **CORRECT:** The plantar grasp is exhibited by infants from birth to the age of 8 months.

    C. INCORRECT: The stepping reflex is exhibited by infants from birth to the age of 4 weeks.

    D. INCORRECT: The tonic neck reflex is exhibited by infants from birth to the age of 3 to 4 months.

    (N) NCLEX® Connection: Health Promotion and Maintenance, Developmental Stages and Transitions

5.   A. **CORRECT:** Clenching teeth together tightly is an appropriate reaction by the adolescent when checking the trigeminal cranial nerve.

    B. INCORRECT: Recognizing sour tastes on the back of the tongue is an appropriate reaction by the adolescent when checking the glossopharyngeal cranial nerve.

    C. INCORRECT: Identifying smells through each nostril is an appropriate reaction by the adolescent when checking the olfactory cranial nerve.

    D. **CORRECT:** Detecting facial touches with eyes closed is an appropriate reaction by the adolescent when checking the trigeminal cranial nerve.

    E. INCORRECT: Looking down and in with the eyes is an appropriate reaction by the adolescent when checking the trochlear cranial nerve.

    (N) NCLEX® Connection: Reduction of Risk Potential, System Specific Assessments

6. *Using the ATI Active Learning Template: Basic Concept*

   A. Underlying Principles
- Child is ready to cooperate
  - Interacting with nurse
  - Making eye contact
  - Permitting physical touch
  - Willingly sitting on examination table
  - Accepting and handling equipment

   B. Nursing Interventions
- Actions to take if child is uncooperative
  - Engage both the child and parent.
  - Be firm and direct about expected behavior.
  - Complete the assessment as quickly as possible.
  - Use a calm voice.
  - Reduce environmental stimuli.
  - Limit the people in the room.
- Actions to enhance child's comfort
  - Perform examination in nonthreatening environment.
  - Take time to play and develop rapport prior to beginning the examination.
  - Keep the room warm and well lit.
  - Keep medical equipment out of sight until needed.
  - Provide privacy.
  - Explain each step of the examination to the child.
  - Examine the child in a secure, comfortable position.
  - Examine the child in an organized sequence when possible.
  - Encourage the child and family to ask questions during the examination.

Ⓝ NCLEX® Connection: Health Promotion and Maintenance, Developmental Stages and Transitions

chapter 3

Expected Growth and Development

- Physical Development
  - The infant's posterior fontanel closes by 6 to 8 weeks of age.
  - The infant's anterior fontanel closes by 12 to 18 months of age.
  - Weight, height, and head circumference measurements are used to track the size of infants.
    - Weight – Infants gain approximately 150 to 210 g (about 5 to 7 oz) per week the first 6 months of life. Birth weight is at least doubled by the age of 6 months, and tripled by the age of 12 months.
    - Height – Infants grow approximately 2.5 cm (1 in) per month the first 6 months of life. Growth occurs in spurts after the age of 6 months, and the birth length increases by 50% by the age of 12 months.
    - Head circumference – The circumference of infants' heads increases approximately 1.5 cm (0.6 in) per month for the first 6 months of life, and then approximately 0.5 cm (0.2 in) between 6 and 12 months of age.
  - Dentition – Six to eight teeth should erupt in infants' mouths by the end of the first year of age. The first teeth typically erupt between the ages of 6 and 10 months.
    - Teething pain can be eased using cold teething rings and over-the-counter teething gels. Acetaminophen (Tylenol) and/or ibuprofen (Advil) are appropriate if irritability interferes with sleeping and feeding, but should not be used for more than 3 days. Ibuprofen should be used only in infants over the age of 6 months.
    - Clean infants' teeth using cool, wet washcloths.
    - Bottles should not be given to infants when they are falling asleep because prolonged exposure to milk or juice can cause early childhood caries.

AGE	GROSS MOTOR SKILLS	FINE MOTOR SKILLS
1 month	› Demonstrates head lag	› Has a grasp reflex
2 months	› Lifts head off mattress when prone	› Holds hands in an open position
3 months	› Raises head and shoulders off mattress when prone › Only slight head lag	› No longer has a grasp reflex › Keeps hands loosely open
4 months	› Rolls from back to side	› Places objects in mouth
5 months	› Rolls from front to back	› Uses palmar grasp dominantly
6 months	› Rolls from back to front	› Holds bottle

AGE	GROSS MOTOR SKILLS	FINE MOTOR SKILLS
7 months	› Bears full weight on feet	› Moves objects from hand to hand
8 months	› Sits unsupported	› Begins using pincer grasp
9 months	› Pulls to a standing position › Creeps on hands and knees instead of crawling	› Has a crude pincer grasp
10 months	› Changes from a prone to a sitting position	› Grasps rattle by its handle
11 months	› Walks while holding onto something	› Places objects into a container › Neat pincer grasp
12 months	› Sits down from a standing position without assistance	› Tries to build a two-block tower without success

 View Video: Fine and Gross Motor Development

- Cognitive Development
  - Piaget – Sensorimotor stage (birth to 24 months)
    - Progress from reflexive to simple repetitive to imitative activities.
    - Separation, object permanence, and mental representation are the three important tasks accomplished in this stage.
      - Separation – Infants learn to separate themselves from other objects in the environment.
      - Object permanence – The process by which infants know that an object still exists when it is out of view. This occurs at approximately 9 months of age.
      - Mental representation – The recognition of symbols.
  - Language Development
    - Crying is the first form of verbal communication.
    - Vocalizes with cooing noises.
    - Responds to noises.
    - Turns head to the sound of a rattle.
    - Laughs and squeals.
    - Pronounces single-syllable words.
    - Begins speaking two-word phrases and progresses to speaking three-word phrases.
    - Says three to five words and comprehends "no" by the age of 1 year.
- Psychosocial Development
  - Erikson – Trust vs. Mistrust (birth to 1 year)
    - Achieving this task is based on the quality of the caregiver-infant relationship and the care received.
    - The infant begins to learn delayed gratification.

- Trust is developed by meeting comfort, feeding, stimulation, and caring needs.
- Mistrust develops if needs are inadequately or inconsistently met, or if needs are continuously met before being vocalized by the infant.
  ○ Social Development
    - Social development is initially influenced by infants' reflexive behaviors and includes attachment, separation, recognition/anxiety, and stranger fear.
    - Attachment is seen when infants begin to bond with their parents. This development is seen within the first month, but it actually begins before birth. The process is enhanced when infants and parents are in good health, have positive feeding experiences, and receive adequate rest.
    - Separation-individuation occurs during the first year of life as infants first distinguish themselves and their primary caregiver as separate individuals, and then develop object permanence.
    - Separation anxiety begins around 4 to 8 months of age. Infants will protest when separated from parents, which can cause considerable anxiety for parents.
    - Stranger fear becomes evident between 6 and 8 months of age, when infants are less likely to accept strangers.
    - Reactive attachment disorder results from maladaptive or absent attachment between the infant and primary caregiver, and continues through childhood and adulthood.
  ○ Body-Image Changes
    - Infants discover that mouths are pleasure producers.
    - Hands and feet are seen as objects of play.
    - Infants discover that smiling causes others to react.

- Age-Appropriate Activities
  ○ Play should provide interpersonal contact and educational stimulation.
  ○ Infants have short attention spans and will not interact with other children during play (solitary play). Appropriate toys and activities that stimulate the senses and encourage development include the following.
    - Rattles
    - Teething toys
    - Nesting toys
    - Playing pat-a-cake
    - Playing with balls
    - Reading books
    - Mirrors
    - Brightly colored toys
    - Playing with blocks

Health Promotion

- Immunizations
  - The Centers for Disease Control and Prevention (CDC) immunization recommendations for healthy infants less than 12 months of age (http://www.cdc.gov) include:
    - Birth – Hepatitis B (Hep B)
    - 2 months – Diphtheria and tetanus toxoids and pertussis (DTaP), rotavirus vaccine (RV), inactivated poliovirus (IPV), Haemophilus influenzae type B (Hib), pneumococcal vaccine (PCV), and Hep B
    - 4 months – DTaP, RV, IPV, Hib, PCV
    - 6 months – DTaP, IPV (6 to 18 months), PCV, and Hep B (6 to 12 months); RV; Hib
    - 6 to 12 months – Seasonal influenza vaccination yearly (the trivalent inactivated influenza vaccine (TIV) is available as an intramuscular injection)
- Nutrition
  - Feeding alternatives
    - Breastfeeding provides a complete diet for infants during the first 6 months.
    - Iron-fortified formula is an acceptable alternative to breast milk. Cow's milk is not recommended.
    - It is recommended to begin vitamin D supplements within the first few days of life.
    - Iron supplements are recommended for infants who are being exclusively breastfed after the age of 4 months.
    - Alternative sources of fluids, such as juice or water, are not needed during the first 4 months of life.
    - After the age of 6 months, 100% fruit juice should be limited to 4 to 6 oz per day.
  - Solids are introduced around 4 to 6 months of age.
    - Indicators for readiness include interest in solid foods, voluntary control of the head and trunk, and disappearance of the extrusion reflex.
    - Iron-fortified cereal is typically introduced first due to its high iron content.
    - New foods should be introduced one at a time, over a 4- to 7-day period, to observe for signs of allergy or intolerance, which may include fussiness, rash, vomiting, diarrhea, and constipation.
    - Vegetables or fruits are started first between 6 and 8 months of age. After both have been introduced, meats may be added.
    - Citrus fruits, meat, and eggs are not started until after 6 months of age.
    - Breast milk/formula should be decreased as intake of solid foods increases, but should remain the primary source of nutrition through the first year.
    - Table foods that are cooked, chopped, and unseasoned are appropriate by 9 months of age.
    - Appropriate finger foods include ripe bananas; toast strips; graham crackers; cheese cubes; noodles; and peeled chunks of apples, pears, or peaches.
  - Weaning can be accomplished when infants show signs of readiness, and are able to drink from a cup (sometime in the second 6 months).
    - One meal may be replaced with breast milk or formula in a cup with handles.
    - Bedtime feedings are the last to be stopped.

- Sleep Patterns
  - Nocturnal sleep pattern is established by 3 to 4 months of age.
  - Infant sleeps 14 to 15 hr daily and 9 to 11 hr at night around the age of 4 months.
  - Infant sleeps through the night and takes one to two naps during the day by the age of 12 months.

- Injury Prevention
  - Aspiration of foreign objects
    - Small objects that can become lodged in the throat (grapes, coins, candy) should be avoided.
    - Age-appropriate toys should be provided.
    - Clothing should be checked for safety hazards (loose buttons).
  - Bodily harm
    - Sharp objects should be kept out of reach.
    - Anchor heavy objects and furniture so they cannot be overturned on top of infant.
    - Infants should not be left unattended with any animals present.
  - Burns
    - The temperature of bath water should be checked.
    - Hot water thermostats should be set at or below 49° C (120° F).
    - Working smoke detectors should be kept in the home.
    - Handles of pots and pans should be kept turned to the back of stoves.
    - Sunscreen should be used when infants are exposed to the sun.
    - Electrical outlets should be covered.
  - Drowning
    - Infants should not be left unattended in bathtubs or around water sources such as toilets, cleaning buckets, or drainage areas.
    - Secure fencing around swimming pools.
    - Close bathroom doors.
  - Falls
    - Crib mattresses should be kept in the lowest position possible with the rails all the way up.
    - Restraints should be used in infant seats.
    - Infant seats should be placed on the ground or floor if used outside of the car, and they should not be left unattended or on elevated surfaces.
    - Place safety gates at the top and bottom of stairs.
  - Poisoning
    - Exposure to lead paint should be avoided.
    - Toxins and plants should be kept out of reach.
    - Safety locks should be kept on cabinets that contain cleaners and other household chemicals.
    - The phone number for a poison control center should be kept near the phone.
    - Medications should be kept in childproof containers, away from the reach of infants.
    - A working carbon monoxide detector should be kept in the home.

- ○ Motor-vehicle injuries
  - ▪ Infant-only and convertible infant-toddler car seats are available.
  - ▪ Infants and toddlers remain in a rear-facing car seat until the age of 2 years or the height recommended by the manufacturer.
  - ▪ Safest area for infants and children is the backseat of the car.
  - ▪ Do not place rear-facing car seats in the front seat of vehicles with passenger airbags.
- ○ Suffocation
  - ▪ Plastic bags should be avoided.
  - ▪ Balloons should be kept away from infants.
  - ▪ Crib mattresses should fit snugly.
  - ▪ Crib slats should be no farther apart than 6 cm (2.375 in).
  - ▪ Crib mobiles or crib gyms should be removed by 4 to 5 months of age.
  - ▪ Pillows should be kept out of the crib.
  - ▪ Infants should be placed on their backs for sleep.
  - ▪ Toys with small parts should be kept out of reach.
  - ▪ Drawstrings should be removed from jackets and other clothing.

APPLICATION EXERCISES

1. A nurse is assessing a 12-month-old infant at a well-child visit. Which of the following findings should the nurse report to the provider?

    A. Closed anterior fontanel

    B. Eruption of six teeth

    C. Birth weight doubled

    D. Birth length increased by 50%

2. A nurse is performing a developmental screening on a 10-month-old infant. Which of the following fine motor skills should the infant be able to perform? (Select all that apply.)

    _____ A. Grasp a rattle by the handle

    _____ B. Try building a two-block tower

    _____ C. Use a crude pincer grasp

    _____ D. Place objects into a container

    _____ E. Move objects from hand to hand

3. A nurse is conducting a well-baby visit with a 4-month-old infant. Which of the following immunizations should the nurse administer to the infant? (Select all that apply.)

    _____ A. Measles, mumps, rubella (MMR)

    _____ B. Polio (IPV)

    _____ C. Pneumococcal vaccine (PCV)

    _____ D. Varicella

    _____ E. Rotavirus vaccine (RV)

4. A nurse is providing education about introducing new foods to the parents of a 4-month-old. To best supply needed nutrients, the nurse should recommend that the parents introduce which of the following foods first?

    A. Strained yellow vegetables

    B. Iron-fortified cereals

    C. Pureed fruits

    D. Whole milk

5. A nurse is providing teaching about dental care and teething to the parent of a 9-month-old infant. Which of the following statements by the parent indicates an understanding of the teaching?

    A. "I can give my baby a frozen, fluid-filled teething ring to relieve discomfort."

    B. "I should clean my baby's teeth with a cool, wet wash cloth."

    C. "I can give Advil for up to 5 days while my baby is teething."

    D. "I should dilute juice with water in the bottle my baby drinks while falling asleep."

6. A nurse is preparing an educational program for a group of parents of infants. Use the ATI Active Learning Template: Growth and Development to complete this item to include the following:

    A. Developmental Stage: Identify the infant's developmental stage according to Piaget and Erikson.

    B. Cognitive Development: List two cognitive developmental tasks the infant should accomplish in the first year of life.

    C. Age-Appropriate Activities: List five activities appropriate for infants.

    D. Injury Prevention: Identify two injury prevention methods in each of the following categories.
- Aspiration
- Drowning
- Suffocation
- Poisoning

APPLICATION EXERCISES KEY

1. A. INCORRECT: By the age of 12 to 18 months, the infant's anterior fontanel should close.

    B. INCORRECT: By the age of 12 months, the infant should have six to eight teeth erupted.

    C. **CORRECT:** By the age of 12 months, the infant's birth weight should have tripled. Therefore, the nurse should report this finding to the provider.

    D. INCORRECT: By the age of 12 months, the infant's birth length should increase by 50%.

    Ⓝ NCLEX® Connection: Management of Care, Collaboration with Interdisciplinary Team

2. A. **CORRECT:** The infant should be able to grasp a rattle by the handle at the age of 10 months.

    B. INCORRECT: The infant should try building a two-block tower at the age of 12 months.

    C. **CORRECT:** The infant should be able to use a crude pincer grasp at the age of 9 months.

    D. INCORRECT: The infant should be able to place objects into a container at the age of 11 months.

    E. **CORRECT:** The infant should be able to move objects from hand to hand at the age of 7 months.

    Ⓝ NCLEX® Connection: Health Promotion and Maintenance, Developmental Stages and Transitions

3. A. INCORRECT: The first MMR vaccine is given between the ages of 12 and 15 months.

    B. **CORRECT:** The nurse should administer an IPV vaccine to a 4-month-old infant.

    C. **CORRECT:** The nurse should administer a PCV vaccine to a 4 month-old infant.

    D. INCORRECT: The first varicella vaccine is given at a minimum age of 12 months.

    E. **CORRECT:** The nurse should administer an RV vaccine to a 4-month-old infant.

    Ⓝ NCLEX® Connection: Health Promotion and Maintenance, Health Promotion/Disease Prevention

4. A. INCORRECT: Strained yellow vegetables are not the best source of needed nutrients and should not be the first food introduced.

    B. **CORRECT:** Iron-fortified cereals are the first solid food introduced due to the high iron content. The order of introducing solid foods after this is variable.

    C. INCORRECT: Pureed fruits are not the best source of needed nutrients and should not be the first food introduced.

    D. INCORRECT: Whole milk is not the best source of needed nutrients and should not be the first food introduced.

    Ⓝ NCLEX® Connection: Basic Care and Comfort, Nutrition and Oral Hydration

5. A. INCORRECT: If fluid-filled, the teething ring is kept cold, not frozen.

    B. **CORRECT:** It is appropriate to use a cool, wet wash cloth for cleaning the infant's teeth.

    C. INCORRECT: Ibuprofen (Advil) should not be used for more than 3 days.

    D. INCORRECT: To prevent early childhood caries, infants should not be given bottles while falling asleep.

    (N) NCLEX® Connection: Health Promotion and Maintenance, Health Promotion/Disease Prevention

6. *Using the ATI Active Learning Template: Growth and Development*

    A. Developmental Stage
        - Piaget: Sensorimotor stage
        - Erikson: Trust vs. mistrust

    B. Cognitive Development
        - Progress from reflexive to simple repetitive to imitative activities.
        - Separation: Learning to separate themselves from other objects in the environment.
        - Object permanence: Understanding that an object still exists when it is out of view.
        - Mental representation: Ability to recognize symbols.

    C. Age-Appropriate Activities
        - Rattles
        - Teething toys
        - Nesting toys
        - Playing pat-a-cake
        - Playing with balls
        - Reading books
        - Mirrors
        - Brightly colored toys
        - Playing with blocks

    D. Injury Prevention
        - Aspiration
            - Avoid small objects.
            - Provide age-appropriate toys.
            - Check clothing for hazards such as loose buttons.
        - Poisoning
            - Keep toxins and plants out of reach.
            - Place safety locks on cabinets where cleaners/chemicals are stored.
            - Use a carbon monoxide detector in the home.
            - Keep medications in childproof containers and out of reach.
        - Drowning
            - Do not leave unattended around any water source.
            - Secure fencing around swimming pool.
            - Keep bathroom door closed.
        - Suffocation
            - Avoid plastic bags.
            - Ensure crib mattress fits snugly.
            - Remove crib mobiles by 4 to 5 months of age.
            - Keep pillows out of the crib.
            - Back to sleep

    (N) NCLEX® Connection: Health Promotion and Maintenance, Health Promotion/Disease Prevention

chapter 4

Expected Growth and Development

- Physical Development
  - Anterior fontanels close by 18 months of age.
  - Weight – At 30 months of age, toddlers should weigh four times their birth weights.
  - Height – Toddlers grow about 7.5 cm (3 in) per year.
  - Head circumference and chest circumference are usually equal by 1 to 2 years of age.

AGE	GROSS MOTOR SKILLS	FINE MOTOR SKILLS
15 months	› Walks without help › Creeps up stairs	› Uses a cup well › Builds a tower of two blocks
18 months	› Assumes a standing position › Throws a ball overhand › Jumps up and down with both feet	› Manages a spoon without rotation › Turns pages in a book, two or three at a time
2 years	› Walks up and down stairs by placing both feet on each step	› Builds a tower of six or seven blocks
2.5 years	› Jumps across the floor using both feet and off a chair or step › Stands on one foot momentarily	› Draws circles › Has good hand-finger coordination

- Cognitive Development
  - Piaget – The sensorimotor stage transitions to the preoperational stage around the age of 19 to 24 months.
    - The concept of object permanence becomes fully developed.
    - Toddlers have and demonstrate memories of events that relate to them.
    - Domestic mimicry (playing house) is evident.
    - Preoperational thought does not allow for toddlers to understand other viewpoints, but it does allow them to symbolize objects and people to imitate previously seen activities.
  - Language
    - Language increases to about 300 words by the age of 2 years.
    - 1 year – use one-word sentences, or holophrases
    - 2 years – use multiword sentences by combining two to three words
    - 3 years – combine several words to create simple sentences using grammatical rules

Q
EBP

- Psychosocial Development
  - Erikson – autonomy versus shame and doubt
    - Independence is paramount for toddlers, who are attempting to do everything for themselves.
    - Toddlers often use negativism, or negative responses, as they begin to express their independence.
    - Ritualism, or maintaining routines and reliability, provides a sense of comfort for toddlers as they begin to explore the environment beyond those most familiar to them.
  - Moral Development
    - Moral development is closely associated with cognitive development.
    - Egocentric – Toddlers are unable to see things from the perspectives of others; they can only view things from their personal points of view.
    - Punishment and obedience orientation begin with a sense that good behavior is rewarded and bad behavior is punished.
  - Self-Concept Development
    - Toddlers progressively see themselves as separate from their parents and increase their explorations away from them.
  - Body-Image Changes
    - Toddlers appreciate the usefulness of various body parts.
    - Toddlers develop gender identity by 3 years of age.
- Age-Appropriate Activities
  - Solitary play evolves into parallel play, in which toddlers observe other children and then may engage in activities nearby.

Q
PCC

  - Appropriate activities
    - Filling and emptying containers
    - Playing with blocks
    - Looking at books
    - Push-pull toys
    - Tossing balls
    - Finger paints
    - Large-piece puzzles
    - Thick crayons
  - Temper tantrums result when toddlers are frustrated with restrictions on independence. Providing consistent, age-appropriate expectations helps toddlers to work through frustration.
  - Toilet training can begin when toddlers have the sensation of needing to urinate or defecate. Parents should demonstrate patience and consistency in toilet training. Nighttime control may develop last.
  - Discipline should be consistent with well-defined boundaries that are established to develop appropriate social behavior.

Health Promotion

- Immunizations
  - The Centers for Disease Control and Prevention (CDC) immunization recommendations for healthy toddlers 12 months to 3 years of age (www.cdc.gov) include
    - 12 to 15 months – Inactivated poliovirus (IPV) (third dose between 6 to 18 months); *Haemophilus influenzae* type B (Hib); pneumococcal vaccine (PCV); measles, mumps, and rubella (MMR); and varicella
    - 12 to 23 months – Hepatitis A (Hep A), given in two doses at least 6 months apart
    - 15 to 18 months – Diphtheria and tetanus toxoids and pertussis (DTaP)
    - 12 to 36 months – Yearly seasonal trivalent inactivated influenza vaccine (TIV); live, attenuated influenza vaccine (LAIV) by nasal spray (at 2 years of age)
- Nutrition
  - Children may establish lifetime eating habits during early childhood.
  - Toddlers begin developing taste preferences, and are generally picky eaters who repeatedly request their favorite foods.
  - Physiologic anorexia occurs, resulting in toddlers becoming fussy eaters because of a decreased appetite.
  - Toddlers should consume 24 to 30 oz of milk per day, and may switch from drinking whole milk to drinking low-fat milk after 2 years of age.
  - Juice consumption should be limited to 4 to 6 oz per day.
  - Trans fatty acids and saturated fats should be avoided.
  - Diet should include 1 cup of fruit daily.
  - Food serving size should be 1 tbsp for each year of age, or ¼ to 1/3 of an adult portion.
  - Toddlers generally prefer finger foods because of increasing autonomy.
  - Regular meal times and nutritious snacks best meet nutrient needs.
  - Snacks or desserts that are high in sugar, fat, or sodium should be avoided.
  - Foods that are potential choking hazards (nuts, grapes, hot dogs, peanut butter, raw carrots, tough meats, popcorn) should be avoided.
  - Adult supervision should always be provided during snack and mealtimes.
  - Foods should be cut into small, bite-size pieces to make them easier to swallow and to prevent choking.
  - Toddlers should not be allowed to engage in drinking or eating during play activities or while lying down.
  - Parents should follow the U.S. Department of Agriculture's guidelines (www.choosemyplate.gov).
- Sleep and Rest
  - Toddlers typically average 11 to 12 hr of sleep per day, including one nap.
  - Naps often are eliminated in older toddlerhood.
  - Resistance to bedtime and expression of fears are common in this age group.
  - Maintaining a regular bedtime and bedtime routines are helpful to promote sleep.

- Dental Health
  - Children should have an established dental home by the age of 1 year.
  - Flossing and brushing should be performed by the adult caregiver, and is the best method of removing plaque.
  - Brushing should occur after meals and at bedtime. Nothing to eat or drink, except water, is given to the child after the bedtime cleaning.
  - Fluoride is supplemented for children living in areas without adequate levels in drinking water.
  - Early childhood caries is a form a tooth decay that develops in toddlers, and is more common in children who are put to bed with a bottle of juice or milk.
  - Consumption of cariogenic foods should be eliminated if possible. If not, the frequency of consumption should be limited.
- Injury Prevention
  - Aspiration of foreign objects
    - Small objects (grapes, coins, candy) that can become lodged in the throat should be avoided.
    - Toys that have small parts should be kept out of reach.
    - Age-appropriate toys should be provided.
    - Clothing should be checked for safety hazards (loose buttons).
    - Balloons should be kept away from toddlers.
    - Parents should know emergency procedures for choking.
  - Bodily harm
    - Sharp objects should be kept out of reach.
    - Firearms should be kept in locked boxes or cabinets.
    - Toddlers should not be left unattended with any animals present.
    - Toddlers should be taught stranger safety.
  - Burns
    - The temperature of bath water should be checked.
    - Thermostats on hot water heaters should be turned down to 49° C (120° F) or below.
    - Working smoke detectors should be kept in the home.
    - Pot handles should be turned toward the back of the stove.
    - Electrical outlets should be covered.
    - Toddlers should wear sunscreen when outside.
  - Drowning
    - Toddlers should not be left unattended in bathtubs.
    - Toilet lids should be kept closed.
    - Toddlers should be closely supervised when near pools or any other body of water.
    - Toddlers should be taught to swim.

- ○ Falls
  - Doors and windows should be kept locked.
  - Crib mattresses should be kept in the lowest position with the rails all the way up.
  - Safety gates should be used across the top and bottom of stairs.
- ○ Motor-vehicle injuries
  - Infants and toddlers remain in a rear-facing car seat until the age of 2 years or the height recommended by the manufacturer.
  - Toddlers over the age of 2 years, or who exceed the height recommendations for rear-facing car seats, are moved to a forward-facing car seat.
  - Safest area for infants and children is the backseat of the car.
  - Do not place rear-facing car seats in the front seat of vehicles with deployable passenger airbags.
- ○ Poisoning
  - Exposure to lead paint should be avoided.
  - Safety locks should be placed on cabinets that contain cleaners and other chemicals.
  - The phone number for a poison control center should be kept near the phone.
  - Medications should be kept in childproof containers, away from the reach of toddlers.
  - A working carbon monoxide detector should be placed in the home.
- ○ Suffocation
  - Plastic bags should be avoided.
  - Crib mattresses should fit tightly.
  - Crib slats should be no farther apart than 6 cm (2.375 in).
  - Pillows should be kept out of cribs.
  - Drawstrings should be removed from jackets and other clothing.

APPLICATION EXERCISES

1. A nurse is assessing a 2½-year-old toddler at a well-child visit. Which of the following findings should the nurse report to the provider?

    A. Height increased by 7.5 cm (3 in) in the past year.

    B. Head circumference exceeds chest circumference.

    C. Anterior and posterior fontanels closed.

    D. Current weight equals four times the birth weight.

2. A nurse is performing a developmental screening on an 18 month-old. Which of the following skills should the toddler be able to perform? (Select all that apply.)

    _____ A. Build a tower with six blocks

    _____ B. Throw a ball overhand

    _____ C. Walk up and down stairs

    _____ D. Draw circles

    _____ E. Use a spoon without rotation

3. A nurse is providing teaching about age-appropriate activities to the parent of a 2-year-old. Which of the following statements by the parent indicates a need for further teaching?

    A. "I send my child's favorite stuffed animal when she will be napping away from home."

    B. "Putting large-piece puzzles together is one of my child's favorite activities."

    C. "The soccer team my child will be playing on starts practicing next week."

    D. "My child likes to ride a straddle truck in the dining room while I am cooking."

4. A nurse is providing anticipatory guidance to the parents of a toddler. Which of the following should the nurse include? (Select all that apply.)

    _____ A. Develop food habits that will prevent dental caries.

    _____ B. Meeting caloric needs results in an increased appetite.

    _____ C. Expression of bedtime fears is common.

    _____ D. Behaviors associated with negativism and ritualism.

    _____ E. Importance of annual screenings for phenylketonuria.

5. A nurse is conducting a well-child visit with a 2-year-old. Use the ATI Active Learning Template: Growth and Development to complete this item to include the following:

A. Developmental Stage: Identify the toddler's developmental stage according to Piaget and Erikson.

B. Nutrition: List three concepts to include in teaching with the family.

C. Injury Prevention: Identify two injury prevention methods to include in teaching with the family for each of the following categories.
- Bodily harm
- Drowning
- Burns
- Falls

APPLICATION EXERCISES KEY

1. A. INCORRECT: Toddler height should increase by 7.5 cm (3 in) each year. Therefore, the nurse should not report this finding to the provider.

   B. **CORRECT:** The head and chest circumference should be equal by 1 to 2 years of age, with the chest circumference continuing to increase in size until it exceeds the head circumference. Therefore, the nurse should report this finding to the provider.

   C. INCORRECT: The posterior fontanel closes by the age of 6 to 8 weeks, and the anterior fontanel closes by 12 to 18 months. Therefore, the nurse should not report this finding to the provider.

   D. INCORRECT: The current weight should be four times the birth weight at the age of 2½ years. Therefore, the nurse should not report this finding to the provider.

   Ⓝ NCLEX® Connection: Management of Care, Collaboration with Interdisciplinary Team

2. A. INCORRECT: The toddler should build a tower with six blocks at the age of 2 years.

   B. **CORRECT:** An 18-month-old should be able to throw a ball overhand.

   C. INCORRECT: The toddler should be able to walk up and down stairs by placing both feet on each step at the age of 2 years.

   D. INCORRECT: The toddler should be able to draw circles at the age of 2½ years.

   E. **CORRECT:** An 18-month-old should be able to use a spoon without rotation.

   Ⓝ NCLEX® Connection: Health Promotion and Maintenance, Developmental Stages and Transitions

3. A. INCORRECT: This statement by the parent does not require additional teaching by the nurse. Transitional objects, such as a favorite stuffed animal, provide a sense of security for toddlers.

   B. INCORRECT: This statement by the parent does not require additional teaching by the nurse. Large-piece puzzles are an age-appropriate activity for toddlers.

   C. **CORRECT:** This statement by the parent indicates a need for further teaching. Toddlers continue to develop gross motor skills, and prefer parallel play, where they play alongside of instead of with other children. This will make the concept of team soccer challenging for the toddler.

   D. INCORRECT: This statement by the parent does not require additional teaching by the nurse. Straddle trucks are an age-appropriate activity for toddlers.

   Ⓝ NCLEX® Connection: Health Promotion and Maintenance, Developmental Stages and Transitions

4. A. **CORRECT:** Because the toddler is developing taste preferences, the development of food habits that will prevent dental caries should be included in the anticipatory guidance.

    B. INCORRECT: Toddlers often experience physiologic anorexia and become fussy eaters because of a decreased appetite.

    C. **CORRECT:** Expression of bedtime fears is common for toddlers and should be included in the anticipatory guidance.

    D. **CORRECT:** Negativism and ritualism are exhibited by toddlers as they seek autonomy, and associated behaviors should be included in the anticipatory guidance.

    E. INCORRECT: Screening for phenylketonuria occurs in the newborn, not the toddler.

    Ⓝ NCLEX® Connection: Health Promotion and Maintenance, Aging Process

5. *Using the ATI Active Learning Template: Growth and Development*
    A. Developmental Stage
       - Piaget: Preoperational stage
       - Erikson: Autonomy vs. shame and doubt
    B. Nutrition
       - May switch from whole milk to low fat milk after the age of 2 years.
       - Trans fatty acids and saturated fats should be avoided.
       - Diet should include 1 cup of fruit daily.
       - Limit fruit juice to 4 to 6 oz per day.
       - Cut food into small, bite-size pieces to prevent choking.
       - Do not allow drinking or eating during play activities or while lying down.
    C. Injury Prevention
       - Bodily harm
          ○ Keep sharp objects out of reach.
          ○ Lock firearms in a cabinet or box.
          ○ Teach toddler stranger safety.
          ○ Do not leave toddler unattended with animals.
       - Drowning
          ○ Do not leave toddler unattended in bathtub.
          ○ Keep toilet lids closed.
          ○ Begin teaching toddler water safety and to swim.
          ○ Keep bathroom doors closed.
       - Burns
          ○ Check bath water temperature prior to toddler contact with water.
          ○ Set hot water heaters to 49° C (120° F) or below.
          ○ Keep pot handles pointed to back of stove when cooking.
          ○ Cover electrical outlets.
          ○ Keep working smoke detectors in the home.
          ○ Apply sunscreen when toddler will be outside.
       - Falls
          ○ Keep doors and windows locked.
          ○ Place crib mattresses in lowest position with rails all the way up.
          ○ Use safety gates at the top and bottom of stairs.

    Ⓝ NCLEX® Connection: Health Promotion and Maintenance, Aging Process

chapter 5

Expected Growth and Development

- Physical Development

  - Weight – Preschoolers should gain about 2 to 3 kg (4.4 to 6.6 lb) per year.

  - Height – Preschoolers should grow about 6.5 to 9 cm (2.6 to 3.5 in) per year.

  - Preschoolers' bodies evolve away from the characteristically unsteady wide stances and protruding abdomens of toddlers, into a more graceful, posturally erect, and sturdy physicality.

  - Fine and gross motor skills

    - Preschoolers should show improvement in fine motor skills, which will be displayed by activities like copying figures on paper and dressing independently.

GROSS MOTOR SKILLS BY AGE		
3-year-old	4-year-old	5-year-old
› Rides a tricycle	› Skips and hops on one foot	› Jumps rope
› Jumps off bottom step	› Throws ball overhead	› Walks backward with heel to toe
› Stands on one foot for a few seconds		› Throws and catches a ball with ease

- Cognitive Development

  - Piaget – The preconceptual phase transitions to the phase of intuitive thought around the age of 4 years. The phase of intuitive thought lasts until the age of 7 years.

    - The preschooler moves from totally egocentric thoughts to social awareness and the ability to understand the viewpoints of others.

  - Preschoolers make judgments based on visual appearances. Variations in thinking during this age include:

    - Magical thinking – Thoughts can cause events to occur.

    - Animism – Inanimate objects are alive.

    - Centration – Focus on one aspect instead of considering the whole.

  - Time – Preschoolers begin to understand the sequence of daily events. By the end of the preschool years, children have a better comprehension of time-oriented words.

  - Language Development

    - The vocabulary of preschoolers increases to more than 2,100 words by the end of the fifth year.

    - Preschoolers speak in sentences of three to four words at the ages of 3 and 4 years, and four to five words at the age of 4 to 5 years.

    - This age group enjoys talking, and language becomes their primary method of communication.

Q
EBP

- Psychosocial Development
    - Erikson – initiative vs. guilt
        - Preschoolers become energetic learners, despite not having all of the physical abilities necessary to be successful at everything.
        - Guilt may occur when preschoolers believe they have misbehaved or when they are unable to accomplish a task.
        - Guiding preschoolers to attempt activities within their capabilities while setting limits is appropriate.
    - Moral Development
        - Early preschoolers continue in the good-bad orientation of the toddler years, and actions are taken based on whether or not it will result in a reward or punishment.
        - Older preschoolers primarily take actions based on satisfying personal needs, yet are beginning to understand the concepts of justice and fairness.
    - Self-Concept Development
        - Preschooler feels good about themselves with regard to mastering skills that allow independence (dressing, feeding). During stress, insecurity, or illness, preschoolers may regress to previous immature behaviors or develop habits (nose picking, bedwetting, thumb sucking).
    - Body-Image Changes
        - Preschoolers begin to recognize differences in appearances, and identify what is considered acceptable and unacceptable.
        - By the age of 5 years, preschoolers begin comparing themselves with peers.
        - Poor understanding of anatomy makes intrusive experiences, such as injections or cuts, frightening to preschoolers.
    - Social Development
        - Preschoolers generally do not exhibit stranger anxiety and have less separation anxiety.
        - Prolonged separation, such as during hospitalization, can provoke anxiety.
            - Favorite toys and appropriate play should be used to help ease preschoolers' fears.
        - Pretend play is healthy and allows preschoolers to determine the difference between reality and fantasy.

Q
PCC

- Age-Appropriate Activities
    - Parallel play shifts to associative play during the preschool years. Play is not highly organized, but cooperation does exist between children. Appropriate activities include:
        - Playing ball
        - Putting puzzles together
        - Riding tricycles
        - Playing pretend and dress-up activities
        - Role playing
        - Painting
        - Simple sewing

- Reading books
- Wading pools
- Skating
- Computer programs
- Electronic games

Health Promotion

- Immunizations
  - The Centers for Disease Control and Prevention (CDC) immunization recommendations for healthy preschoolers 3 to 6 years of age (www.cdc.gov) include:
    - 4 to 6 years – diphtheria and tetanus toxoids and pertussis (DTaP); measles, mumps, and rubella (MMR); varicella; and inactivated poliovirus (IPV)
    - 3 to 6 years – yearly seasonal influenza vaccine; trivalent inactivated influenza vaccine (TIV); or live, attenuated influenza vaccine (LAIV) by nasal spray
- Nutrition
  - Preschoolers consume about half the amount of energy that adults do (1,800 kcal).
  - Picky eating may remain a behavior in preschoolers, but often by 5 years of age they become more willing to sample different foods.
  - Preschoolers need 13 to 19 g/day of protein in addition to adequate calcium, iron, folate, and vitamins A and C.
  - Saturated fats should be less than 10% of preschoolers' total caloric intake, and total fat over several days should be 20% to 30% of total caloric intake.
    - Parents should follow the United States Department of Agriculture's healthy diet recommendations (www.choosemyplate.gov).
- Sleep and Rest
  - On average, preschoolers need about 12 hr of sleep per day. Some still require a daytime nap.
  - Sleep disturbances frequently occur during early childhood, and problems range from difficulty going to bed to sleep terrors. Appropriate interventions vary, but may include the following:
    - Keep a consistent bedtime routine.
    - Use a night-light.
    - Reassure preschoolers who are frightened, but avoid allowing preschoolers to sleep with their parents.
- Dental health
  - Eruption of primary teeth is finalized by the beginning of the preschool years.
  - Parents need to assist and supervise brushing and flossing to ensure performed appropriately and prevent dental caries.
  - Trauma to teeth is common in preschool-age children and should be immediately assessed by a dentist.

Q
S

- Injury Prevention
  - Bodily harm
    - Firearms should be kept in locked cabinets or containers.
    - Preschoolers should be taught stranger safety.
    - Preschoolers should be taught to wear protective equipment (helmet, pads).
  - Burns
    - Thermostats should be turned down on hot water heaters.
    - Working smoke detectors should be kept in the home.
    - Preschoolers should have sunscreen applied when outside.
  - Drowning
    - Preschoolers should not be left unattended in bathtubs.
    - Preschoolers should be closely supervised when near the pool or any other body of water.
    - Preschoolers should be taught to swim.
  - Motor-vehicle injuries
    - Preschoolers should use a federally approved car restraint according to the manufacturer recommendations.

Q
EBP

    - When the forward-facing car seat is outgrown, the preschooler transitions to a booster seat.
    - It is recommended that children use an approved car restraint system until they achieve a height of 145 cm (4 feet, 9 in).
    - Safest area for children is the backseat of the car.
    - Supervise preschool-age children when playing outside, and do not allow them to play near a curb or parked cars.
    - Teach pedestrian safety rules to preschool-age children.
      - Stand back from curb while waiting to cross the street.
      - Before crossing the street look left, then right, then left again.
      - Walk on the left, facing traffic, when there are no sidewalks.
      - At night, wear light-colored clothing with fluorescent materials attached.

APPLICATION EXERCISES

1. A nurse is providing teaching about methods to promote sleep to the parent of a preschool-age child. Which of the following statements by the parent indicates an understanding of the teaching?

    A. "I will sleep in the bed with my child if she wakes up during the night."

    B. "I will let my child stay up an additional two hours on weekend nights."

    C. "I will let my child watch television for 30 minutes just before bedtime each night."

    D. "I will keep a dim lamp on in my child's room during the night."

2. A nurse is conducting a well-child visit with a child who is scheduled to receive the recommended immunizations for 4- to 6-year-olds. Which of the following immunizations should the nurse administer? (Select all that apply.)

    _____ A. Diphtheria, tetanus, pertussis (DTaP)

    _____ B. Inactivated poliovirus (IPV)

    _____ C. Measles, mumps, rubella (MMR)

    _____ D. Pneumococcal (PCV)

    _____ E. Haemophilus influenzae type b (Hib)

3. A nurse is preparing an education program about nutrition for preschool-age children for a group of parents. Which of the following should the nurse include?

    A. Saturated fats should equal 20% of total caloric intake.

    B. Average daily intake should be 1,800 calories.

    C. Finicky eating habits develop around 5 years of age.

    D. Healthy diets include 8 g of protein each day.

4. A nurse is performing a developmental screening on a 3-year-old child. Which of the following skills should the child be able to perform?

    A. Ride a tricycle

    B. Hop on one foot

    C. Jump rope

    D. Throw a ball overhead

5. A nurse is caring for a preschool-age child who says she needs to leave the hospital because her doll is scared to be at home alone. Which of the following characteristics of preoperational thought is the child exhibiting?

   A. Egocentrism

   B. Centration

   C. Animism

   D. Magical thinking

6. A nurse is providing anticipatory guidance to the parents of a preschool-age child. Use the ATI Active Learning Template: Growth and Development to complete this item to include the following:

   A. Physical Development: Identify general expectations for height and weight during the preschool years.

   B. Cognitive Development: List two concepts related to language development in preschool-age children.

   C. Age-Appropriate Activities: List five activities appropriate for preschool-age children.

   D. Injury Prevention: Identify two pedestrian safety rules parents should teach children.

APPLICATION EXERCISES KEY

1. A. INCORRECT: The child should not be allowed to sleep in the same bed as the parent. This statement by the parent does not indicate an understanding of the teaching.

    B. INCORRECT: The parent should maintain a consistent bedtime routine and avoid allowing the child to stay up past a reasonable hour. This statement by the parent does not indicate an understanding of the teaching.

    C. INCORRECT: Watching television prior to bed can cause the child to resist and delay sleep. This statement by the parent does not indicate an understanding of the teaching.

    D. **CORRECT:** Leaving a light on in the child's room is an appropriate method to promote sleep for a preschool-age child. This statement by the parent indicates an understanding of the teaching.

    (N) NCLEX® Connection: Basic Care and Comfort, Rest and Sleep

2. A. **CORRECT:** DTaP is a recommended immunization for 4- to 6-year-olds, and should be administered by the nurse.

    B. **CORRECT:** IPV is a recommended immunization for 4- to 6-year-olds, and should be administered by the nurse.

    C. **CORRECT:** MMR is a recommended immunization for 4- to 6-year-olds, and should be administered by the nurse.

    D. INCORRECT: PCV is given as a series of immunizations in the first 15 months of life, and is not recommended for 4- to 6-year-olds.

    E. INCORRECT: Hib is given as a series of immunizations in the first 15 months of life, and is not recommended for 4- to 6-year-olds.

    (N) NCLEX® Connection: Health Promotion and Maintenance, Health Promotion/Disease Prevention

3. A. INCORRECT: Saturated fats should be less than 10% of total caloric intake.

    B. **CORRECT:** Preschool-age children should consume an average of 1,800 calories each day.

    C. INCORRECT: Finicky eating habits are more common during the toddler years, but children often become more willing to try new foods by the age of 5 years.

    D. INCORRECT: Healthy diets include 13 to 19 g of protein each day.

    (N) NCLEX® Connection: Basic Care and Comfort, Nutrition and Oral Hydration

4. A. **CORRECT:** A 3-year-old child should be able to ride a tricycle.

   B. INCORRECT: A 4-year-old child should be able to hop on one foot.

   C. INCORRECT: A 5-year-old child should be able to jump rope.

   D. INCORRECT: A 4-year-old child should be able to throw a ball overhead.

   (N) NCLEX® Connection: Health Promotion and Maintenance, Developmental Stages and Transitions

5. A. INCORRECT: Egocentrism occurs when the child is unable to see another person's perspective.

   B. INCORRECT: Centration occurs when the child focuses on one aspect of something instead of considering the whole.

   C. **CORRECT:** Animism occurs when the child gives living qualities to inanimate objects, such as a doll feeling scared.

   D. INCORRECT: Magical thinking occurs when the child believes their thoughts cause an event to occur.

   (N) NCLEX® Connection: Health Promotion and Maintenance, Developmental Stages and Transitions

6. *Using the ATI Active Learning Template: Growth and Development*

   A. Physical Development
   - Height: Preschoolers should gain about 2 to 3 kg (4.4 to 6.6 lb) per year.
   - Weight: Preschoolers should grow about 6.5 to 9 cm (2.6 to 3.5 in) per year.

   B. Cognitive Development
   - Vocabulary increases to more than 2,100 words by the end of the fifth year.
   - Speak in sentences of three to four words at the ages of 3 and 4 years.
   - Speak in sentences of four to five words at the age of 4 to 5 years.
   - Enjoy talking, and language becomes primary method of communication.

   C. Age-Appropriate Activities
   - Putting puzzles together
   - Playing pretend and dress-up activities
   - Painting
   - Simple sewing
   - Reading books
   - Wading pools
   - Skating
   - Electronic games

   D. Injury Prevention
   - Stand back from curb while waiting to cross the street.
   - Before crossing the street look left, then right, then left again.
   - Walk on the left, facing traffic, when there are no sidewalks.
   - At night, wear light-colored clothing with fluorescent materials attached.

   (N) NCLEX® Connection: Health Promotion and Maintenance, Aging Process

chapter 6

Expected Growth and Development

- Physical Development
  - Weight – School-age children will gain about 2 to 3 kg (4.4 to 6.6 lb) per year.
  - Height – School-age children will grow about 5 cm (2 inches) per year.
  - Prepubescence
    - Preadolescence is typically when prepubescence occurs.
    - Onset of physiologic changes begins around the age of 9 years, particularly in girls.
    - Rapid growth in height and weight occurs.
    - Differences in the rate of growth and maturation between boys and girls becomes apparent.
    - Visible sexual maturation is minimal in boys during preadolescence.
  - Permanent teeth erupt.
    - Bladder capacity differs, but remains greater in girls than boys.
    - Immune system improves.
    - Bones continue to ossify.
- Cognitive Development
  - Piaget – Concrete operations
    - Transitions from perceptual to conceptual thinking
    - Masters the concept of conservation
      - Conservation of mass is understood first, followed by weight, and then volume
    - Learns to tell time
    - Classifies more complex information
    - Able to see the perspective of others
    - Able to solve problems
- Psychosocial Development
  - Erikson– industry vs. inferiority
    - A sense of industry is achieved through the development of skills and knowledge that allows the child to provide meaningful contributions to society.
    - A sense of accomplishment is gained through the ability to cooperate and compete with others.
    - Children should be challenged with tasks that need to be accomplished, and be allowed to work through individual differences in order to complete the tasks.

- Creating systems that reward successful mastery of skills and tasks can create a sense of inferiority in children unable to complete the tasks or acquire the skills.
- Children should be taught that not everyone will master every skill.
  - Moral Development
    - Early school-age years
      - Do not understand the reasoning behind rules and expectations for behavior.
      - Believe what they think is wrong, and what others tell them is right.
      - Judgment is guided by rewards and punishment.
      - Sometimes interpret accidents as punishment.
    - Later school-age years
      - Able to judge the intentions of an act rather than just its consequences.
      - Understand different points of view instead of just whether or not an act is right or wrong.
      - Conceptualizes treating others as they like to be treated.
  - Self-Concept Development
    - School-age children develop an awareness of themselves in relation to others, as well as an understanding of personal values, abilities, and physical characteristics.
    - Confidence is gained through establishing a positive self-concept, which leads to feelings of worthiness and the ability to provide significant contributions.
    - Parents continue to influence the school-age child's self-ideals, but by middle childhood the opinions of peers and teachers become more valuable.
  - Body-Image Changes
    - Solidification of body image occurs.
    - Curiosity about sexuality should be addressed with education regarding sexual development and the reproductive process.
    - School-age children are more modest than preschoolers and place more emphasis on privacy issues.
  - Social Development
    - Peer groups play an important part in social development. Peer pressure begins to take effect.
    - Clubs and best friends are popular.
    - Bullying actions are intended to cause harm or to control someone, and are sometimes attributed to poor relationships with peers and difficulty identifying with a group.
    - Children prefer the company of same-gender companions, but begin developing an interest in the opposite sex toward the end of the school-age years.
    - Most relationships come from school associations.
    - Conformity becomes evident.

- Age-Appropriate Activities
  - Competitive and cooperative play is predominant.
  - Children from 6 to 9 years of age
    - Play simple board and number games.
    - Play hopscotch.

- Jump rope.
- Collect rocks, stamps, cards, coins, or stuffed animals.
- Ride bicycles.
- Build simple models.
- Join organized sports (for skill building).
○ Children from 9 to 12 years of age
  - Make crafts.
  - Build models.
  - Collect things/engage in hobbies.
  - Solve jigsaw puzzles.
  - Play board and card games.
  - Join organized competitive sports.

Health Promotion

- Immunizations
  ○ The Centers for Disease Control and Prevention (CDC) immunization recommendations for healthy school-age children 6 to 12 years of age (www.cdc.gov) include:
    - If not given between 4 and 5 years of age, children should receive the following vaccines by 6 years of age – diphtheria and tetanus toxoids and pertussis (DTaP); inactivated poliovirus (IPV); measles, mumps, and rubella (MMR); and varicella
    - Yearly seasonal influenza vaccine – trivalent inactivated influenza vaccine (TIV) or live, attenuated influenza vaccine (LAIV) by nasal spray
    - 11 to 12 years – tetanus and diphtheria toxoids and pertussis vaccine (Tdap); human papillomavirus vaccine – HPV2 or HPV4 in three doses for females, HPV4 for males; and meningococcal (MCV4).
- Health Screenings
  ○ Scoliosis – School-age children should be screened for scoliosis by examining for a lateral curvature of the spine before and during growth spurts. Screening may take place at schools or at a health care facilities.

 View Video: Scoliosis Screening

- Nutrition
  ○ By the end of the school-age years, children should eat adult portions of food. They need quality nutritious snacks.
  ○ Obesity is an increasing concern of this age group that predisposes children to low self-esteem, diabetes, heart disease, and high blood pressure. Advise parents to:
    - Avoid using food as a reward.
    - Emphasize physical activity.

- Ensure that a balanced diet is consumed by following the U.S. Department of Agriculture's healthy diet recommendations (www.choosemyplate.gov).
- Teach children to make healthy food selections for meals and snacks.
- Avoid eating fast-food frequently.
- Avoid skipping meals.
- Model healthy behaviors.
- Sleep and rest
  - Required sleep is highly variable in the school-age years, and is dependent on the following:
    - Age
    - Level of activity
    - Health status
  - Approximately 9 hours of sleep is needed each night at the age of 12 years.
  - Resistance to bedtime is sometimes experienced around the age of 8 and 9 years, and again around the age of 11 years, but is typically resolved by the age of 12 years.
- Dental health
  - Brush after meals and snacks, and at bedtime.
  - Floss daily.
  - Have regular checkups.
  - If necessary, have regular fluoride treatments.
- Injury Prevention
  - Bodily harm
    - Firearms should be kept in locked cabinets or boxes.
    - Safe play areas should be identified.
    - Stranger safety should be taught.
    - Children should be taught to wear helmets and/or pads when rollerskating, skateboarding, bicycling, riding scooters, skiing, and snowboarding.
  - Burns
    - Children should be taught fire safety and potential burn hazards.
    - Working smoke detectors should be kept in the home.
    - Children should use sunscreen when outside.
    - Teach child safety precautions to take while cooking.
  - Drowning
    - Children should be supervised when swimming or when near a body of water.
    - Children should be taught to swim.
    - Check depth of water before allowing child to dive.
    - Encourage breaks to prevent child from becoming over-tired.

- ○ Motor-vehicle injuries
  - It is recommended that children use an approved car restraint system until they achieve a height of 145 cm (4 feet, 9 inches).
  - Teach children appropriate seat belt use when no longer using a car restraint system or booster seat.
  - Safest area for children is the backseat of the car.
  - Never let child ride in the bed of a pickup truck.
  - Reinforce safe pedestrian behaviors.
- ○ Poisoning/substance abuse
  - Cleaners and chemicals should be kept in locked cabinets or out of reach of younger children.
  - Children should be taught to say "no" to substance abuse.

APPLICATION EXERCISES

1. A nurse is discussing prepubescence and preadolescence with a group of parents of school-age children. Which of the following information should the nurse include in the discussion?

   A. Initial physiologic changes appear during early childhood.

   B. Changes in height and weight occur slowly during this period.

   C. Growth differences between boys and girls become evident.

   D. Signs of sexual maturation become highly visible in boys.

2. A nurse is conducting a well-child visit with a child who is scheduled to receive the recommended immunizations for 11- to 12-year-olds. Which of the following immunizations should the nurse administer? (Select all that apply.)

   _____ A. Trivalent inactivated influenza (TIV)

   _____ B. Pneumococcal (PCV)

   _____ C. Meningococcal (MCV4)

   _____ D. Tetanus and diphtheria toxoids and pertussis (Tdap)

   _____ E. Rotavirus (RV)

3. A nurse is providing education about sleep and rest to a group of parents of school-age children. Which of the following statements by a parent indicates a need for further teaching?

   A. "My child's age influences the number of hours of sleep he needs."

   B. "My child's level of activity during the day influences the number of hours of sleep he needs."

   C. "My child's health status influences the number of hours of sleep he needs."

   D. "My child's family history of sleep apnea influences the number of hours of sleep he needs."

4. A nurse is teaching a course about safety during the school-age years to a group of parents. Which of the following information should the nurse include in the course? (Select all that apply.)

   _____ A. Gating stairs at the top and bottom

   _____ B. Wearing helmets when riding bicycles or skateboarding

   _____ C. Riding safely in bed of pickup trucks

   _____ D. Implementing firearm safety

   _____ E. Wearing seat belts

5. A nurse is providing anticipatory guidance to the parents of a school-age child. Use the ATI Active Learning Template: Growth and Development to complete this item to include the following:

   A. Developmental Stage: Identify the child's developmental stage according to Piaget and Erikson.

   B. Physical Development: Identify three facts relevant to the child's physical development.

   C. Nutrition: List three strategies the family can implement to reduce the risk of obesity.

APPLICATION EXERCISES KEY

1. A. INCORRECT: Initial physiologic changes appear toward the end of middle childhood, around the age of 9 years.

    B. INCORRECT: Changes in height and weight occur rapidly during this time period.

    C. **CORRECT:** The nurse should include in the discussion that growth differences between boys and girls become evident.

    D. INCORRECT: Visible signs of sexual maturation are minimal in boys.

     NCLEX® Connection: Health Promotion and Maintenance, Developmental Stages and Transitions

2. A. **CORRECT:** TIV is a recommended immunization for 11- to 12-year-olds, and should be administered by the nurse.

    B. INCORRECT: PCV is recommended as a series of immunizations in the first 15 months of life, and is not recommended for 11- to 12-year-olds.

    C. **CORRECT:** MCV4 is a recommended immunization for 11- to 12-year-olds, and should be administered by the nurse.

    D. **CORRECT:** Tdap is a recommended immunization for 11- to 12-year-olds, and should be administered by the nurse.

    E. INCORRECT: RV is recommended as a series of immunizations in the first 6 months of life, and is not recommended for 11- to 12-year-olds.

    NCLEX® Connection: Health Promotion and Maintenance, Health Promotion/Disease Prevention

3. A. INCORRECT: The child's age influences the number of hours of sleep he needs. This statement by a parent does not indicate a need for further teaching.

    B. INCORRECT: The child's level of activity during the day influences the number of hours of sleep he needs. This statement by a parent does not indicate a need for further teaching.

    C. INCORRECT: The child's health status influences the number of hours of sleep he needs. This statement by a parent does not indicate a need for further teaching.

    D. **CORRECT:** The child's family history of sleep apnea does not contribute to the number of hours of sleep he needs. This statement by the parent indicates a need for further teaching.

    NCLEX® Connection: Basic Care and Comfort, Rest and Sleep

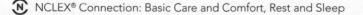

4. A. INCORRECT: Gating stairs at the top and bottom should not be included in the teaching. This is appropriate information to include when teaching about safety during infant and toddler years.

    B. **CORRECT:** The nurse should include information about wearing helmets when riding bicycles or skateboarding when teaching about safety in the school-age years.

    C. INCORRECT: Riding safely in the bed of trucks should not be included in the teaching. The nurse should teach that it is never safe to ride in the bed of a pickup truck.

    D. **CORRECT:** The nurse should include information about implementing firearm safety when teaching about safety in the school-age years.

    E. **CORRECT:** The nurse should include information about wearing seat belts when teaching about safety in the school-age years.

    (N) NCLEX® Connection: Safety and Infection Control, Accident/Error/Injury Prevention

5. *Using the ATI Active Learning Template: Growth and Development*

    A. Developmental Stage
    - Piaget: concrete operations
    - Erikson: industry vs. inferiority

    B. Physical Development
    - Will gain 2 to 3 kg (4.4 to 6.6 lb) per year.
    - Will grow about 5 cm (2 in) per year.
    - Bladder capacity is variable with each child.
    - Immune system improves.
    - Bones continue to ossify.

    C. Nutrition
    - Avoid using food as a reward.
    - Emphasize physical activity.
    - Ensure a balanced diet is consumed.
    - Teach children to select healthy foods and snacks.
    - Avoid eating fast foods frequently.
    - Avoid skipping meals.
    - Model healthy behaviors.

    (N) NCLEX® Connection: Health Promotion and Maintenance, Aging Process

chapter 7

Expected Growth and Development

- Physical Development
  - The final 20% to 25% of height is achieved during puberty.
  - Acne may appear during adolescence.
  - Girls stop growing at about 2 to 2.5 years after the onset of menarche. They grow 5 to 20 cm (2 to 8 in) and gain 7 to 25 kg (15.5 to 55 lb).
  - Boys stop growing at around 18 to 20 years of age. They grow 10 to 30 cm (4 to 12 inches) and gain 7 to 30 kg (15.5 to 66 lb).
  - In girls, sexual maturation occurs in the following order:
    - Breast development
    - Pubic hair growth (some girls experience hair growth before breast development)
    - Axillary hair growth
    - Menstruation
  - In males, sexual maturation occurs in the following order:
    - Testicular enlargement
    - Pubic hair growth
    - Facial hair growth
    - Vocal changes
- Cognitive Development
  - Piaget – formal operations
    - Able to think through more than two categories of variables concurrently
    - Capable of evaluating the quality of their own thinking
    - Able to maintain attention for longer periods of time
    - Highly imaginative and idealistic
    - Increasingly capable of using formal logic to make decisions
    - Think beyond current circumstances
    - Able to understand how the actions of an individual influence others

- Psychosocial Development
  - Erikson – identity vs. role confusion
    - Adolescents develop a sense of personal identity, and come to view themselves as unique individuals.
      - Group identity – Adolescents become part of a peer group that greatly influences behavior.
  - Sexual identity
    - Begins with close, same-sex friendships during early adolescence, which sometimes involve sexual experimentation driven by curiosity.
    - Self-exploration occurs through masturbation.
    - Transition from same-sex friendships to intimate relationships with the opposite sex during middle adolescence.
    - In late adolescence, sexual identity typically is formed through the integration of sexual experiences, feelings, and knowledge.
  - Health perceptions – Adolescents may view themselves as invincible to bad outcomes of risky behaviors.
  - Moral Development
    - Solve moral dilemma using internalized moral principles.
    - Question relevance of existing moral values to society and individuals.
  - Self-Concept Development
    - View themselves in relation to similarities with peers during younger adolescence.
    - View themselves according to their unique characteristics as the adolescent years progress.
  - Body-Image Changes
    - Base their own normality on comparisons with peers.
    - The image established during adolescence is retained throughout life.
  - Social Development
    - Peer relationships develop. These relationships act as a support system for adolescents.
    - Best-friend relationships are more stable and longer-lasting than they were in previous years.
    - Parent-child relationships change to allow a greater sense of independence.

Q PCC
- Age-Appropriate Activities
  - Nonviolent video games
  - Nonviolent music
  - Sports
  - Caring for a pet
  - Career-training programs
  - Reading
  - Social events (going to movies, school dances)

Health Promotion

- Immunizations
  - The Centers for Disease Control and Prevention (CDC) recommendations for healthy adolescents 13 to 18 years of age (www.cdc.gov) include catch-up doses of any recommended immunizations not received at 11 to 12 years of age.
    - Yearly seasonal influenza vaccine – Trivalent inactivated influenza vaccine (TIV) or live, attenuated influenza vaccine (LAIV) by nasal spray.
    - 16 to 18 years – Meningococcal (MCV4) booster is recommended if first dose was received between the ages of 13 and 15 years. A booster dose is not needed if the first dose is received at age 16 or older.
- Health Screenings
  - Screenings for scoliosis should continue during the adolescent years. These screenings should include an examination for a lateral curvature of the spine before and during growth spurts. Screenings may take place at school or at a health care facility.
- Nutrition
  - Rapid growth and high metabolism require increases in quality nutrients, and make adolescents unable to tolerate caloric restrictions.
    - During times of rapid growth, additional calcium, iron, and zinc are needed.
    - Inadequate intake of folic acid, vitamin B_6, vitamin A, iron, calcium, and zinc is common.
  - Both overeating and undereating present special challenges during the adolescent years.
    - Yearly assessments of height, weight, and BMI for age are needed in order to identify nutritional issues and intervene early.
  - Advise parents to:
    - Avoid using food as a reward.
    - Emphasize physical activity.
    - Ensure that a balanced diet is consumed by following the U.S. Department of Agriculture's healthy diet recommendations (www.choosemyplate.gov).
    - Encourage adolescents to make healthy food selections for meals and snacks.
- Sleep and Rest
  - Sleep habits change with puberty due to increased metabolism and rapid growth.
  - Adolescents tend to stay up late, sleep in later in the morning, and sleep more than during the school-age years.
  - During periods of active growth, the need for sleep increases.
- Dental health
  - Corrective appliances are most common with this age group.
  - Brush after meals and snacks, and at bedtime.
  - Floss daily.
  - Have regular checkups.
  - If necessary, have regular fluoride treatments.

- Sexuality
  - Provide adolescents with accurate information and discuss what is heard from peers.
  - Emphasize abstinence and practicing safe sex.
  - Provide information about preventing sexually transmitted infections and pregnancy.
  - Promote an atmosphere where adolescents are comfortable asking questions.
  - Assist adolescents with problem-solving and decision-making skills.

- Injury Prevention
  - Bodily harm
    - Keep firearms unloaded and in a locked cabinet or box.
    - Teach proper use of sporting equipment prior to use.
    - Insist on helmet use and/or pads when roller skating, skateboarding, bicycling, riding scooters, skiing, and snowboarding.
    - Be aware of changes in mood. Monitor for self-harm in adolescents who are at risk. Watch for:
      - Poor school performance
      - Lack of interest in things that were of interest to the adolescent in the past
      - Social isolation
      - Disturbances in sleep or appetite
      - Expression of suicidal thoughts
  - Burns
    - Teach fire safety.
    - Apply sunscreen when outside.
    - Avoid tanning beds.
  - Drowning
    - Teach adolescents to swim.
    - Teach adolescents not to swim alone.
  - Motor-vehicle injuries
    - Encourage attendance at drivers' education courses. Emphasize the need for adherence to seat belt use.
    - Insist on helmet use with bicycles, motorcycles, skateboards, roller skates, and snowboards.
    - Discourage use of cell phones while driving and enforce laws regarding use.
    - Teach the dangers of combining substance abuse with driving.
    - Role model desired behavior.
  - Substance abuse
    - Monitor for signs of substance abuse in adolescents who are at risk.
    - Teach adolescents to say "no" to harmful substances and alcohol.
    - Present a no-tolerance attitude.

APPLICATION EXERCISES

1. A nurse is providing teaching about expected changes during puberty to a group of parents of early adolescent girls. Which of the following statements by one of the parents indicates an understanding of the teaching?

    A. "Girls usually stop growing about 2 years after menarche."

    B. "Girls are expected to gain about 65 pounds during puberty."

    C. "Girls experience menstruation prior to breast development."

    D. "Girls typically grow more than 10 inches during puberty."

2. A nurse is providing anticipatory guidance to the parent of a 13-year-old. The nurse should recommend which of the following screenings for the adolescent? (Select all that apply.)

    _____ A. Body mass index

    _____ B. Blood lead level

    _____ C. Height

    _____ D. Weight

    _____ E. Scoliosis

3. A nurse is caring for an adolescent whose mother expresses concerns about her son sleeping such long hours. The nurse should inform the mother that additional sleep is needed during adolescence due to which of the following?

    A. Sleep terrors

    B. Rapid growth

    C. Elevated zinc levels

    D. Slowed metabolism

4. A nurse is teaching a class about puberty in males. Which of the following should the nurse include as the first manifestation of sexual maturation?

    A. Pubic hair growth

    B. Vocal changes

    C. Testicular enlargement

    D. Facial hair growth

5. A nurse is preparing an educational program for a group of parents of adolescents. Use the ATI Active Learning Template: Growth and Development to complete this item to include the following:

A. Developmental Stage: Identify adolescent developmental stages according to Piaget and Erikson.

B. Cognitive Development: List five cognitive developmental tasks the adolescent should accomplish.

C. Injury Prevention: Identify three injury prevention methods in each of the following categories:
   • Bodily harm
   • Motor vehicle injuries

APPLICATION EXERCISES KEY

1. A. **CORRECT:** Girls usually stop growing about 2 years after menarche. This statement by the parent indicates and understanding of the teaching.

    B. INCORRECT: Girls are expected to gain 7 to 25 kg (15.5 to 55 lb) during puberty. This statement by the parent does not indicate an understanding of the teaching.

    C. INCORRECT: Breast development is usually the first manifestation of sexual maturity in girls, and appears before menstruation. This statement by the parent does not indicate an understanding of the teaching.

    D. INCORRECT: Girls typically grow 5 to 20 cm (2 to 8 in) during puberty. This statement by the parent does not indicate an understanding of the teaching.

    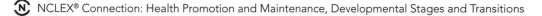 NCLEX® Connection: Health Promotion and Maintenance, Developmental Stages and Transitions

2. A. **CORRECT:** The nurse should recommend that the adolescent have a body mass index screening annually.

    B. INCORRECT: Blood lead level screenings are recommended for children at the age of 1 and 2 years, and for children between the ages of 3 and 6 years who have not previously been screened.

    C. **CORRECT:** The nurse should recommend that the adolescent have a height screening annually.

    D. **CORRECT:** The nurse should recommend that the adolescent have a weight screening annually.

    E. **CORRECT:** The nurse should recommend that the adolescent have a scoliosis screening annually.

    NCLEX® Connection: Health Promotion and Maintenance, Health Screening

3. A. INCORRECT: Sleep terrors occur most often in preschool-age children, and do not contribute to the adolescent's need for additional sleep.

    B. **CORRECT:** Rapid growth during the adolescent years results in the need for additional sleep.

    C. INCORRECT: Zinc levels do not typically elevate during the adolescent years, and do not contribute to the adolescent's need for additional sleep. Zinc is often identified as a deficient due to inadequate dietary intake during adolescence.

    D. INCORRECT: An increased metabolism contributes to the adolescent's need for additional sleep.

    NCLEX® Connection: Basic Care and Comfort, Rest and Sleep

4.   A. INCORRECT: Pubic hair appears during early puberty, but is not the first manifestation of sexual maturation in males.

   B. INCORRECT: Vocal changes occur after the appearance of pubic hair, typically in early to midpuberty, and are not the first manifestation of sexual maturation in males.

   C. **CORRECT:** Testicular enlargement is the first manifestation of sexual maturation in males.

   D. INCORRECT: Facial hair growth typically appears about 2 years after pubic hair, and is not the first manifestation of sexual maturation in males.

   Ⓝ NCLEX® Connection: Health Promotion and Maintenance, Developmental Stages and Transitions

5.   *Using the ATI Active Learning Template: Growth and Development*

   A. Developmental Stage
   • Piaget: formal operations
   • Erikson: identity vs. role confusion

   B. Cognitive Development
   • Able to think through more than two categories of variables concurrently
   • Capable of evaluating the quality of own thinking
   • Able to maintain attention for longer periods of time
   • Highly imaginative and idealistic
   • Increasingly capable of using formal logic to make decisions
   • Think beyond current circumstances
   • Understand how the actions of an individual influence others

   C. Injury Prevention
   • Bodily injury
     ○ Keep firearms unloaded and in a locked cabinet or box.
     ○ Teach proper use of sporting equipment prior to use.
     ○ Insist on helmet use and/or pads when roller skating, skateboarding, bicycling, riding scooters, skiing, and snowboarding.
     ○ Be aware of changes in mood. Continuously monitor adolescents at risk for self harm.
   • Motor vehicle injuries
     ○ Encourage attendance at drivers' education courses.
     ○ Emphasize the need for adherence to seat belt use.
     ○ Discourage use of cell phones while driving and enforce laws regarding use.
     ○ Teach the dangers of combining substance abuse with driving.
     ○ Role model desired behavior.

   Ⓝ NCLEX® Connection: Health Promotion and Maintenance, Aging Process

UNIT 1   FOUNDATIONS OF NURSING CARE OF CHILDREN

SECTION: SPECIAL CONSIDERATIONS OF NURSING CARE OF CHILDREN

› Safe Administration of Medication
› Pain Management
› Hospitalization, Illness, and Play
› Death and Dying

NCLEX® CONNECTIONS

When reviewing the chapters in this unit, keep in mind the relevant sections of the NCLEX® outline, in particular:

Client Needs: Psychosocial Integrity

› Relevant topics/tasks include:
  » End-of-Life Care
    › Recognize the need for and provide psychosocial support to family/caregiver.
  » Grief and Loss
    › Evaluate the client's coping and fears related to grief and loss.

Client Needs: Basic Care and Comfort

› Relevant topics/tasks include:
  » Nonpharmacological Comfort Interventions
    › Assess client need for pain management.

Client Needs: Pharmacological and Parenteral Therapies

› Relevant topics/tasks include:
  » Dosage Calculation
    › Perform calculations needed for medication administration.
  » Medication Administration
    › Educate the client about medications.
  » Pharmacological Pain Management
    › Administer and document pharmacological pain management appropriate for the client's age and diagnoses.

Client Needs: Health Promotion and Maintenance

› Relevant topics/tasks include:
  » Developmental Stages and Transitions
    › Assess impact of change on family system.

chapter 8

Overview

- Growth and organ system maturity affect the metabolism and excretion of medications in infants and children.

- Administration of medications to the pediatric population can be challenging, and requires that a nurse be patient and creative.

- Pediatric dosages are based on age, body weight, and body surface area (BSA).

Assessment

- Medication and food allergies

- Appropriateness of medication dose for the child's age and weight

- Child's developmental age

- Tissue and skin integrity when administering IM, subcutaneous, and topical medications

- IV patency when administering IV medications

Nursing Interventions

- Medication Administration

  - Calculate the safe dosage for medication.

  - Notify the provider if medication dosage is determined to be outside the safe dosage range, and for any questions about medication preparation or route.

  - Double-check high-risk and facility-regulated medications with a second nurse.

  - Perform the six rights of medication administration.

  - Use two client identifiers prior to administration: client name and date of birth. Use parent(s) for verification of infants or nonverbal children. However, two identifiers from the ID band must be confirmed: client name, date of birth, or hospital identification number.

  - Determine parental involvement with administration.

  - Allow the child to make appropriate choices regarding administration (choosing the left or right leg, whether the parent or nurse will administer the medication).

  - Prepare the child according to the developmental stage and age.

- Oral Medication
  - This route of medication administration is preferred for children.
  - Determine the child's ability to swallow pills.
  - Use the smallest measuring device for doses of liquid medication. Use an oral medication syringe for smaller amounts, and a medication cup for larger amounts.
  - Avoid measuring liquid medication in a teaspoon or tablespoon.
  - Avoid mixing medication with formula or putting it in a bottle of formula because the infant may not take the entire feeding, and the medication may alter the taste of the formula.
  - Hold the infant in a semireclining position similar to a feeding position.
  - Hold the small child in an upright position to prevent aspiration.
  - Administer the medication in the side of the mouth in small amounts. This allows the infant or child to swallow.
  - Only use the droppers that come with the medication for measurement.
  - Stroke the infant under the chin to promote swallowing while holding cheeks together.
  - Teach the child to swallow tablets that aren't available in liquid form and can't be crushed.
    - Teach in short sessions using verbal instruction, demonstration, and positive reinforcement.
  - Provide atraumatic care.
    - Mix the medication in a small amount of sweet fluid.
    - Offer juice, a soft drink, or snack after administration.
    - Have the child pinch her nose before, during, and shortly after administration.
    - Add flavoring to medications.
    - Use a nipple to allow the infant to suck the medication.
  - Administer medications via a feeding tube.
    - Confirm placement.
    - Use liquid formulation.
    - Do not add medication to the formula bag.
    - Flush with water to clear tubing of residual medication.
- Optic Medication
  - Place the child in a supine or sitting position.
  - Extend head and ask the child to look up.
  - Pull the lower eye lid downward and apply medication in the pocket.
  - Administer ointments before nap or bedtime.
  - Provide atraumatic care.
    - If infants clinch their eyes closed, place the drops in the nasal corner. When the infant opens his eyes, the medication will enter the eye.
    - Apply light pressure to the lacrimal punctum for 1 minute to prevent unpleasant taste.
    - Play games with younger children.

- Otic Medication
  - Place the child in a prone or supine position with the affected ear upward.
  - Children younger than 3 years: pull the pinna downward and straight back.
  - Children older than 3 years: pull the pinna upward and back.
  - Provide atraumatic care.
    - Allow refrigerated medications to warm to room temperature prior to administration.
    - Massage the outer area for a few minutes following administration.
    - Play games with younger children.
- Nasal Medication
  - Position the child with the head extended.
  - Use a football hold for infants.
  - Provide atraumatic care.
    - Insert the tip into the naris vertically, then angle it prior to administration.
    - Play games with younger children.
- Aerosol Medication
  - Use mask for younger children.
  - Provide atraumatic care.
    - Allow parents to hold during treatment.
    - Use distraction.
- Rectal Medication
  - Insert beyond both rectal sphincters.
  - Hold the buttocks gently together for 5 to 10 minutes.
  - Halve the medication lengthwise, if necessary.
  - Provide atraumatic care.
    - Perform the procedure quickly.
    - Use distraction.
- Injection Medications
  - Change needle if it pierced a rubber stopper on a vial.
  - Secure the infant and child prior to injections.
  - Assess the need for assistance.
  - Avoid tracking of medication.
  - When selecting sites, consider:
    - Medication amount, viscosity, and type.
    - Muscle mass, condition, access of site, and potential for contamination.
    - Treatment course and number of injections.
    - Age and size of child.

- Intradermal
  - ○ Administer on the inside surface of the forearm.
  - ○ Use a TB syringe with a 26- to 30-gauge needle with an intradermal bevel.
  - ○ Insert needle at a 15° angle.
  - ○ Do not aspirate.
- Subcutaneous (SQ)
  - ○ Give anywhere there is SQ tissue. Common sites are the lateral aspect of the upper arm, abdomen, and anterior thigh.
  - ○ Inject volumes of less than 0.5 mL.
  - ○ Use a 1 mL syringe with a 26- to 30-gauge needle.
  - ○ Insert at a 90° angle. Use a 45° angle for children who are thin.
  - ○ Check policy for aspiration practices.
- Intramuscular (IM)
  - ○ Use a 22- to 25-gauge, ½- to 1-inch needle.
  - ○ Vastus lateralis is the recommended site in infants and small children.
    - Position the child supine, side lying, or sitting.
    - Inject up to 0.5 mL for infants.
    - Inject up to 2 mL in children.
  - ○ Ventrogluteal
    - Position the child supine, side lying, or prone.
    - Inject 0.5 to 1.0 mL depending on muscle size of infant.
    - Inject up to 2 mL in children.
  - ○ Deltoid
    - Position the child sitting or standing.
    - Inject up to 1 mL.
  - ○ Provide atraumatic care
    - Apply eutectic mixture of lidocaine and prilocaine (EMLA) to the site for 60 min prior to injection.
    - Change needle after puncturing a rubber stopper.
    - Use the smallest gauge of needle possible.
    - Secure the child firmly to decrease movement of the needle while injecting.
    - Use distraction.
    - Use play therapy.
    - Offer sucrose pacifiers to infants.

View Video: Pediatric IM Injections

- Intravenous (IV) Medications
  - Peripheral venous access devices
    - Use a 24- to 20-gauge catheter.
    - Use for continuous and intermittent IV medication administration.
    - A child who requires short-term IV therapy may complete it at home with the assistance of a home health nurse.
  - Central venous access devices
    - Short term: nontunneled catheter or peripherally inserted central catheters (PICC)
    - Long term: tunneled catheter or implanted infusion ports
  - Provide atraumatic care
    - Decide to insert a PICC before multiple peripheral attempts.
    - Use a transilluminator to assist in vein location.
    - Avoid terminology such as a "bee sting" or "stick."
    - Attach an extension tubing to decrease movement of the catheter.
    - Use play therapy.
    - Apply EMLA to the site for 60 minutes prior to attempt.
    - Keep equipment out of site until procedure begins.
    - Perform procedure in a treatment room.
    - Use nonpharmacologic therapies.
    - Allow parents to stay if they prefer.
    - Use therapeutic holding.
    - Avoid using the dominant or sucking hand.
    - Cover site with a colorful wrap.
    - Swaddle infants.
    - Offer nonnutritive sucking to infants before, during, and after the procedure.

APPLICATION EXERCISES

1. A nurse is planning to administer the influenza vaccination to a toddler. Which of the following is an appropriate action for the nurse to take?

    A. Administer subcutaneously in the abdomen.

    B. Use a 20-gauge needle.

    C. Divide the medication into two injections.

    D. Place the child in the supine position.

2. A nurse is preparing to administer an intramuscular (IM) injection to a child. Which of the following muscle groups is contraindicated?

    A. Deltoid

    B. Ventrogluteal

    C. Vastus lateralis

    D. Dorsal gluteal

3. A nurse is teaching a parent of an infant about administration of oral medications. Which of the following should the nurse include in the teaching? (Select all that apply.)

    _____ A. Use a universal dropper for medication administration.

    _____ B. Ask the pharmacy to add flavoring to the medication.

    _____ C. Add the medication to the formula bottle before feeding.

    _____ D. Use the nipple of the bottle to administer the medication.

    _____ E. Hold the infant in an semireclining position.

4. A nurse is preparing to administer medication to a toddler. Which of the following are appropriate actions for the nurse to take? (Select all that apply.)

    _____ A. Identify the toddler by asking the parent.

    _____ B. Tell the parent to administer the medication.

    _____ C. Calculate the safe dosage.

    _____ D. Ask the toddler what toy he wants to hold during administration.

    _____ E. Offer juice after the medication.

5. A nurse is caring for an infant who needs otic medication. Which of the following is an appropriate action for the nurse to take?

    A. Hold the infant in an upright position.

    B. Pull the pinna downward and straight back.

    C. Hyperextend the infant's neck.

    D. Ensure that the medication is cool.

6. A nurse is planning to initiate IV access for a toddler. What actions should the nurse plan to take? Use the ATI Active Learning Template: Basic Concepts to complete this item to include Nursing Interventions: Describe 10 atraumatic care interventions.

APPLICATION EXERCISES KEY

1. A. INCORRECT: The influenza vaccination is administered IM.

    B. INCORRECT: A 22- to 25-gauge needle is recommended for IM injections.

    C. INCORRECT: The total volume of the influenza vaccination is 0.5 mL, which can be administered in the vastus lateralis.

    D. **CORRECT:** The vastus lateralis is recommended for administering IM medications. Therefore, placing the toddler in a supine position is the appropriate action for the nurse to take.

    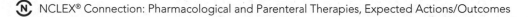 NCLEX® Connection: Pharmacological and Parenteral Therapies, Expected Actions/Outcomes

2. A. INCORRECT: The deltoid muscle can be used once developed for IM injections in children for medication containing up to 1 mL of fluid.

    B. INCORRECT: The ventrogluteal muscle can be used for IM injections in children for medication containing up to 2 mL of fluid.

    C. INCORRECT: The vastus lateralis muscle can be used for intramuscular injections in children for medication containing up to 2 mL of fluid.

    D. **CORRECT:** The dorsal gluteal site has major nerves and blood vessels and is not a recommended site for IM injections for children.

    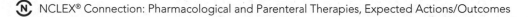 NCLEX® Connection: Pharmacological and Parenteral Therapies, Expected Actions/Outcomes

3. A. INCORRECT: Medication has different viscosities, and droppers do not have a standard opening. Therefore, a universal dropper is not an accurate way to measure medications.

    B. **CORRECT:** Multiple flavorings are available to add to medications and can assist in masking the taste.

    C. INCORRECT: Because an infant may not finish an entire bottle of formula, it is not recommended to add medication to the bottle.

    D. **CORRECT:** Administering medications through an empty nipple may assist with successful administration of the medication.

    E. **CORRECT:** For successful medication administration, the infant should be held in a semireclining position, similar to feeding.

    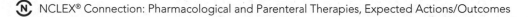 NCLEX® Connection: Pharmacological and Parenteral Therapies, Medication Administration

4. A. INCORRECT: For safe medication administration, confirm two identifiers by looking at the identification band or having the toddler state his name and date of birth.

    B. INCORRECT: The nurse should assess the preferred level of involvement of the parents prior to medication administration.

    C. **CORRECT:** For safe medication administration, the nurse should calculate safe dosage prior to administering medication.

    D. **CORRECT:** Offering choices to the toddler is an example of atraumatic care.

    E. **CORRECT:** Offering juice after the medication is an example of atraumatic care.

    (N) NCLEX® Connection: Pharmacological and Parenteral Therapies, Medication Administration

5. A. INCORRECT: Position the infant supine or prone for administration of otic medication.

    B. **CORRECT:** Pulling the pinna downward and straight back will straighten the ear canal to allow medication to flow into the ear.

    C. INCORRECT: Hyperextending the infant's neck could occlude the airway and should not be performed during otic medication administration.

    D. INCORRECT: Allowing the otic medication to warm up to room temperature is recommended to provide atraumatic care.

    (N) NCLEX® Connection: Pharmacological and Parenteral Therapies, Medication Administration

6. *Using the ATI Active Learning Template: Basic Concepts*

    - Nursing Interventions
        - Decide to insert a peripherally inserted catheter before multiple peripheral attempts.
        - Use a transilluminator to assist in vein location.
        - Avoid terminology such as a "bee sting" or "stick."
        - Attach extension tubing to decrease movement of the catheter.
        - Use play therapy.
        - Apply eutectic mixture of lidocaine and prilocaine (EMLA) to the site for 60 minutes prior to attempts.
        - Keep equipment out of sight until procedure begins.
        - Perform the procedure in a treatment room.
        - Use nonpharmacologic therapies.
        - Allow parents to stay if they prefer.
        - Use therapeutic holding.
        - Avoid using the dominant or sucking hand.
        - Cover site with a colorful wrap.
        - Swaddle infants.
        - Offer nonnutritive sucking to infants before, during, and after the procedure.

    (N) NCLEX® Connection: Basic Care and Comfort, Non-Pharmacological Comfort Interventions

UNIT 1   FOUNDATIONS OF NURSING CARE OF CHILDREN
         SECTION: SPECIAL CONSIDERATIONS OF NURSING CARE OF CHILDREN

CHAPTER 9   Pain Management

Overview

- Assessment of pain depends on the child's cognitive, emotional, and physical development.
- Atraumatic care is the use of interventions that minimize or eliminate physical and psychological distress.
- Pain is managed by atraumatic, nonpharmacological, and pharmacological interventions.

Influential Factors

- Influential factors that can have a positive or negative effect on pain perception include:
  - Age
  - Development stage
  - Chronic or acute disease
  - Prior experiences with pain
  - Personality
  - Family dynamics
  - Culture
  - Socioeconomic status

Nursing Assessment

 View Video: Pain Assessment in Children

- Subjective and Objective Data
  - Developmental Characteristics
    - Young infant
      - Loud cry
      - Rigid body or thrashing
      - Local reflex withdrawal from pain stimulus
      - Expressions of pain (eyes tightly closed, mouth open in a squarish shape, eyebrows lowered and drawn together)
      - Lack of association between stimulus and pain

- Older infant
  - Loud cry
  - Deliberate withdrawal from pain
  - Facial expression of pain
- Toddler
  - Loud cry or screaming
  - Verbal expressions of pain
  - Thrashing of extremities
  - Attempt to push away or avoid stimulus
  - Noncooperation
  - Clinging to significant person
  - Behaviors occur in anticipation of painful stimulus
- School-age child
  - Stalling behavior
  - Muscular rigidity
  - Any behaviors of the toddler, but less intense in the anticipatory phase and more intense with painful stimulus
- Adolescent
  - More verbal expressions of pain with less protest
  - Muscle tension with body control
- Pain Intensity
  - Assessment includes behavioral measures, physiologic measures, and self-report.
  - Self-report is used for children older than 4 years of age. Children under 4 are unable to accurately report their pain.
  - Multiple tools have been developed and researched as reliable.
  - A nurse should choose an appropriate pain tool that will adequately assess the infant or child's pain.
  - Include the parent or caregiver in rating the infant or child's pain.
  - Assess the location, quality, and severity of pain.

PAIN ASSESSMENT TOOL FOR EVALUATION BY AGE

FLACC (2 months to 7 years)

> Pain rated on a scale of 0 to 10.

> Assess behaviors of the child.

> Face (F)

0 – Smile or no expression	1 – Occasional frown or grimace, withdrawn	2 – Frequent or constant frown, clenched jaw, quivering chin

> Legs (L)

0 – Relaxed or normal position	1 – Uneasy, restless, tense	2 – Kicking or legs drawn up

> Activity (A)

0 – Lying quietly, moves easily, normal position	1 – Squirming, shifting, tense	2 – Arched, ridged, or jerking

> Cry (C)

0 – No cry	1 – Moans or whimpers, occasional complaints	2 – Crying, screaming, sobbing, frequent complaints

> Consolability (C)

0 – Content or relaxed	1 – Reassured by occasional touching, or hugging. Able to distract	2 – Difficult to console or comfort

FACES (3 years and older)

> Pain rated on a scale of 0 to 5 using a diagram of six faces.

> Substitute 0, 2, 4, 6, 8, 10 for 0 to 5 to convert to the 0 to 10 scale.

> Explain each face to the child; ask the child to choose a face that best describes how they are feeling.

0 – No hurt	2 – Hurts a little more	4 – Hurts a whole lot
1 – Hurts a bit	3 – Hurts even more	5 – Hurts worst

Oucher (3 to 13 years)

> Pain rated on a scale of 0 to 5 using six photographs.

> Substitute 0, 2, 4, 6, 8, 10 for 0 to 5 to convert to the 0 to 10 scale.

> Have the child organize the photographs in order of no pain to the worst pain; ask the child to choose a picture that best describes how they are feeling.

0 – No hurt	2 – Hurts a little more	4 – Hurts a whole lot
1 – Hurts a bit	3 – Hurts even more	5 – Hurts worst

PAIN ASSESSMENT TOOL FOR EVALUATION BY AGE			
Numeric scale (5 years and older)			
› Pain rated on a scale of 0 to 10.			
› Explain to the child that 0 means "no pain" and 10 means "worst pain."			
› Have the child verbally report a number or point to their level of pain on a visual scale.			
Non-communicating children's pain checklist (3 to 18 years)			
› Behaviors are observed for 10 min.			
› Six subcategories are scored on a scale 0 to 3.			
› Subcategories are vocal, social, facial, activity, body and limbs, and physiological, each with observable behaviors to be scored.			
0 – Not at all	1 – Just a little	2 – Fairly often	3 – Very often
› Cutoff scores			
11 or higher indicates moderate to severe pain.		6 to 10 indicates mild pain.	

Nursing Interventions

- Reassess the child's pain level frequently.
- Use nonpharmacological, pharmacological, or both approaches to manage pain.
- Ask parent or caregiver to reassess the child's pain level.
- Ask the parent or caregiver their satisfaction of the pain management.
- Assess child for adverse reactions to pain medications.
- Review laboratory reports.
- Assess child's physical functioning following pain management intervention.
- Assess for negative affect or distress the child might be experiencing related to the pain, such as anxiety, withdrawal, fear, depression, or unhappiness.
- Atraumatic measures
  - Use a treatment room for painful procedures.
  - Avoid procedures in "safe places" such as the play room and the child's bed.
  - Use developmentally appropriate terminology when explaining procedures.
  - Offer choices to the child.
  - Allow parents to stay with child during painful procedures.
  - Use play therapy to explain procedures, allowing the child to perform the procedure on a doll or toy.
- Pharmacological measures
  - Optimal dosage of medications will control pain without causing severe adverse effects.
  - Select the least traumatic route for medication administration.
  - Give medications routinely, versus PRN (as needed), to manage pain that is expected to last for an extended period of time.
  - Combine adjuvant medications (steroids, antidepressants, sedatives, antianxiety medications, muscle relaxants, anticonvulsants) with other analgesics.

○ Use nonopioid and opioid medications.

■ Acetaminophen (Tylenol) and NSAIDs are acceptable for mild to moderate pain.

■ Opioids are acceptable for moderate to severe pain. Medications used include morphine sulfate, oxycodone (OxyContin), and fentanyl (Duragesic).

■ Combining a nonopioid and an opioid medication treats pain peripherally and centrally. This offers greater analgesia with less adverse effects (respiratory depression, constipation, nausea).

○ IM injections are not recommended for pain control in children.

○ Intranasal medications are not recommended for children younger than 18 years.

○ Rectal medications have variable absorption rates, and children dislike them.

○ Intradermal medications are used for skin anesthesia prior to procedures.

• Appropriate Routes

ROUTE	NURSING IMPLICATIONS
Oral	› Route is preferred due to convenience, cost, and ability to maintain steady blood levels. › Take 1 to 2 hr to reach peak analgesic effects. Oral medications are not suited for children experiencing pain that requires rapid relief or pain that is fluctuating in nature.
Topical/ transdermal	› Eutectic mixture of local anesthetics (EMLA) contains equal quantities of lidocaine and prilocaine in the form of a cream or disk. » Used for any procedure in which the skin will be punctured (IV insertion, biopsy) 60 min prior to a superficial puncture and 2.5 hr prior to a deep puncture. » Place an occlusive dressing over the cream after application. » Prior to procedure, remove the dressing or disk and clean the skin. Indication of an adequate response is reddened or blanched skin. » Demonstrate to the child that the skin is not sensitive by tapping or scratching lightly. » Instruct parents to apply EMLA at home prior to coming to a health care facility for the procedure. › Fentanyl » Use for children older than 12 years of age. » Use to provide continuous pain control. Onset of 12 to 24 hr and a duration of 72 hr. » Use an immediate-release opioid for breakthrough pain. » Treat respiratory depression with naloxone (Narcan).
Intravenous IV	› Bolus » Rapid pain control in approximately 5 min » Use for medications such as morphine, hydromorphone › Continuous = provides steady blood levels › Patient-controlled analgesia (PCA) » Self-administration of pain medication » Can be basal, bolus, or combination » Has lockouts to prevent overdosing › Family-controlled analgesia » Same concept as PCA » Parent or caregiver manages the child's pain

Q
PCC

- Nonpharmacological Measures
  - Strategies
    - Distraction
      - Use play, radio, computer game, movie.
      - Tell jokes or a story to the child.
    - Relaxation
      - Hold or rock the infant or young child.
      - Assist older children into a comfortable position.
      - Assist with breathing techniques.
    - Guided imagery
      - Assist the child in an imaginary experience.
      - Have the child describe the details.
    - Positive self-talk
      - Have the child say positive things during a procedure or through a painful episode.
    - Behavioral contracting
      - Use stickers or tokens as rewards.
      - Give time limits for the child to cooperate.
      - Reinforce cooperation with a reward.
    - Containment
      - Swaddle the infant.
      - Place rolled blankets around the child.
      - Maintain proper positioning.
    - Nonnutritive sucking
      - Offer pacifier with sucrose before, during, and after painful procedures.
      - Offer nonnutritive sucking during episodes of pain.
    - Kangaroo care – skin-to-skin contact between infants and parents
    - Complementary and alternative medicine
      - Offer foods, vitamins, or supplements.
      - Offer massage or chiropractic option.
      - Review energy based treatments such as magnets.
      - Discuss mind-body techniques such as hypnosis, homeopathy, naturopathy.
- Complications
  - Chronic pain syndromes – Poorly controlled pain predisposes children to chronic pain conditions.
- Nursing Actions
  - Assess pain thoroughly and adequately.
  - Administer medications in a timely manner.
  - Evaluate and monitor the child's response to treatments.
  - Titrate analgesic medications to achieve optimal dosing.
  - Make recommendations for alternate medications if needed.

APPLICATION EXERCISES

1. A nurse is completing a pain assessment of an infant. Which of the following pain scales should the nurse use?

    A. FACES

    B. FLACC

    C. Oucher

    D. Non-communicating children's pain checklist

2. A nurse is planning care for a child following a surgical procedure. Which of the following interventions should be included in the plan of care?

    A. Administer NSAIDs for pain greater than 7.

    B. Administer intranasal analgesics PRN.

    C. Administer IM analgesics for pain.

    D. Administer IV analgesics on a schedule.

3. A nurse is assessing an infant. Which of the following are clinical manifestations of pain in an infant? (Select all that apply.)

    _____ A. Pursed lips

    _____ B. Loud cry

    _____ C. Lowered eyebrows

    _____ D. Rigid body

    _____ E. Pushes away stimulus

4. A nurse is preparing a toddler for an intravenous catheter insertion using atraumatic care. Which of the following are appropriate interventions? (Select all that apply.)

    _____ A. Explain the procedure using the child's favorite toy.

    _____ B. Ask the parents to leave during the procedure.

    _____ C. Perform the procedure with the child in his bed.

    _____ D. Allow the child to make one choice regarding the procedure.

    _____ E. Apply EMLA cream to three potential insertion sites.

5. A nurse is planning care for an infant who is experiencing pain. Which of the following should be included in the plan of care? (Select all that apply.)

_____ A. Offer a pacifier.

_____ B. Use guided imagery.

_____ C. Use swaddling.

_____ D. Initiate a behavioral contract.

_____ E. Encourage kangaroo care.

6. A nurse educator is reviewing pain assessment tools with a group of pediatric nurses. What should be included in this discussion? Use the ATI Active Learning Template: Nursing Skill to describe four different pain tools used with pediatric clients.

APPLICATION EXERCISES KEY

1.   A. INCORRECT: The FACES pain assessment scale is recommended for children 3 years or older.

   B. **CORRECT:** The FLACC pain assessment scale is recommended for infants and children between 2 months and 7 years of age.

   C. INCORRECT: The Oucher pain assessment scale is recommended for children between the ages of 3 and 13 years.

   D. INCORRECT: The non-communicating children's pain checklist is recommended for non-communicating children between the ages of 3 and 18 years.

   Ⓝ NCLEX® Connection: Pharmacological and Parenteral Therapies, Pharmacological Pain Management

2.   A. INCORRECT: NSAIDs are used for mild to moderate pain.

   B. INCORRECT: Intranasal analgesics are used for clients older than 18 years.

   C. INCORRECT: IM analgesics are not recommended for pain management in children.

   D. **CORRECT:** IV analgesics should be administered on a schedule to achieve optimal pain management.

   Ⓝ NCLEX® Connection: Pharmacological and Parenteral Therapies, Pharmacological Pain Management

3.   A. INCORRECT: Infant who experience pain will have their mouth open in a squarish shape.

   B. **CORRECT:** Infants who experience pain will exhibit a loud cry.

   C. **CORRECT:** Infants who experience pain will lower and draw together their eyebrows.

   D. **CORRECT:** Infants who experience pain will exhibit a rigid body.

   E. INCORRECT: Infants who experience pain will exhibit a local reflex to withdraw from the stimulus.

   Ⓝ NCLEX® Connection: Pharmacological and Parenteral Therapies, Pharmacological Pain Management

4. A. **CORRECT:** Explaining the procedure using the child's favorite toy can assist the child to manage fears and provides atraumatic care.

   B. INCORRECT: The parents should be allowed to remain for procedures to offer comfort to the child.

   C. INCORRECT: Safe places such as the child's bed should be avoided.

   D. **CORRECT:** Allowing the child to make choices offers a sense of control over the situation and should be used to provide atraumatic care.

   E. **CORRECT:** A topical analgesic, such as EMLA, decreases pain and should be used to provide atraumatic care.

    NCLEX® Connection: Pharmacological and Parenteral Therapies, Parenteral/Intravenous Therapies

5. A. **CORRECT:** Nonnutritive sucking is a therapeutic nonpharmacological strategy for pain management with infants.

   B. INCORRECT: Guided imagery is a nonpharmacological strategy used with children.

   C. **CORRECT:** Swaddling the infant is a therapeutic nonpharmacological strategy for pain management.

   D. INCORRECT: Behavioral contracts are a nonpharmacological strategy used with children.

   E. **CORRECT:** Skin-to-skin touch is a relaxation technique and should be encouraged for infants who have pain.

    NCLEX® Connection: Basic Care and Comfort, Non-Pharmacological Comfort Interventions

6. *Using the ATI Active Learning Template: Nursing Skill*
  - FLACC (2 months to 7 years)
    - Pain rated on a scale of 0 to 10.
    - Assess behaviors of the child.
    - Face (F)
      - 0 – Smile or no expression
      - 1 – Occasional frown or grimace, withdrawn
      - 2 – Frequent or constant frown, clenched jaw, quivering chin
    - Legs (L)
      - 0 – Relaxed or normal position
      - 1 – Uneasy, restless, tense
      - 2 – Kicking or legs drawn up
    - Activity (A)
      - 0 – Lying quietly, moves easily, normal position
      - 1 – Squirming, shifting, tense
      - 2 – Arched, ridged, or jerking
    - Cry (C)
      - 0 – No cry
      - 1 – Moans or whimpers, occasional complaints
      - 2 – Crying, screaming, sobbing, frequent complaints
    - Consolability (C)
      - 0 – Content or relaxed
      - 1 – Reassured by occasional touching, or hugging. Able to distract
      - 2 – Difficult to console or comfort
  - FACES (3 years and older)
    - Pain rated on a scale of 0 to 5 using a diagram of six faces.
    - Substitute 0, 2, 4, 6, 8, 10 for 0 to 5 to convert to the 0 to 10 scale.
    - Explain each face to the child.
      - 0 – No hurt
      - 1 – Hurts a bit
      - 2 – Hurts a little more
      - 3 – Hurts even more
      - 4 – Hurts a whole lot
      - 5 – Hurts worst
    - Ask the child to choose a face that best describes how they are feeling
  - Oucher (3 to 13 years)
    - Pain rated on a scale of 0 to 5 using six photographs.
    - Substitute 0, 2, 4, 6, 8, 10 for 0 to 5 to convert to the 0 to 10 scale.
    - Have the child organize the photographs in order of no pain to the worst pain.
      - 0 – No hurt
      - 1 – Hurts a bit
      - 2 – Hurts a little more
      - 3 – Hurts even more
      - 4 – Hurts a whole lot
      - 5 – Hurts worst
    - Ask the child to choose a picture that best describes how they are feeling.
  - Numeric scale (5 years and older)
    - Pain rated on a scale of 0 to 10.
    - Explain to the child that 0 means "no pain" and 10 means "worst pain."
    - Have the child verbally report a number or point on a visual scale their pain level.
  - Non-communicating children's pain checklist (3 to 18 years)
    - Behaviors are observed for 10 min.
    - Six subcategories are scored on a scale 0 to 3.
    - Subcategories are vocal, social, facial, activity, body and limbs, and physiological, each with observable behaviors to be scored.
      - 0 – Not at all
      - 1 – Just a little
      - 2 – Fairly often
      - 3 – Very often
    - Cutoff scores:
      - 11 or more indicates moderate to severe pain.
      - 6 to 10 indicates mild pain.

Ⓝ NCLEX® Connection: Pharmacological and Parenteral Therapies, Pharmacological Pain Management

chapter 10

Overview

- A nurse is likely to encounter children who are ill and/or hospitalized. When caring for these children, it is important to know what play activities are considered appropriate.

HOSPITALIZATION AND ILLNESS

Overview

- Families and children may experience major stress related to hospitalization. The nurse should be alert to evidence of stress and intervene as appropriate.
- Families should be considered clients when children are ill.
- Separation anxiety during hospitalization manifests in three behavioral responses.
  - Protest (screaming, clinging to parents, verbal and physical aggression toward strangers)
  - Despair (withdrawl from others, depression, decreased communication, developmental regression)
  - Detachment (interacts with strangers, forms new relationships, appears happy)
- Each child's understanding of illnesses and hospitalization is dependent on the child's stage of development and cognitive ability.

Impact Based on Development

INFANT	
Level of Understanding	› Inability to describe illness and follow directions › Lack of understanding of the need of therapeutic procedures
Impact of Hospitalization	› Experiences stranger anxiety between 6 to 18 months of age › Displays physical behaviors as expressions of discomfort due to inability to verbalize › May experience sleep deprivation due to strange noises, monitoring devices, and procedures
TODDLER	
Level of Understanding	› Limited ability to describe illness › Poorly developed sense of body image and boundaries › Limited understanding of the need for therapeutic procedures › Limited ability to follow directions
Impact of Hospitalization	› Experiences separation anxiety › May exhibit an intense reaction to any type of procedure due to the intrusion of boundaries › Behavior may regress

PRESCHOOLER	
Level of Understanding	› Limited understanding of the cause of illness but knows what illness feels like › Limited ability to describe clinical manifestations › Fears related to magical thinking › Ability to understand cause and effect inhibited by concrete thinking
Impact of Hospitalization	› May experience separation anxiety › May harbor fears of bodily harm › May believe illness and hospitalization are a punishment
SCHOOL-AGE CHILD	
Level of Understanding	› Beginning awareness of body functioning › Ability to describe pain › Increasing ability to understand cause and effect
Impact of Hospitalization	› Fears loss of control › Seeks information as a way to maintain a sense of control › May sense when not being told the truth › May experience stress related to separation from peers and regular routine
ADOLESCENT	
Level of Understanding	› Increasing ability to understand cause and effect › Perceptions of illness severity are based on the degree of body image changes
Impact of Hospitalization	› Develops body image disturbance › Attempts to maintain composure but is embarrassed about losing control › Experiences feelings of isolation from peers › Worries about outcome and impact on school/activities › May not adhere to treatments/medication regimen due to peer influence

Family Responses

- Fear and guilt regarding not bringing the child in for care earlier.
- Frustration due to the perceived inability to care for the child.
- Altered family roles.
- Worry regarding finances if work is missed.
- Worry regarding care of other children within the household.
- Fear related to lack of knowledge regarding illness or treatments.
- Siblings experience loneliness, jealousy, guilt, fear, or anger.

Assessment

- Child's and family's understanding of the illness or the reason for hospitalization
- Stressors unique to the child and family (needs of other children in the family, socioeconomic situation, health of other extended family members)
- Past experiences with hospitalization and illness
- Developmental level and needs of child/family
- Parenting role and the family's perception of role changes
- Support available to the child/family

Nursing Interventions

- Teach the child and family what to expect during hospitalization.
- Encourage parents or family members to stay with the child during the hospital experience to reduce the stress.
- Attempt to maintain routine as much as possible.
- Encourage independence and choices.
- Explain treatments, procedures, and cares to the child.
- Provide developmentally appropriate activities.

AGE-RELATED INTERVENTIONS	
AGE	INTERVENTIONS
Infant	› Place infants whose parents are not in attendance close to nurses' stations so that their needs may be quickly met. › Provide consistency in assigning caregivers.
Toddler	› Encourage parents to provide routine care for the child, such as changing diapers and feeding. › Encourage the child's autonomy by offering appropriate choices. › Provide consistency in assigning caregivers.
Preschooler	› Explain procedures using simple, clear language. Avoid medical jargon and terms that can be misinterpreted. › Encourage independence by letting the child provide self-care. › Encourage the child to express feelings. › Validate the child's fears and concerns. › Provide toys that allow for emotional expression, such as a pounding board to release feelings of protest. › Provide consistency in assigning caregivers. › Give choices when possible, such as, "Do you want your medicine in a cup or a spoon?" › Allow younger children to handle equipment if it is safe.

AGE-RELATED INTERVENTIONS	
AGE	INTERVENTIONS
School-age	› Provide factual information. › Encourage the child to express feelings. › Try to maintain a normal routine for long hospitalizations, including time for school work. › Encourage contact with peer group.
Adolescent	› Provide factual information. › Include the adolescent in the planning of care to relieve feelings of powerlessness and lack of control. › Encourage contact with peer group.

M View Video: Interventions for Hospitalization

PLAY

Overview

- Play allows children to express feelings and fears.
- Play facilitates mastery of developmental stages and assists in the development of problem solving abilities.
- Play allows children to learn socially acceptable behaviors.
- Play activities should be specific to each child's stage of development.
- Play can be used to teach children.
- Play is a means of protection from everyday stressors.

Content of Play

- Social affective – taking pleasure in relationships
- Sense-pleasure – objects in the environment catching the child's attention
- Skill – demonstrating new abilities
- Unoccupied behavior – focusing attention on something of interest
- Dramatic – pretending and fantasizing
- Games – imitative, formal, or competitive

Social Character of Play

- Onlooker – the child observing others
- Solitary – the child playing alone
- Parallel – children playing independently but among other children, which is characteristic of toddlers
- Associative – children playing together without organization, which is characteristic of preschoolers
- Cooperative play – organized playing in groups, which is characteristic of school-age children

Functions of Play

- Play helps in the development of the following types of skills:
  - Intellectual
  - Sensorimotor
  - Social
  - Self-awareness
  - Creativity
  - Therapeutic and moral values

Play Activities Related to Age

- Infants
  - Birth to 3 months – colorful moving mobiles, music/sound boxes
  - 3 to 6 months – noise-making objects and soft toys
  - 6 to 9 months – teething toys and social interaction
  - 9 to 12 months – large blocks, toys that pop apart, and push-and-pull toys
- Toddlers
  - Cloth books, puzzles with large pieces
  - Large crayons and paper
  - Push-and-pull toys, balls
  - Tricycles
  - Educational television
  - Videos for children
- Preschoolers
  - Imitative and imaginative play
  - Drawing, painting, riding a tricycle, swimming, jumping, and running
  - Educational television and videos

- School-age children
  - Games that can be played alone or with another person
  - Team sports
  - Musical instruments
  - Arts and crafts
  - Collections
- Adolescents
  - Team sports
  - School activities
  - Reading and listening to music
  - Peer interactions

Therapeutic Play

- Makes use of dolls and/or stuffed animals
- Encourages the acting out of feelings of fear, anger, hostility, and sadness
- Enables the child to learn coping strategies in a safe environment
- Assists in gaining cooperation for medical treatment

Assessment

- Developmental level of the child
- Motor skills
- Level of activity tolerance
- Child's preferences

Nursing Interventions

- Select toys that are safe for the child.
- Consider isolation precautions and the child's illness in relation to toy selection.
- Select activities that enhance development.
- Observe the child's play for clues to the child's fears or anxieties.
- Encourage parents to bring one favorite toy from home.
- Use dolls and/or stuffed animals to demonstrate a procedure before it is done.
- Provide play opportunities that meet the child's level of activity tolerance.
- Allow the child to go to the play room if able.
- Encourage the adolescent's peers to visit.
- Involve a child life specialist in planning activities.

APPLICATION EXERCISES

1. A nurse is caring for a preschooler. Which of the following is an expected behavior of a preschool-age child?

    A. Describing manifestations of illness

    B. Relating fears to magical thinking

    C. Understanding cause of illness

    D. Awareness of body functioning

2. A nurse on a pediatric unit is caring for a toddler. Which of the following toddler behaviors is an effect of hospitalization? (Select all that apply.)

    _____ A. Believes the experience is a punishment

    _____ B. Experiences separation anxiety

    _____ C. Displays intense emotions

    _____ D. Exhibits regressive behaviors

    _____ E. Manifests disturbance in body image

3. A nurse is teaching a parent about parallel play in children. Which of the following statements by the nurse should be included in the teaching?

    A. "Children sit and observe others playing."

    B. "Children exhibit organized play when in a group."

    C. "The child plays alone."

    D. "The child plays independently when in a group."

4. A nurse is teaching a group of parents about separation anxiety. Which of the following should be included in the teaching?

    A. It is often observed in the school-age child.

    B. Detachment is the stage exhibited in the hospital.

    C. It results in prolonged issues of adaptability.

    D. Kicking a stranger is an example.

5. A nurse on a pediatric unit is caring for a group of children of different ages and planning play activities. What activities should the nurse include in the plan of care? Use the ATI Active Learning Template: Basic Concept to complete this item to identify appropriate toys and activities for children in three age groups.

APPLICATION EXERCISES KEY

1. A. INCORRECT: Preschool-age children have limited ability to describe manifestations of illness.

    B. **CORRECT:** Preschool-age children are egocentric and relate fears to magical thinking.

    C. INCORRECT: Preschool-age children have limited understanding of cause-and-effect relationship, but understand what illness feels like.

    D. INCORRECT: Awareness of body functioning is a behavior of an adolescent.

    Ⓝ NCLEX® Connection: Health Promotion and Maintenance, Developmental Stages and Transitions

2. A. INCORRECT: Preschool children believe hospitalization is a punishment.

    B. **CORRECT:** Separation anxiety is a potential effect of hospitalization in a toddler.

    C. **CORRECT:** Intense emotions are a potential impact of hospitalization in a toddler.

    D. **CORRECT:** Behavior regression is a potential impact of hospitalization in a toddler.

    E. INCORRECT: Body image disturbances can be seen in adolescents who are hospitalized.

    Ⓝ NCLEX® Connection: Health Promotion and Maintenance, Developmental Stages and Transitions

3. A. INCORRECT: Onlooker play is when a child sits and observes others playing.

    B. INCORRECT: Cooperative play is when a child exhibits organized play in a group.

    C. INCORRECT: Solitary play is when a child plays alone.

    D. **CORRECT:** Parallel play is when the toddler plays independently but is among other children in a group.

    Ⓝ NCLEX® Connection: Health Promotion and Maintenance, Aging Process

4. A. INCORRECT: Separation anxiety is commonly observed in the toddler.

    B. INCORRECT: The detachment stage is rarely seen in the hospital setting.

    C. INCORRECT: Children are adaptable and permanent issues are rare.

    D. **CORRECT:** Physical aggression toward strangers is a behavior seen in the protest stage of separation anxiety.

    Ⓝ NCLEX® Connection: Health Promotion and Maintenance, Developmental Stages and Transitions

5. *Using the ATI Active Learning Template: Basic Concept*
- Infants
  - Birth to 3 months – colorful moving mobiles, music/sound boxes
  - 3 to 6 months – noise-making objects and soft toys
  - 6 to 9 months – teething toys and social interaction
  - 9 to 12 months – large blocks, toys that pop apart, and push-and-pull toys
- Toddlers
  - Cloth books
  - Large crayons and paper
  - Push-and-pull toys
  - Tricycles
  - Balls
  - Puzzles with large pieces
  - Educational television
  - Videos for children
- Preschoolers
  - Imitative and imaginative play
  - Drawing, painting, riding a tricycle, swimming, jumping, and running
  - Educational television and videos
- School-age children
  - Games that can be played alone or with another person
  - Team sports
  - Musical instruments
  - Arts and crafts
  - Collections
- Adolescents
  - Team sports
  - School activities
  - Reading and listening to music
  - Peer interactions

Ⓝ NCLEX® Connection: Health Promotion and Maintenance, Developmental Stages and Transitions

chapter 11

Overview

- A nurse is tasked with meeting the physical, psychological, spiritual, and emotional needs of a client and the family during illness and at the time of death.

- Palliative care is a multidisciplinary approach that focuses on the process of dying rather than prolonging life in cases in which cures are no longer possible.

  ○ Focus on control of managing the client's manifestations and offering supportive care.

- Hospice care specializes in the care of a client who is dying.

  ○ Family members are the primary caregivers.

  ○ Nursing focus is on pain control and comfort.

  ○ Family and client needs are equal.

  ○ Provide support for the family grieving process, which can continue after the client's death.

- End-of-life decisions require honest information regarding prognosis, disease progression, treatment options, and the impact of treatments. These decisions are made during a highly stressful time. It is important that all health care personnel are aware of the child and family's decisions.

- Nurses may experience personal grief when caring for children with whom they have developed rapport and intimacy.

Factors Influencing Loss, Grief, and Coping Ability

- Interpersonal relationships and social support networks
- Type and significance of loss
- Culture and ethnicity
- Spiritual and religious beliefs and practices
- Prior experience with loss
- Socioeconomic status
- Grief and mourning

  ○ Anticipatory grief: when death is expected or a possible outcome

  ○ Complicated grief: extends for more than a year following the loss

    ▪ Intense thoughts
    ▪ Distressing yearning
    ▪ Feelings of loneliness
    ▪ Distressing emotions and feelings
    ▪ Disturbances in personal activities such as sleep
    ▪ May require referral to an expert in grief counseling

○ Parental grief

■ Intense, long-lasting, and complex

■ Secondary losses related to the death of the child such as absence of hope and dreams, disruption of the family unit, loss of identity as a parent

■ Differences in maternal and paternal grief

○ Sibling grief

■ Differs from adult/parental grief

■ Reactions depend on age and developmental stage

• Current stage of development

AGE	RELEVANT FACTORS
Infants/toddlers (birth to 3 years)	› Have little to no concept of death › Egocentric thinking prevents their understanding death (toddlers) › Mirror parental emotions (sadness, anger, depression, anxiety) › React in response to the changes brought about by being in the hospital (change of routine, painful procedures, immobilization, less independence, separation from family) › May regress to an earlier stage of behavior
Preschool children (3 to 6 years)	› Egocentric thinking › Magical thinking allows for the belief that thoughts can cause an event such as death (as a result, child may feel guilt and shame) › Interpret separation from parents as punishment for bad behavior › View dying as temporary because of the lack of a concept of time and because the dead person may still have attributes of the living (sleeping, eating, breathing)
School-age children (6 to 12 years)	› Start to respond to logical or factual explanations › Begin to have an adult concept of death (inevitable, irreversible, universal), which generally applies to older school-age children (9 to 12 years) › Experience fear of the disease process, the death process, the unknown, and loss of control » Fear often displayed through uncooperative behavior › May be curious about funeral services and what happens to the body after death
Adolescents (12 to 20 years)	› May have an adultlike concept of death › May have difficulty accepting death because they are discovering who they are, establishing an identity, and dealing with issues of puberty › Rely more on peers than the influence of parents, which may result in the reality of a serious illness causing adolescents to feel isolated › May be unable to relate to peers and communicate with parents › May become increasingly stressed by changes in physical appearance due to medications or illness than the prospect of death › May experience guilt and shame

- Factors that may increase the family's potential for dysfunctional grieving following the death of a child
  - Lack of a support system
  - Presence of inadequate coping skills
  - Association of violence or suicide with the death of a child
  - Sudden and unexpected death of a child
  - Lack of hope or presence of pre-existing mental health issues

Assessment

- Physical manifestations of death
  - Sensation of heat when the body feels cool
  - Decreased sensation and movement in the lower extremities
  - Loss of senses (hearing is the last to be lost)
  - Confusion or loss of consciousness (LOC)
  - Decreased appetite and thirst
  - Swallowing difficulties
  - Loss of bowel and bladder control
  - Bradycardia, hypotension
  - Cheyne-Stokes respirations
- Knowledge regarding diagnosis, prognosis, and care
- Perceptions and desires regarding diagnosis, prognosis, and care
- Nutritional status, as well as growth and development patterns
- Activity and energy level of the child
- Parents' wishes regarding the child's end-of-life care
- Presence of a do-not-resuscitate (DNR) order
- Family coping and available support
- The stage of grief the child and family are experiencing

Nursing Interventions

- Allow an opportunity for anticipatory grieving, which impacts the way a family will cope with the death of a child.
- Provide consistency among nursing personnel who are caring for the client/family.
- Encourage parents to remain with the client.
- Attempt to maintain a normal environment.
- Communicate with the client honestly and respectfully.
- Encourage independence.

- Stay with the client as much as possible.
- Administer analgesics to control pain.
- Provide privacy.
- Soften lights.
- Offer soft music if desired.
- Assist with arranging religious or cultural rituals desired by the client and family.
- Assist the client with unfinished tasks.
- Provide support for the family and client.
- Palliative care

  ○ Consider the client, siblings, and parents as the units of care.
  ○ Provide an environment that is as close to being like home as possible.
  ○ Consult with the client and family for desired measures.
  ○ Respect the family's cultural and religious preferences and rituals.
  ○ Provide and clarify information and explanations.
  ○ Encourage physical contact; address feelings; and show concern, empathy, and support.
  ○ Provide comfort measures (warmth, quiet, noise control, dry linens).
  ○ Provide adequate nutrition and hydration.
  ○ Control pain.
    - Give medications on a regular schedule.
    - Treat breakthrough pain.
    - Increase doses as necessary to control pain.
    - Encourage use of relaxation, imagery, and distraction to help manage pain.
- Care for grieving families during the dying process.
  ○ Provide information to the client and family about the disease, medications, procedures, and expected events.
  ○ Encourage and support parents to participate in caring for the client.
  ○ Encourage parents to remain near the child as much as possible.
  ○ Encourage the client's independence and control as developmentally and physically appropriate.
  ○ Allow for visitation of family and friends as desired.
  ○ Emphasize open, honest communication among the client, family, and health care team.
  ○ Provide support to the client and family with decision-making.
  ○ Provide opportunities for the client and family to ask questions.
  ○ Assist parents to cope with their feelings and help them to understand the client's behaviors.
  ○ Use books, movies, art, music, and play therapy to stimulate discussions and provide an outlet for emotions.
  ○ Provide and encourage professional support and guidance from a trusted member of the health care team.

  ○ Remain neutral and accepting.

  ○ Give reassurance that the client is not in pain and that all efforts are being made to maintain comfort and support of the client's life.

  ○ Recognize and support the individual differences of grieving. Advise families that each member may react differently on any given day.

  ○ Give families privacy, unlimited time, and opportunities for any cultural or religious rituals. Respect the family's decisions regarding care of the client.

  ○ Encourage discussion of special memories and people, reading of favorite books, providing favorite toys/objects, physical contact, sibling visits, and continued verbal communication, even if the client seems unconscious.

- After death

  ○ Allow family to stay with the body as long as they desire.

  ○ Allow family to rock the infant/toddler, if desired.

  ○ Remove tubes and equipment.

  ○ Offer family the option to assist with the preparation of the body.

  ○ Assist with preparations involving the death ritual.

  ○ Encourage parents to prepare siblings for the funeral and related death rituals.

  ○ Remain with the family and offer support.

  ○ Allow family to share stories about the client's life.

  ○ Refer to the client by name.

  ○ Allow all family members to communicate feelings.

- Nurses caring for a client who is dying should:

  ○ Express personal feelings of loss to someone who can offer support.

  ○ Maintain good general health.

  ○ Develop the ability for empathy.

  ○ Take time off from work as needed.

  ○ Develop well-rounded interests.

  ○ Develop professional and social support systems.

  ○ Focus on the positive aspects of caring for children who are dying.

  ○ Attend funeral services if desired.

  ○ Maintain contact with the family.

APPLICATION EXERCISES

1. A nurse is caring for a child. Which of the following are physical manifestations of impending death? (Select all that apply.)

_____ A. Heightened sense of hearing

_____ B. Tachycardia

_____ C. Difficulty swallowing

_____ D. Sensation of being cold

_____ E. Cheyne-Stokes respirations

2. A nurse is teaching a parent about complicated grief. Which of the following statements by the nurse is appropriate?

A. "It is considered complicated grief if you are still grieving 6 months after your loss."

B. "Personal activities are affected when experiencing complicated grief."

C. "Parents will experience complicated grief together."

D. "Complicated grief self-resolves in 12 months."

3. A nurse is teaching a parent of a preschool child about factors that affect the child's perception of death. Which of the following should be included in the teaching?

A. Preschool children have no concept of death.

B. Preschool children perceive death as temporary.

C. Preschool children often regress to an earlier stage of behavior.

D. Preschool children experience fear related to the disease process.

4. A nurse often cares children who are dying. Which of the following is an appropriate action for a nurse to take to maintain their effectiveness? (Select all that apply.)

_____ A. Remain in contact with the family after their loss.

_____ B. Develop a professional support system.

_____ C. Take time off from work.

_____ D. Suggest that a hospital representative attend the funeral.

_____ E. Demonstrate feelings of sympathy toward the family.

5. A nurse is caring for a child who has a terminal illness and reviews palliative care with an assistive personnel (AP). Which of the following statements by the AP indicates understanding of this review?

    A. "I'm sure the family is hopeful that the new medication will stop the illness."

    B. "I'll miss working with this client, now that only nurses will be caring for him."

    C. "I will get all the client's personal objects out of his room."

    D. "I will listen and respond as the family talks about their child's life."

6. A nurse is planning care for a client who is nearing the end of life. What interventions should the nurse include in the plan of care? Use the ATI Active Learning Template: Basic Concept to complete this item to describe at least eight nursing interventions to be used.

APPLICATION EXERCISES KEY

1. A. INCORRECT: A decrease in the senses of smell, sight, and hearing are physical manifestations of approaching death.

   B. INCORRECT: Bradycardia is a physical manifestation of approaching death.

   C. **CORRECT:** Difficulty swallowing is a physical finding of approaching death.

   D. INCORRECT: A client's sensation of heat when the body feels cool is a physical manifestation of approaching death.

   E. **CORRECT:** Cheyne-Stokes respirations are an abnormal breathing pattern with periods of apnea that is a physical finding of impending death.

    NCLEX® Connection: Physiological Adaptations, Alterations in Body Systems

2. A. INCORRECT: A parent who is still experiencing intense grieving after 1 year is evaluated for complicated grief.

   B. **CORRECT:** A parent who is experiencing complicated grief experiences intense emotions that affect personal activities.

   C. INCORRECT: Parents grieve differently, and not all parents experience complicated grief.

   D. INCORRECT: A nurse should refer the parent to an expert in grief counseling if complicated grief is identified.

    NCLEX® Connection: Psychosocial Integrity, Grief and Loss

3. A. INCORRECT: Toddlers have no concept of death.

   B. **CORRECT:** Preschool children perceive death as temporary because they have no concept of time.

   C. INCORRECT: Toddlers often regress to an earlier stage of behavior.

   D. INCORRECT: School-age children experience fear related to the disease process.

    NCLEX® Connection: Psychosocial Integrity, Grief and Loss

4. A. **CORRECT:** Maintaining contact with the family after their loss is an act of support for the family.

    B. **CORRECT:** Developing professional support systems is a strategy the nurse can use to maintain effectiveness when working with the client who is dying and their family.

    C. **CORRECT:** Taking time off from work is a strategy the nurse can use to maintain effectiveness when working with the client who is dying and their family.

    D. INCORRECT: Nurses should be encouraged to participate in funeral rituals as an act of support for the family.

    E. INCORRECT: A nurse should develop the ability for empathy when dealing with dying clients.

    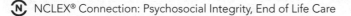 NCLEX® Connection: Psychosocial Integrity, End of Life Care

5. A. INCORRECT: Palliative care is provided when there is no longer hope for a disease cure.

    B. INCORRECT: Palliative care focuses on providing consistency among the multidisciplinary team and nursing personnel to offer supportive care and a normal environment.

    C. INCORRECT: Palliative care focuses on offering support and a normal environment as the dying process occurs.

    D. **CORRECT:** Palliative care focuses on the process of dying and grieving, which includes using therapeutic communication.

    NCLEX® Connection: Basic Care and Comfort, Non-Pharmacological Comfort Interventions

6. *Using the ATI Active Learning Template: Basic Concept*
    - Nursing Interventions
      - Allow an opportunity for anticipatory grieving, which affects the way a family will cope with the death of a child.
      - Provide consistency among nursing staff caring for the client/family.
      - Encourage parents to remain with the client.
      - Attempt to maintain a normal environment.
      - Communicate with the client honestly and respectfully.
      - Encourage independence.
      - Stay with the client as much as possible.
      - Administer analgesics to control pain.
      - Provide privacy.
      - Soften lights.
      - Offer soft music if desired.
      - Assist with arranging religious or cultural rituals desired by the client and family.
      - Assist the client with unfinished tasks.
      - Provide support for the family and client.

    NCLEX® Connection: Psychosocial Integrity, End of Life Care

UNIT 2   Nursing Care of Children with System Disorders

SECTION: NEUROSENSORY DISORDERS

› Meningitis and Reye Syndrome
› Seizures
› Head Injury
› Visual and Hearing Impairments

NCLEX® CONNECTIONS

When reviewing the chapters in this unit, keep in mind the relevant sections of the NCLEX® outline, in particular:

Client Needs: Pharmacological and Parenteral Therapies

› Relevant topics/tasks include:
  » Adverse Effects/ Contraindications/Side Effects/Interactions
    › Notify the provider of side effects, adverse effects, and contraindications of medications and parenteral therapy.
  » Expected Actions/Outcomes
    › Evaluate client response to medication.

Client Needs: Health Promotion and Maintenance

› Relevant topics/tasks include:
  » Diagnostic Tests
    › Monitor the results of diagnostic testing and intervene as needed.
  » Potential for Alterations in Body Systems
    › Compare current client data to baseline client data.
  » Potential for Complications of Diagnostic Tests/ Treatments/Procedures
    › Use precautions to prevent injury and/or complications associated with a procedure or diagnosis.

Client Needs: Physiological Adaptation

› Relevant topics/tasks include:
› Alterations in Body Systems
  » Provide care to the client who has experienced a seizure.
› Illness Management
  » Evaluate the effectiveness of the treatment regimen for a client with an acute or chronic diagnosis.
› Unexpected Response to Therapies
  » Assess the client for an unexpected adverse response to therapy.

chapter 12

Overview

- Meningitis is an inflammation of the cerebrospinal fluid (CSF) and meninges, which are the connective tissues that cover the brain and spinal cord.

- Reye syndrome is a life-threatening disorder that involves acute encephalopathy and fatty changes of the liver.

- Meningitis and Reye syndrome have similar manifestations and are both sometimes preceded by viral infections. Testing is necessary to differentiate between the two.

MENINGITIS

Overview

- Viral (or aseptic) meningitis usually requires only supportive care for recovery.

- Bacterial (or septic) meningitis is a contagious infection. The prognosis depends on how quickly care is initiated.

Assessment

- Risk Factors

  ○ Viral Meningitis

    ▪ Many viral illnesses, such as cytomegalovirus, adenovirus, mumps, herpes simplex virus, and arbovirus

  ○ Bacterial Meningitis

    ▪ Infections caused by bacterial agents (*Neisseria meningitidis* [meningococcal], *Streptococcus pneumoniae* [pneumococcal], *Haemophilus influenzae* type B [Hib], *Escherichia coli*)

      □ Incidence of bacterial meningitis has decreased in all age groups except infants under the age of 2 months since the introduction of the Hib and pneumococcal conjugate vaccines (PCV).

    ▪ Injuries that provide direct access to CSF (skull fracture, penetrating head wound)

    ▪ Crowded living conditions

- Subjective Data

  ○ Photophobia

  ○ Nausea

  ○ Irritability

  ○ Headache

- Objective Data
  - ○ Physical Assessment Findings
    - ▪ Manifestations of viral and bacterial meningitis are similar.
    - ▪ Newborns
      - □ No illness is present at birth, but it progresses within a few days.
      - □ Clinical manifestations are vague and difficult to diagnose.
        - ‣ Poor muscle tone, weak cry, poor suck, refuses feeding, and vomiting or diarrhea
        - ‣ Possible fever or hypothermia
      - □ Neck is supple without nuchal rigidity.
      - □ Bulging fontanels are a late sign.
    - ▪ 3 months to 2 years
      - □ Seizures with a high-pitched cry
      - □ Fever and irritability
      - □ Bulging fontanels
      - □ Possible nuchal rigidity
      - □ Poor feeding
      - □ Vomiting
      - □ Brudzinski's and Kernig's signs not reliable for diagnosis
    - ▪ 2 years through adolescence
      - □ Seizures (often initial sign)
      - □ Nuchal rigidity
      - □ Positive Brudzinski's sign (flexion of extremities occurring with deliberate flexion of the child's neck)
      - □ Positive Kernig's sign (resistance to extension of the child's leg from a flexed position)

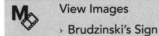

 View Images	
› Brudzinski's Sign	› Kernig's Sign

      - □ Fever and chills
      - □ Headache
      - □ Vomiting
      - □ Irritability and restlessness that may progress to drowsiness, delirium, stupor, and coma
      - □ Petechia or purpuric type rash (seen with meningococcal infection)
      - □ Involvement of joints (seen with meningococcal and HIb)
      - □ Chronic draining ear (seen with pneumococcal infection)

- Laboratory Tests
  - Blood cultures are sometimes positive when the CSF culture is negative.
  - Collect complete blood counts.
  - CSF analysis indicative of meningitis.
    - Bacterial
      - Cloudy color
      - Elevated WBC count
      - Elevated protein content
      - Decreased glucose content
      - Positive Gram stain
    - Viral
      - Clear color
      - Slightly elevated WBC count
      - Normal or slightly elevated protein content
      - Normal glucose content
      - Negative Gram stain
- Diagnostic Procedures
  - Lumbar puncture
    - This is the definitive diagnostic test for meningitis.
    - Insertion of a spinal needle into the subarachnoid space between L3 and L4 or L4 and L5 vertebral spaces.
    - Measures spinal fluid pressure and collects CSF for analysis.
    - Nursing Actions
      - Have the child empty his bladder.
      - Assist the provider with the procedure.
      - A topical anesthetic (EMLA cream) may be applied over the biopsy area 45 min to 1 hr prior to the procedure.
      - Place the child in the side-lying position with the head flexed and knees drawn up toward the chest, and assist in maintaining the position. Distraction may need to be used.
      - The child may be sedated with fentanyl (Sublimaze) and midazolam (Versed).
      - The provider will clean the skin and inject a local anesthetic.
      - The provider will take pressure readings and collect three to five test tubes of CSF.
      - Pressure and an elastic bandage will be applied to the puncture site after the needle is removed.
      - Label specimens appropriately, and deliver them to the laboratory.
      - Monitor the site for bleeding, hematoma, or infection.
    - Client Education
      - Instruct the client to remain in bed for 4 to 8 hr in a flat position to prevent leakage and a resulting spinal headache. This may not be possible for an infant, toddler, or preschooler.

- CT scan or MRI
  - □ These may be performed to identify increased ICP and/or an abscess.
  - □ Nursing Actions
    - ▸ Assist with positioning.
    - ▸ Administer sedatives as prescribed.

Patient-Centered Care

- Nursing Care
  - ○ The presence of petechia or a purpuric-type rash requires immediate medical attention.
  - ○ Isolate the client as soon as meningitis is suspected, and maintain droplet precautions per facility protocol. Droplet precautions require:
    - A private room or a room with other clients who have the same infectious disease, ensuring that each client have their own equipment.
    - Masks for providers and visitors.
  - ○ Monitor vital signs, urine output, fluid status, pain level, neurologic status, and head circumference (for infants).
  - ○ Correct fluid volume deficits and then restrict fluids until no evidence of increased ICP and serum sodium levels within the expected range.
  - ○ Maintain NPO status if the client has a decreased level of consciousness. As the client's condition improves, advance to clear liquids and then to a diet that the client can tolerate.
  - ○ Decrease environmental stimuli.
    - Provide a quiet environment.
    - Minimize exposure to bright light (natural and electric).
  - ○ Provide comfort measures.
    - Keep the client's room cool.
    - Position the client without a pillow and slightly elevate the head of the bed. The client can also be positioned side-lying to reduce neck discomfort.
  - ○ Maintain safety (keep the bed in a low position, implement seizure precautions).
  - ○ Keep the family informed of the client's condition.
- Medications
  - ○ Antibiotics
    - Administer for bacterial infections IV. Length of therapy is determined by the client's condition and CSF results (normal blood glucose levels, negative culture). Therapy may last as long as 10 days.
    - Nursing Considerations
      - □ Assess for allergies.
    - Client Education
      - □ Provide support for the client and family.
      - □ Educate the family about the need to complete the entire course of medication.

- ○ Corticosteroids – dexamethasone (Decadron)
  - Not indicated for viral meningitis.
  - Assists with initial management of increased ICP, but may not be effective for long-term complications.
  - Most effective for reducing neurologic complications in children with infections caused by Hib.
  - Nursing Considerations
    - □ Assess for effectiveness of medication.
  - Client Education
    - □ Provide support for the client and family.
    - □ Educate on administration and possible adverse effects of the medication.
- ○ Analgesics
  - Acetaminophen (Tylenol) with codeine may be used to relieve discomfort.
  - Nursing Considerations
    - □ Assess the client's temperature prior to administering acetaminophen or ibuprofen (Advil) because these medications can mask a fever.
    - □ Monitor respiratory status.
    - □ Monitor level of consciousness.
  - Client Education
    - □ Provide support for the client and family.
- • Care After Discharge
  - ○ Client Education
    - Early and complete treatment is necessary for upper respiratory infections.
    - Encourage parents to maintain appropriate immunizations for the client. Children should receive the Hib and PCV vaccines at 2, 4, and 6 months of age, then again between 12 and 15 months of age.

Complications

- • Increased ICP
  - ○ Could lead to neurological dysfunction
  - ○ Nursing Actions
    - Monitor for signs of increased ICP.
      - □ Infants – bulging or tense fontanels, increased head circumference, high-pitched cry, distended scalp veins, irritability, bradycardia, and respiratory changes
      - □ Children – increased irritability, headache, nausea, vomiting, diplopia, seizures, bradycardia, and respiratory changes
    - Provide interventions to reduce ICP (positioning; avoidance of coughing, straining, and bright lights; minimizing environmental stimuli).

REYE SYNDROME

Overview

- Reye syndrome primarily affects the liver and brain, causing:
  - Liver dysfunction
  - Cerebral edema
- The cause of Reye syndrome is not understood.
- Peak incidence of Reye syndrome occurs when influenza is most common, typically January, February, and March.
- Reye syndrome can be mistaken for other disorders, including encephalitis, meningitis, poisoning, sudden infant death syndrome (SIDS), diabetes mellitus, and psychiatric illness.
- The prognosis for the client who has Reye syndrome is best with early recognition and treatment.

Assessment

- Risk Factors
  - There is a potential association between using aspirin (salicylate) products for treating fevers caused by viral infections and the development of Reye syndrome.
  - Reye syndrome typically follows a viral illness (influenza, gastroenteritis, varicella).
- Subjective Data
  - Recent viral illness or use of aspirin (Bayer Children's).
- Objective Data
  - Physical Assessment Findings
    - Reye syndrome presents in clinical stages based on the severity of liver and neurologic findings.
      - Lethargy
      - Irritability
      - Combativeness
      - Confusion
      - Delirium
      - Profuse vomiting
      - Convulsions
      - Loss of consciousness
  - Laboratory Tests
    - Liver enzymes (alanine aminotransferase [ALT], aspartate aminotransferase [AST]) – elevated.
    - Serum ammonia level – elevated.
    - Serum electrolytes – altered due to cerebral edema and liver changes.
    - Coagulation times may be extended.

○ Diagnostic Procedures

- Liver biopsy

  □ A liver biopsy consists of taking a piece of liver tissue via a large-bore needle, and sending this tissue to the pathology department. Care should be taken to ensure that the clotting studies are within normal limits prior to the procedure.

  □ Nursing Actions

    ▸ Maintain NPO status prior to the procedure.

    ▸ Monitor for hemorrhage postprocedure.

    ▸ Assess vital signs frequently postprocedure.

  □ Client Education

    ▸ Encourage the parents to limit the client's postprocedure activities to decrease the risk of hemorrhage.

- CSF analysis

  □ A lumbar puncture should be performed to collect CSF and rule out meningitis.

Patient-Centered Care

- Nursing Care

  ○ Maintain hydration while preventing cerebral edema.

    - Administer IV fluids as prescribed.

    - Maintain accurate I&O.

    - Insert indwelling urinary catheter as ordered.

  ○ Position the client.

    - Avoid extreme flexion, extension, or rotation.

    - Maintain the head in a midline neutral position.

    - Keep the head of the bed elevated 30°.

  ○ Monitor coagulation and prevent hemorrhage.

    - Note unexplained or prolonged bleeding.

    - Apply pressure after procedures that cause bleeding.

  ○ Monitor pain status and response to painful stimuli. Administer pain medications when appropriate.

  ○ Assist with intubation and maintain a ventilator if required.

  ○ Implement seizure precautions.

  ○ Keep the family informed of the client's status.

  ○ Provide private time for the family to be with the client if death is imminent.

  ○ Initiate referrals to support resources for family.

- Medications
  - Osmotic diuretic – mannitol (Osmitrol)
    - To decrease cerebral swelling, administer as prescribed.
    - Nursing Considerations
      - Monitor the client for increased ICP.
  - Vitamin K
    - Improves synthesis of blood clotting factors in the liver
    - Nursing Considerations
      - Subcutaneous is preferred route.
      - Identify client sensitivity to benzyl alcohol or castor oil.
    - Client Education
      - Teach about dietary intake of vitamin K.
- Teamwork and Collaboration
  - The client who has neurologic deficits post-Reye syndrome will require interventions from other members of the health care team.
  - Occupational therapy and physical therapy may be needed to help the client adapt to neurologic deficits.
  - A dietician may also be needed to assist in maintaining adequate nutrition.
- Care After Discharge
  - Client Education
    - Teach parents to avoid giving salicylates for pain or fever in children.
    - Teach parents to read labels of over-the-counter medications to check for the presence of salicylates.
    - Clients regain full liver function, but may have some neurological deficits.

Complications

- Neurologic Sequelae
  - Neurologic complications vary by degree of severity, and sometimes include speech and/or hearing impairment, and developmental delays based on the length and severity of illness.
  - Nursing Actions
    - Explain the client's condition and needs to the family.
  - Client Education
    - Help the family identify support services for home care.
- Death
  - Nursing Actions
    - Support the family in grief.
    - Make referrals to spiritual support as appropriate.

APPLICATION EXERCISES

1. A nurse is caring for a client who has suspected meningitis and a decreased level of consciousness. Which of the following actions by the nurse is appropriate?

    A. Place the client on NPO status.

    B. Prepare the client for a liver biopsy.

    C. Position the client dorsal recumbent.

    D. Put the client in a protective environment.

2. A nurse is caring for a 4-month-old infant who has meningitis. Which of the following findings is associated with this diagnosis?

    A. Depressed anterior fontanel

    B. Constipation

    C. Presence of the rooting reflex

    D. High-pitched cry

3. A nurse is reviewing cerebrospinal fluid analysis for a client who has suspected meningitis. Which of the following results indicate viral meningitis? (Select all that apply.)

    _____ A. Negative gram stain

    _____ B. Normal glucose content

    _____ C. Cloudy color

    _____ D. Decreased WBC count

    _____ E. Normal protein content

4. A nurse is developing an in-service about viral and bacterial meningitis. The nurse should include that the introduction of which of the following immunizations decreased the incidence of bacterial meningitis in children? (Select all that apply.)

    _____ A. Inactivated polio vaccine (IPV)

    _____ B. Pneumococcal conjugate vaccine (PCV)

    _____ C. Diphtheria and tetanus toxoids and acellular pertussis vaccine (DTaP)

    _____ D. *Haemophilus influenzae* type B (Hib) vaccine

    _____ E. Trivalent inactivated influenza vaccine (TIV)

5. A nurse is caring for a school-age client who possibly has Reye syndrome. Which of the following is a risk factor for developing Reye syndrome?

    A. Recent history of infectious cystitis caused by *Candida*

    B. Recent history of bacterial otitis media

    C. Recent episode of gastroenteritis

    D. Recent episode of *Haemophilus influenzae* meningitis

6. A nurse is admitting a client who has Reye Syndrome. Use the ATI Active Learning Template: Systems Disorder complete this item to include the following:

    A. Description of Disorder/Disease Process

    B. Objective and Subjective Data: Identify five.

    C. Laboratory Tests: List two results indicative of Reye syndrome.

APPLICATION EXERCISES KEY

1. A. **CORRECT:** Due to the client's decreased level of consciousness, placing the client on NPO status is an appropriate action by the nurse.

    B. INCORRECT: This is not an appropriate action by the nurse. Liver biopsies are used to diagnose Reye syndrome.

    C. INCORRECT: This is not an appropriate action by the nurse. Position the client without a pillow and slightly elevate the head of the bed.

    D. INCORRECT: This is not an appropriate action by the nurse. Clients who have undergone allogeneic hematopoietic stem cell transplants are put in protective environments. This client should be placed on droplet precautions.

    N NCLEX® Connection: Physiological Adaptations, Alterations in Body Systems

2. A. INCORRECT: A bulging anterior fontanel is a finding associated with meningitis in a 4-month-old infant.

    B. INCORRECT: Vomiting is a finding associated with meningitis in a 4-month-old infant.

    C. INCORRECT: The rooting reflex is expected in infants until the age of 3 to 4 months, and can remain until the age of 12 months.

    D. **CORRECT:** A high-pitched cry is a finding associated with meningitis in a 4-month-old infant.

    N NCLEX® Connection: Physiological Adaptations, Alterations in Body Systems

3. A. **CORRECT:** A negative gram stain indicates viral meningitis.

    B. **CORRECT:** Normal glucose content indicates viral meningitis.

    C. INCORRECT: A clear color indicates viral meningitis.

    D. INCORRECT: A slightly elevated WBC count indicates viral meningitis.

    E. **CORRECT:** Normal protein content indicates viral meningitis.

    N NCLEX® Connection: Reduction of Risk Potential, Diagnostic Tests

4. A. INCORRECT: The introduction of the IPV did not decrease the incidence of bacterial meningitis.

   B. **CORRECT:** The introduction of the PCV decreased the incidence of bacterial meningitis in children, as it provides immunity against bacteria that causes the illness.

   C. INCORRECT: The introduction of the DTaP vaccine did not decrease the incidence of bacterial meningitis.

   D. **CORRECT:** The introduction of the Hib vaccine decreased the incidence of bacterial meningitis in children, as it provides immunity against bacterium that cause the illness.

   E. INCORRECT: The introduction of the TIV did not decrease the incidence of bacterial meningitis.

   Ⓝ NCLEX® Connection: Health Promotion and Maintenance, Health Promotion/Disease Prevention

5. A. INCORRECT: A recent history of infectious cystitis caused by *Candida*, a fungal infection, is not a risk factor for Reye syndrome.

   B. INCORRECT: A recent history of bacterial otitis media is not a risk factor for Reye syndrome.

   C. **CORRECT:** A recent episode of gastroenteritis, a viral illness, is a risk factor for Reye syndrome. Reye syndrome typically follows a viral illness, such as influenza, gastroenteritis, or varicella.

   D. INCORRECT: A recent episode of *Haemophilus influenzae* meningitis, a bacterial infection, is not a risk factor for Reye syndrome.

   Ⓝ NCLEX® Connection: Health Promotion and Maintenance, Health Promotion/Disease Prevention

6. *Using the ATI Active Learning Template: Systems Disorder*

   A. Description of Disorder/Disease Process
      • Reye syndrome is a life-threatening disorder involving acute encephalopathy and fatty changes of the liver.

   B. Objective and Subjective Data
      • Recent viral illness
      • Recent use of aspirin (Bayer Children's)
      • Lethargy
      • Irritability
      • Combativeness
      • Confusion
      • Delirium
      • Profuse vomiting
      • Convulsions
      • Loss of consciousness

   C. Laboratory Tests
      • Altered serum electrolytes due to cerebral edema and liver changes
      • Possibly extended coagulation times
      • Elevated liver enzymes
      • Elevated serum ammonia levels

   Ⓝ NCLEX® Connection: Physiological Adaptations, Pathophysiology

Overview

- Seizures are abnormal, excessive electrical discharges of neurons within the brain caused by a disease process.
- Seizures are classified according to their type and etiology.
- Epilepsy is chronic, recurring, and diagnosed after all other possible etiologies for the seizures have been ruled out.

Assessment

- Risk Factors for Seizures
  - Some seizures have no known etiology
  - Febrile episode
  - Cerebral edema
  - Intracranial infection or hemorrhage
  - Brain tumors or cysts
  - Anoxia
  - Toxins or drugs
  - Lead poisoning
  - Tetanus, *Shigella*, or *Salmonella*
  - Hypoglycemia, hypocalcemia, alkalosis, hyponatremia, hypernatremia, or hypomagnesemia
- Risk Factors for Epilepsy
  - Trauma
  - Hemorrhage
  - Congenital defects
  - Anoxia
  - Infection
  - Toxins
  - Hypoglycemic injury
  - Uremia
  - Migraine
  - Cardiovascular dysfunction

- Subjective and Objective Data
  - Generalized
    - Tonic-clonic seizure (previously referred to as grand mal)
      - Onset without warning
      - Tonic phase (10 to 20 seconds)
        - Eyes roll upward
        - Loss of consciousness
        - Tonic contraction of entire body, with arms flexed and legs, head and neck extended
        - Possible piercing cry
        - Increased salivation
        - Loss of swallowing reflex
        - Apnea leading to cyanosis
      - Clonic phase (time varies)
        - Violent jerking movements of the body
        - May having foaming in the mouth
        - May be incontinent
        - Gradual slowing of movements until cessation
      - Postictal state
        - Arouses with difficulty
        - Confused for several hours
        - Impairment of fine motor movements
        - Lack of coordination
        - Possible vomiting, headache, visual or speech difficulties
        - Sleeps for several hours
        - No recollection of the seizure
    - Absence seizure (previously referred to petit mal)
      - Onset between age 4 to 12 years and ceases by puberty
      - Loss of consciousness lasting 5 to 10 seconds
      - Minimal or no change in behavior
      - Resembles daydreaming or inattentiveness
      - May drop items being held
      - Lip smacking, twitching of eyelids or face, or slight hand movements
      - Unable to recall episodes
    - Myoclonic seizure
      - Variety of seizure episodes
      - Symmetric or asymmetric involvement
      - Brief contractions of muscle or groups of muscle
      - No postictal state
      - May or may not lose consciousness

- Atonic or akinetic seizure
  - Muscle tone is lost for a few seconds.
  - A period of confusion follows.
  - Loss of muscle tone frequently results in falling.
- Infantile Spasms
  - Most common during first 8 months of life
  - Sudden, brief, symmetric muscle contractions
  - Flexed head, extended arms with legs drawn up
  - Possible eyes rolling upward and inward
  - Possible loss of consciousness
  - Possible flushing, pallor or cyanosis
  - Possible cry or giggle before or after
- Partial (focal/local)
  - Simple partial seizures with motor signs
    - Aversive seizure: eyes and head turn away from the side of focus, with or without loss of consciousness
    - Rolandic seizure: tonic-clonic movements involving the face and most common during sleep
  - Simple partial seizure with sensory signs
    - Tingling, numbness or pain in one area of the body then spreading to other parts, with visual sensations.
  - Complex partial seizures
    - Altered behavior
    - Inability to respond to the environment
    - Impaired consciousness
    - Confusion and unable to recall event
    - Complex sensory aura: strange feeling in stomach that rises to the throat, auditory or visual hallucinations, feelings of fear, distorted sense of time and self
- Laboratory tests depend on age, history, and physical condition.
  - Lead level
  - WBC
  - Blood glucose
  - Serum electrolytes
  - Metabolic panel
  - Chromosomal analysis
  - Toxicology screen

- ○ Diagnostic Procedures
  - ▪ Electroencephalogram (EEG) records electrical activity and may identify the origin of seizure activity.
    - □ Can be monitored during sleep, when awake, and with stimulation and hyperventilation.
    - □ Test can last 1 hr to multiple periods and days of monitoring.
    - □ Can be performed with video monitoring.
    - □ Client Education
      - ▸ Abstain from caffeine for several hours prior to the procedure.
      - ▸ Wash hair before (no oils or sprays) and after the procedure to remove electrode gel.
      - ▸ Inform the client that he may be asked to take deep breaths and/or exposed to flashes of light during the procedure.
      - ▸ If prescribed, instruct parent to withhold sleep from child prior to test.
        - ▹ Inform the client that he may be allowed to sleep during the test. Sleep may be withheld prior to test and may be induced during the test.
      - ▸ Inform the client that the test will not be painful.
  - ▪ Magnetic resonance imaging (MRI) is used to detect malformations, cortical dysplasia, or tumors.
  - ▪ Lumbar puncture (LP) detects infection.
  - ▪ Computed tomography (CT) scan detects hemorrhage, infarction or malformations.

Patient-Centered Care

- • Nursing Care
  - ○ Initiate seizure precautions for any child at risk.
    - ▪ Pad side rails of bed, crib, and wheelchair.
    - ▪ Keep bed free of objects that could cause injury.
    - ▪ Have suction and oxygen equipment available.
  - ○ During a seizure
    - ▪ Protect from injury (move furniture away, hold head in lap if on the floor).
    - ▪ Maintain a position to provide a patent airway.
    - ▪ Be prepared to suction oral secretions.
    - ▪ Turn client to the side (decreases risk of aspiration).
    - ▪ Loosen restrictive clothing.
    - ▪ Do not attempt to restrain the child.
    - ▪ Do not attempt to open the jaw or insert an airway during seizure activity (this may damage teeth, lips, or tongue). Do not use padded tongue blades.
    - ▪ Remove glasses.
    - ▪ Administer oxygen.
    - ▪ Remain with the child.
    - ▪ Note onset, time, and characteristics of seizure.
    - ▪ Allow the seizure to end spontaneously.

- ○ Postseizure

  - Maintain in a side-lying position to prevent aspiration and to facilitate drainage of oral secretions.

  - Check vital signs.

  - Assess for injuries, including the mouth (tongue, teeth).

  - Perform neurologic checks.

  - Allow for rest if necessary.

  - Reorient and calm the client (due to agitation or confusion).

  - Maintain seizure precautions, including placing the bed in the lowest position and padding the side rails to prevent future injury.

  - Note the time of the postictal period.

  - Remain with the client.

  - Do not offer food or liquids until completely awake and swallow reflex is present.

  - Encourage client to describe the period before, during, and after the seizure activity.

  - Determine if the client experienced an aura, which may indicate the origin of seizure in the brain.

  - Try to determine the possible trigger, such as fatigue or stress.

  - Document the onset and duration of seizure and client findings/observations prior to, during, and following the seizure (level of consciousness, apnea, cyanosis, motor activity, incontinence).

- • Medications

  - ○ Antiepileptic drugs (AEDs) – diazepam (Valium), phenytoin (Dilantin), carbamazepine (Tegretol), valproic acid (Depakene), and fosphenytoin sodium (Cerebyx)

    - Medication selection is based on the client's age, type of seizure, and other medical factors.

    - A single medication is initiated at low dosage and gradually increased until seizures are controlled.

    - A second medication can be added to achieve seizure control.

    - Nursing Considerations

      - □ Monitor for seizure control.

      - □ Monitor for adverse affects.

      - □ Monitor therapeutic serum medication levels.

    - Client Education

      - □ Medications should be taken at the same time every day to enhance effectiveness.

      - □ Be aware of medication and food interactions that are specific to each medication.

      - □ Teach the child and family about adverse affects of the medications.

- • Teamwork and Collaboration

  - ○ The school nurse should be involved in providing for the child's safety in the school setting. This may include implementation of an individualized education plan or another specialized program.

  - ○ Referral to nutrition services if a ketogenic diet (high-fat, low-carbohydrate, and adequate protein) is prescribed.

- Surgical Interventions
  - Removal of a tumor, lesion, or hematoma
  - Focal resection of an area of the brain to remove epileptogenic zone
  - Hemispherectomy: removal of one hemisphere of the brain
  - Corpus callosotomy: separation of the two hemispheres in the brain
- Vagal nerve stimulator
  - Under general anesthesia, the stimulator is implanted into the left chest wall and connected to an electrode that is placed at the left vagus nerve. The device is then programmed to administer intermittent vagal nerve stimulation at a rate specific to the client's needs.
  - In addition to routine stimulation, the client may initiate vagal nerve stimulation by holding a magnet over the implantable device at the onset of seizure activity. This will either abort the seizure or lessen its severity.
- Client Education
  - Educate the client/family about the importance of periodic laboratory testing to monitor AED levels.
  - Encourage medication adherence.
  - Inform the client about possible medication interactions (decreased effectiveness of oral contraceptives).
  - Encourage wearing of a medical alert bracelet or necklace at all times.
  - Refer the family to the state's Department of Motor Vehicles to determine laws regarding driving for clients who have seizure disorders.
  - Teach the child to wear safety devices, such as helmets, with activities.
  - Teach the family not to leave the child unattended in water.
  - Avoid triggering factors.

Complications

- Status epilepticus is prolonged seizure activity that lasts longer than 30 min or continuous seizure activity in which the client does not enter a postictal phase. This acute condition requires immediate treatment to prevent loss of brain function, which may become permanent.
  - Nursing Actions
    - Maintain airway, administer oxygen, establish IV access, perform ECG monitoring, and monitor pulse oximetry and ABG results.
    - As prescribed, administer a loading dose of diazepam (Valium) or lorazepam (Ativan). If seizures continue after the loading dose is given, fosphenytoin followed by phenobarbital should be administered.
  - Client Education – Provide support for the client/family.
- Developmental delays
  - Nursing Actions
    - Promote optimal development.
    - Make appropriate referrals.
    - Provide support for the family.

APPLICATION EXERCISES

1. A nurse is caring for a child who has absence seizures. Which of the following findings can the nurse expect? (Select all that apply.)

_____ A. Loss of consciousness

_____ B. Appearance of daydreaming

_____ C. Dropping held objects

_____ D. Falling to the floor

_____ E. Having a piercing cry

2. A nurse is caring for a child who just experienced a generalized seizure. Which of the following is the priority action for the nurse to take?

A. Maintain in a side-lying position.

B. Monitor vital signs.

C. Reorient the child to the environment.

D. Assess for injuries.

3. A nurse is providing teaching to the parent of a child who is to have an electroencephalogram (EEG). Which of the following should be included in the teaching?

A. "Decaffeinated beverages should offered on the morning of the procedure."

B. "Do not wash your child's hair the night before the procedure."

C. "Withhold all foods the morning of the procedure."

D. "Give your child an analgesic the night before the procedure."

4. A nurse is teaching a group of parents about the risk factors for seizures. Which of the following should be included in the teaching? (Select all that apply.)

_____ A. Febrile episodes

_____ B. Hypoglycemia

_____ C. Sodium imbalances

_____ D. Low serum lead levels

_____ E. Presence of diphtheria

5. A nurse is reviewing treatment options with the parent of a child who has worsening seizures. Which of the following should be included in the discussion? (Select all that apply.)

_____ A. Vagal nerve stimulator

_____ B. Additional antiepileptic medications

_____ C. Corpus callosotomy

_____ D. Focal resection

_____ E. Radiation therapy

6. A nurse is planning care for a child who has tonic-clonic seizures. What nursing actions should be included in the plan of care? Use the ATI Active Learning Template: Systems Disorder to complete this item to include Nursing Care: Describe nursing actions during and after a seizure.

APPLICATION EXERCISES KEY

1. A. **CORRECT:** Loss of consciousness for 5 to 10 seconds is a clinical manifestation of an absence seizure.

    B. **CORRECT:** Behavior that resembles daydreaming is a clinical manifestation of an absence seizure.

    C. **CORRECT:** A child who is having absence seizures may drop a held object.

    D. INCORRECT: Falling to the floor is a clinical manifestation of a tonic-clonic seizure.

    E. INCORRECT: The presence of a piercing cry is a clinical manifestation of a tonic-clonic seizure.

    (N) NCLEX® Connection: Physiological Adaptations, Alterations in Body Systems

2. A. **CORRECT:** Using the airway, breathing, circulation priority-setting framework, the first action is to place the child in a side-lying position to maintain a patent airway and prevent aspiration of secretions.

    B. INCORRECT: Monitoring the child's vital signs is an appropriate action. However, it is not the priority action.

    C. INCORRECT: Reorienting the child to the environment following a generalized seizure is an appropriate action. However, it is not the priority action.

    D. INCORRECT: Assessing for injuries is an appropriate action. However, it is not the priority action.

    (N) NCLEX® Connection: Physiological Adaptations, Alterations in Body Systems

3. A. **CORRECT:** Caffeine can alter the results of an EEG and should be avoided prior to the test.

    B. INCORRECT: The child's hair should be washed to remove oils that permit adherence of the EEG electrodes.

    C. INCORRECT: Foods are not withheld prior to an EEG.

    D. INCORRECT: Analgesics may alter the results of an EEG and should be avoided prior to the test.

    (N) NCLEX® Connection: Reduction of Risk Potential, Diagnostic Tests

4. A. **CORRECT:** Febrile episodes can cause general tonic-clonic seizures in infants and young children.

    B. **CORRECT:** Seizure activity is a late manifestation of hypoglycemia.

    C. **CORRECT:** Seizure activity is a manifestation of hyponatremia and hypernatremia.

    D. INCORRECT: High serum lead levels is a risk factor for seizure activity.

    E. INCORRECT: Diphtheria is a respiratory illness causing difficulty breathing and is not a risk factor for seizures.

    (N) NCLEX® Connection: Physiological Adaptations, Alterations in Body Systems

5. A. **CORRECT:** The implantation of a vagal nerve stimulator is an option to provide seizure control.

    B. **CORRECT:** Additional antiepileptic medication can be added to the current medication regime to control seizures.

    C. **CORRECT:** A corpus callosotomy can be performed for uncontrolled seizures.

    D. **CORRECT:** A focal resection can be performed for uncontrolled seizures.

    E. INCORRECT: Radiation therapy is used in cancer treatment and is not used to control seizures.

    (N) NCLEX® Connection: Reduction of Risk Potential, Therapeutic Procedures

6. *Using the ATI Active Learning Template: Systems Disorder*

    - During a seizure
      - Protect the child from injury. (Move furniture away, hold head in lap if on the floor.)
      - Position the child to maintain a patent airway.
      - Be prepared to suction oral secretions.
      - Turn the child to the side (decreases risk of aspiration).
      - Loosen restrictive clothing.
      - Do not attempt to restrain the child.
      - Do not attempt to open the jaw or insert an airway during seizure activity. (This may damage teeth, lips, or tongue.) Do not use padded tongue blades.
      - Remove glasses.
      - Administer oxygen.
      - Remain with the child.
      - Note the onset, time, and characteristics of the seizure.
      - Allow the seizure to end spontaneously.

    - Postseizure
      - Maintain the child in a side-lying position to prevent aspiration and to facilitate drainage of oral secretions.
      - Check vital signs.
      - Assess for injuries, including the mouth.
      - Perform neurologic checks.
      - Allow the child to rest if necessary.
      - Reorient and calm the child (she may be agitated or confused).
      - Maintain seizure precautions, including placing the bed in the lowest position and padding the side rails to prevent future injury.
      - Note the time of the postictal period.
      - Remain with the child.
      - Do not offer food or liquids until completely awake and has a swallow reflex.
      - Encourage the child to describe the period before, during, and after the seizure activity.
      - Determine if the child experienced an aura, which may indicate the origin of seizure in the brain.
      - Try to determine the possible trigger, such as fatigue or stress.
      - Document the onset and duration of seizure and client findings/observations prior to, during, and following the seizure (level of consciousness, apnea, cyanosis, motor activity, incontinence).

    (N) NCLEX® Connection: Physiological Adaptations, Alterations in Body Systems

chapter 14

Overview

- Concussion is a injury to the brain that alters the way the brain functions.
- Contusion is bruising of the cerebral tissue.
- Laceration is tearing of the cerebral tissue.
- Fractures can be linear, depressed, comminuted, basilar, open, or growing.

Health Promotion and Disease Prevention

- Wear helmets when skateboarding, riding a bike or motorcycle, skiing, playing football, and participating in any other sport that may lead to head injury.
- Wear seat belts when driving or riding in a car.
- Avoid dangerous activities (riding a bicycle at night without a light, driving faster than the speed limit or while under the influence of alcohol or drugs).
- Never shake a baby.

Assessment

- Risk Factors
  - Lack of supervision
  - Inappropriate/absent safety practices
  - Improper use of safety devices (helmets, seat belts)
- Subjective Data
  - History of events leading up to the injury, including any reports of dizziness, headache, diplopia, and/or vomiting
  - Amnesia (loss of memory) before or after injury
  - Alcohol or drug ingestion
- Objective Data
  - Physical Assessment Findings
    - Loss of consciousness – The length of time the client is unconscious is significant.
    - Minor Injury
      - Possible loss of consciousness
      - Confusion
      - Vomiting

- Pallor
- Irritability
- Drowsiness
  - Progression of Injury
    - Changes in vital signs
    - Altered mental status
  - Severe Injury
    - Increased intracranial pressure (ICP)
      - Infants: bulging fontanel, separation of cranial sutures, irritability, increased sleeping, high-pitched cry, poor feeding, setting-sun sign
      - Children: nausea, headache, vomiting, blurred vision, increased sleeping, inability to follow simple commands, seizures
      - Late Signs: alterations in pupillary response, posturing (decorticate and decerebrate), bradycardia, decreased motor response, decreased sensory response, Cheyne-Stokes respirations, coma
        - Decorticate (dysfunction of the cerebral cortex) – Demonstrates the arms, wrists, and fingers flexed and bent inward onto the chest and the legs extended and adducted.
        - Decerebrate (dysfunction at the midbrain) – Demonstrates a backward arching of the head and arms with legs rigidly extended and toes pointing downward.

 View Images
> Decorticate Posturing   > Decerebrate Posturing

- Laboratory Tests
  - Arterial blood gases (ABGs)
  - Blood alcohol and toxicology screening
  - CBC with differential
- Diagnostic Procedures
  - Cervical spine x-rays to rule out cervical spine injury.
  - Computerized tomography (CT) and/or magnetic resonance imaging (MRI) of head and/or neck may be performed with and without contrast if indicated.
  - Measurement of ICP
    - The expected reference range is 10 to 15 mm Hg.
    - Client Education – Provide support to the client and family.

Patient-Centered Care

- Nursing Care (determined by the extent of the brain trauma)
  - Ensure the spine is stabilized until spinal cord injury is ruled out.
  - Monitor vital signs, level of consciousness, pupils, ICP, motor activity, sensory perception, and verbal responses at frequent intervals. Use the Glasgow Coma Scale as indicated.

- ○ Maintain a patent airway. Provide mechanical ventilation as indicated.

- ○ Administer oxygen as indicated to maintain an oxygen saturation level greater than 95%.

- ○ Use padded restraints for clients who have agitation to prevent injury.

- ○ Assess for clear fluid drainage from ears or nose (cerebral spinal fluid) and report to the provider.

- ○ Implement actions that will decrease ICP.

  - Keep the head of the bed elevated to 30°, which will also promote venous drainage.

  - Avoid extreme flexion, extension, or rotation of the head and maintain in midline neutral position.

  - Keep the client's body in alignment, avoiding hip flexion/extension.

  - Minimize endotracheal or oral suctioning.

  - Instruct the client to avoid coughing and blowing her nose, because these activities increase ICP.

- ○ Implement measures to prevent complications of immobility (turn every 2 hr, maintain footboard and splints). Specialty beds may be used.

- ○ Insert and maintain an indwelling urinary catheter.

- ○ Administer stool softener to prevent straining (Valsalva maneuver).

- ○ Provide a calm, restful environment (limit visitors, minimize noise).

- ○ Use energy conservation measures. Alternate activities with rest periods.

- ○ Implement seizure precautions.

- ○ Monitor fluid and electrolyte values and osmolarity to detect changes in sodium regulation, the onset of diabetes insipidus, or severe hypovolemia.

- ○ Provide adequate fluids to maintain cerebral perfusion. When a large amount of IV fluids is ordered, monitor the client for excess fluid volume, which may increase ICP.

- ○ Maintain the client's safety (side rails up, padded side rails, call light within reach).

- ○ Provide nutritional support (total parenteral nutrition, enteral nutrition).

- ○ Maintain ongoing communication with the client and family.

- ○ Instruct the family on effective ways to communicate with the child (touching, talking, assisting with care as appropriate).

- • Medications

  - ○ Corticosteroids – dexamethasone (Decadron) and methylprednisolone (Solu-Medrol) – used to decrease cerebral edema

  - ○ Mannitol (Osmitrol) – osmotic diuretic used to treat cerebral edema

  - ○ Antiepileptics – used to prevent or treat seizures that may occur

  - ○ Antibiotics – in cases of CSF leakage, lacerations, or penetrating injuries

  - ○ Analgesics – acetaminophen (Tylenol) – used for headache/pain management

- Teamwork and Collaboration

  - Care for the client who has a head injury should include professionals from other disciplines as indicated. These may include physical, occupational, recreational, and/or speech therapists.

  - Social services should be contacted to provide links to social service agencies and schools.

  - Rehabilitation facilities are frequently used to compress the time required to recover from a head injury.

- Surgical Interventions

  - Craniotomy

    - Involves removal of part of the skull.

    - The bone is replaced once the edema has resolved.

Complications

- Epidural Hemorrhage

  - Bleeding between the dura and the skull

  - Clinical manifestations: short period of unconsciousness followed by a normal period leading to herniation, coma, and death

- Subdural Hemorrhage

  - Bleeding between the dura and the arachnoid membrane

  - May be a result of birth injury, falls or violent shaking

  - Clinical manifestations: irritability, vomiting, seizures

- Cerebral Edema

  - Can develop within 24 to 72 hr posttrauma

  - Clinical manifestations: increased ICP

- Brain Herniation

  - Downward shift of brain tissue

  - Clinical manifestations: loss of blinking, loss of gag reflex, pupils fail to react to light, coma, and respiratory arrest

APPLICATION EXERCISES

1. A nurse is caring for a child who was admitted to the emergency department after a motor-vehicle crash. The child is unresponsive, has spontaneous respirations of 22/min, and has a laceration on the forehead that is bleeding. Which of the following is the priority nursing action at this time?

    A. Keep the neck stabilized.

    B. Insert a nasogastric tube.

    C. Obtain vital signs.

    D. Establish IV access.

2. A nurse is caring for an adolescent who has sustained a closed head injury. Which of the following are clinical manifestations of increased intracranial pressure (ICP)? (Select all that apply.)

_____ A. Report of headache

_____ B. Alteration in pupillary response

_____ C. Increased motor response

_____ D. Increased sleeping

_____ E. Increased sensory response

3. A nurse is caring for a child who has increased intracranial pressure. Which of the following are appropriate actions by the nurse? (Select all that apply.)

_____ A. Suction the endotracheal tube every 2 hr.

_____ B. Maintain a quiet environment.

_____ C. Use two pillows to elevate the head.

_____ D. Administer a stool softener.

_____ E. Maintain body alignment.

4. A nurse is assessing a child who has a concussion. Which of the following are clinical manifestations of a minor head injury? (Select all that apply.)

_____ A. Vomiting

_____ B. Delayed pupillary response

_____ C. Drowsiness

_____ D. Pallor

_____ E. Confusion

5. A nurse is teaching a parent about dexamethasone (Decadron) to treat head injury. Which of the following should be included in the teaching?

      A. "It decreases cerebral edema."

      B. "It promotes control of seizures."

      C. "It promotes improved pain management."

      D. "It is used to treat an infection."

6. A nurse is teaching a parent of a child about complications of a head injury. What should be included in the teaching? Use the ATI Active Learning Template: Systems Disorder to complete this item to include Potential Complications: Identify three and their corresponding clinical manifestation.

APPLICATION EXERCISES KEY

1. A. **CORRECT:** The greatest risk to a child following a motor vehicle crash is cervical injury. Therefore, keeping the neck stabilized until cervical injury can be ruled out is the priority action.

    B. INCORRECT: Inserting a nasogastric tube in is important. However, this is not the priority action.

    C. INCORRECT: Obtaining vital signs is important. However, this is not the priority action.

    D. INCORRECT: Establishing IV access is important. However, this is not the priority action.

    Ⓝ NCLEX® Connection: Safety and Infection Control, Accident/Error/Injury Prevention

2. A. **CORRECT:** A headache is a clinical manifestation of ICP.

    B. **CORRECT:** Alterations in pupillary response are a clinical manifestation of ICP.

    C. INCORRECT: Decreased motor response is a clinical manifestation of ICP.

    D. **CORRECT:** Increased sleeping is a clinical manifestation of ICP.

    E. INCORRECT: Decreased sensory response is a clinical manifestation of ICP.

    Ⓝ NCLEX® Connection: Physiological Adaptations, Unexpected Response to Therapies

3. A. INCORRECT: Routine suctioning of the endotracheal tube is poorly tolerated, not recommended, and raises intracranial pressure.

    B. **CORRECT:** Stimulation can cause increased intracranial pressure, and maintaining a quiet environment is an appropriate action for the nurse to take.

    C. INCORRECT: Pillows under the head cause flexion of the neck and increase intracranial pressure.

    D. **CORRECT:** Increased pressure in the abdomen with the Valsalva maneuver can increase intracranial pressure. Administering a stool softener is an appropriate action by the nurse.

    E. **CORRECT:** Flexion and extension of the neck or hips increase intracranial pressure. Therefore, maintaining body alignment is an appropriate action by the nurse.

    Ⓝ NCLEX® Connection: Physiological Adaptations, Alterations in Body Systems

4. A. **CORRECT:** Vomiting is a clinical manifestation of a minor head injury.

    B. INCORRECT: Alterations in pupillary response are a clinical manifestation of a major injury.

    C. **CORRECT:** Drowsiness is a clinical manifestation of a minor head injury.

    D. **CORRECT:** Pallor is a clinical manifestation of a minor head injury.

    E. **CORRECT:** Confusion is a clinical manifestation of a minor head injury.

    Ⓝ NCLEX® Connection: Physiological Adaptations, Pathophysiology

5. A. **CORRECT:** Dexamethasone is a corticosteroid and is used to decrease cerebral edema associated with a head injury.

    B. INCORRECT: Antiepileptics control seizures.

    C. INCORRECT: Analgesics are used for pain management.

    D. INCORRECT: Antibiotics treat infections.

    Ⓝ NCLEX® Connection: Pharmacological and Parenteral Therapies, Medication Administration

6. *Using the ATI Active Learning Template: Systems Disorder*
    - Potential Complications
        - Epidural hemorrhage
            - Bleeding between the dura and the skull
            - Clinical manifestations: short period of unconsciousness followed by a normal period leading to herniation, coma, and death
        - Subdural hemorrhage
            - Bleeding between the dura and the arachnoid membrane
            - Results from birth injury, falls, or violent shaking
            - Clinical manifestations: irritability, vomiting, seizures
        - Cerebral edema
            - Develops 24 to 72 hr posttrauma
            - Clinical manifestations: increased ICP
        - Brain herniation
            - Downward shift of brain tissue
            - Clinical manifestations: loss of blinking, loss of gag reflex, decreased pupillary response, coma, and respiratory arrest

    Ⓝ NCLEX® Connection: Physiological Adaptations, Unexpected Response to Therapies

UNIT 2   **NURSING CARE OF CHILDREN WITH SYSTEM DISORDERS**
        SECTION: NEUROSENSORY DISORDERS

CHAPTER 15   Visual and Hearing Impairments

Overview

- Sensory impairments in children most commonly affect the eyes and ears. Adequate vision and hearing are necessary for normal growth and development. Therefore, it is important to identify any impairments early in life.

VISUAL IMPAIRMENTS

Overview

- Visual impairments encompass both partial sight and legal blindness.
- Common visual impairments in children include myopia, hyperopia, astigmatism, anisometropia, amblyopia, strabismus, cataracts, and glaucoma.

Health Promotion and Disease Prevention

- Encourage the family to work with the child's school to meet educational needs.
- Screen children for visual impairments yearly.

Assessment

- Risk Factors
  - Prenatal or postnatal conditions such as retinopathy of prematurity, trauma, and postnatal infections.
  - Perinatal infections such as herpes, rubella, syphilis, chlamydia, and toxoplasmosis.
  - Chronic illness such as sickle cell disease, rheumatoid arthritis, retinoblastoma, and Tay-Sachs disease.
- Subjective and Objective Data
  - Visual screening
    - This is completed using the Snellen letter, tumbling E, or picture chart.
      - Place the client 10 feet from the chart with heels on the 10-foot mark.
      - Client should be wearing glasses, if appropriate, and keep both eyes open during the screening.
      - While covering one eye, the client reads each line on the chart, starting at the bottom of the chart, until he can pass a line. The client needs to identify four of the six characters in the line correctly to pass.
      - The client is then asked to start at the top and move down until he can no longer pass a line.
      - The procedure is repeated with the other eye.

- Partial visual impairment is classified as visual acuity of 20/70 to 20/200.
- Legal blindness is classified as visual acuity of 20/200 or worse.

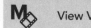 View Video: Vision and Hearing Screening

○ Ocular alignment is observed using the corneal light reflex test.
  - A flashlight is shone directly into the client's eye, from a distance of 16 inches.
  - Reflected light should be observed in the same location on both corneas.
○ Cover test – Client is asked to cover each eye and observe an object at a distance of 13 inches.
  - The cover is removed and the eye is observed for movement, which should not occur.
○ Peripheral vision is evaluated by having the client fixate on an object.
  - A pencil is moved from beyond the field of vision into the range of peripheral vision.
  - The client is asked to say stop when the object is noted in the peripheral vision. This angle is then measured.
  - Each quadrant of peripheral vision is tested. The test is repeated in the other eye.
  - Normal findings are 50° upward, 70° downward, 60° nasalward, and 90° temporally.
○ Color vision is evaluated using the Ishihara or Hardy-Rand-Rittler test.
  - The client is shown a set of cards and asked to identify the number embedded in the confusion of colors.
  - The client should identify all of the numbers on the cards with correct color vision.

VISUAL IMPAIRMENT SYMPTOMS	
Myopia (nearsightedness)	
› Sees close objects clearly, but not objects in the distance › Headaches and vertigo › Eye rubbing	› Difficulty reading › Clumsiness (frequently walking into objects) › Poor school performance
Hyperopia (farsightedness)	
› Sees distant objects clearly, but not objects that are close	› Because of accommodation, not usually detected until age 7
Astigmatism	
› Uneven vision in which only parts of letters on a page may be seen › Headache and vertigo	› The appearance of normal vision because tilting the head enables all letters to be seen
Strabismus – Esotropia (inward deviation of eye); Exotropia (outward deviation of eye)	
› Abnormal corneal light reflex or cover test › Misaligned eyes › Frowning or squinting › Difficulty seeing print clearly	› One eye closed to enable better vision › Head tilted to one side › Headache, dizziness, diplopia, photophobia, and crossed eyes

VISUAL IMPAIRMENT SYMPTOMS	
Amblyopia (lazy eye)	
› Reduced visual acuity in one eye	
Anisometropia	
› Different refractive strength in each eye	› Excessive eye rubbing
› Headache and vertigo	› Poor school performance
Cataracts	
› Decreased ability to see clearly	› Strabismus
› Possible loss of peripheral vision	› Gray opacity of the lens
› Nystagmus	› Absence of red reflex
Glaucoma	
› Loss of peripheral vision	› Spasmodic winking (blepharospasm)
› Perception of halos around objects	› Corneal haziness
› Red eye	› Enlargement of the eyeball (buphthalmos)
› Excessive tearing (epiphora)	› Possible pain
› Photophobia	

Patient-Centered Care

- Nursing Care

  - Maintain normal to bright lighting for the child when reading, writing, or participating in any activity that requires close vision.

  - Assess infants and children for visual impairments, and identify children that are high-risk.

  - Observe for behaviors that suggest vision loss or decrease.

  - Promote child's optimal development and parent-child attachment.

  - Identify safety hazards, and prevent injury to the eyes (helmets, safety glasses).

  - Provide information regarding laser surgery for clients who have myopia, hyperopia, or astigmatism.

  - Inform the child and family about corrective measures.

    - Myopia

      □ Biconcave lenses

      □ Laser surgery

    - Hyperopia

      □ Convex lenses

      □ Laser surgery

- Astigmatism
  - Special lenses that compensate for refractive errors
  - Laser surgery
- Anisometropia
  - Special lenses that compensate for the refractive errors
  - Preferably corrective contacts
  - Laser surgery
- Amblyopia
  - Treat primary visual defect
- Strabismus
  - Occlusion therapy (patch stronger eye)
  - Surgery
- Cataracts and glaucoma
  - Surgery
- Caring for a child who has lost her vision
  - Reassure the child and family.
  - Orient the child to the surroundings and provide a safe environment.
  - Promote independence and meeting developmental milestones while assisting with play and socialization.
  - Referr to educational services for visual impairment (Braille, audio tapes, special computers).

HEARING IMPAIRMENTS

Overview

- Hearing impairments affect the ability to clearly process linguistic sounds and affect speech.

Health Promotion and Disease Prevention

- Screen for hearing impairments.
- Help families identify community resources for children who are hearing impaired.
- Teach children and families to avoid further damage and hearing loss.
  - Avoid exposing children to hazardous noise.
  - Encourage children to wear ear protection if loud environmental noise cannot be avoided.

Assessment

- Risk Factors

  ○ Exposure to loud environmental sounds.

  ○ Hearing defects may be caused by a variety of conditions, including anatomic malformation, maternal ingestion of toxic substances during pregnancy, perinatal asphyxia, perinatal infection, chronic ear infection, and/or ototoxic medications.

  ○ Hearing defects are associated with chronic conditions such as Down syndrome and/or cerebral palsy.

    ▪ Conductive losses involve interference of sound transmission, which may result from otitis media, external ear infection, foreign bodies, or excessive ear wax.

    ▪ Sensorineural losses involve interference of the transmission along the nerve pathways, which may result from congenital defects or secondary to acquired conditions (infection, ototoxic medication, exposure to constant noise – as in a NICU).

    ▪ Central auditory imperception involves all other hearing losses (aphasia, agnosia [inability to interpret sounds]).

Subjective and Objective Data

- Infants

  ○ Lack of startle reflex

  ○ Failure to respond to noise

  ○ Absence of vocalization by 7 months

  ○ Lack of response to the spoken word

- Older children

  ○ Using gestures rather than talking after 15 months

  ○ Failure to develop understood speech by 24 months

  ○ Yelling to express emotions

  ○ Irritability due to inability to gain attention

  ○ Seeming shy or withdrawn

  ○ Inattentive to surroundings

  ○ Speaking in monotone

  ○ Need for repeated conversation

  ○ Speaking loudly for situation

Patient-Centered Care

- Nursing Care
  - Assess children for hearing impairment.
  - Promote speech development, lipreading, and use of cued speech (hand gestures with verbal communication).
  - Use sign language.
  - Encourage socialization and use of aids to promote independence (flashing light when the door bell or phone rings, telecommunication devices, closed captioning on the television).
  - Refer to community support groups for child and family.
  - Use a sign language interpreter when working with a child who is hearing impaired. Always talk to the child, not the interpreter.
  - Assess gait/balance for instability.
  - Adjust environment for physiologic symptoms.
  - Identify safety hazards.
  - Assist with the use of hearing aids.

Complications

- Delayed growth and development
  - Visual and hearing impairments may prevent the child from appropriate speech and motor development. Identifying the impairment early may minimize this.

  - Nursing Actions
    - Encourage self-care and optimal independence.
    - Make interprofessional referrals as needed (social services, speech therapy, physical therapy, occupational therapy, teachers).
  - Client Education
    - Assist the family to obtain and access appropriate assistive devices.

APPLICATION EXERCISES

1. A nurse is planning to perform a peripheral vision test on a child. Which of the following is an appropriate action for the nurse to take?

    A. Place the child 10 feet away from the chart.

    B. Show a set of cards to the child one at a time.

    C. Cover the child's eye while performing the test on the other eye.

    D. Have the child focus on an object while performing the test.

2. A nurse is teaching the parent of a child who has strabismus. Which of the following should be included in the teaching?

    A. "Your child should be fitted for contact lenses."

    B. "Wearing glasses with convex lenses will correct this problem."

    C. "Placing a patch over the strong eye is needed."

    D. "Special lenses can correct the vision."

3. A nurse is assessing a child. Which of the following are clinical manifestations of myopia? (Select all that apply.)

    _____ A. Headaches

    _____ B. Photophobia

    _____ C. Difficult reading

    _____ D. Difficulty focusing on close objects

    _____ E. Poor school performance

4. A nurse is assessing a toddler for possible hearing loss. Which of the following are clinical manifestations of a hearing impairment? (Select all that apply.)

    _____ A. Uses telegraphic speech

    _____ B. Speaks loudly

    _____ C. Repeats sentences

    _____ D. Appears shy

    _____ E. Is overly attentive to the surroundings

5. A nurse is completing a physical assessment of a child with suspected glaucoma. Which of the following findings confirm this diagnosis? (Select all that apply.)

_____ A. Epiphora

_____ B. Absent red reflex

_____ C. Strabismus

_____ D. Blepharospasm

_____ E. Report of pain

6. A nurse is planning to perform a visual screening test on a child. What nursing actions should the nurse include? Use the ATI Active Learning Template: Nursing Skill to complete this item to include the following sections:

A. Nursing Actions: Explain the procedure.

B. Client Outcomes: Describe findings that indicate visual impairment.

APPLICATION EXERCISES KEY

1. A. INCORRECT: A nurse should place the child 10 feet away from the chart when performing a visual acuity test.

    B. INCORRECT: A nurse should show a set of cards to the child one at a time when performing a color test.

    C. INCORRECT: A nurse should cover the child's eye while performing the test on the other eye when performing a cover test.

    D. **CORRECT:** When performing a peripheral vision test, the nurse asks the child to focus on an object while bringing a pencil into the child's peripheral vision.

    (N) NCLEX® Connection: Health Promotion and Maintenance, Health Screening

2. A. INCORRECT: Contact lenses are used for children who have anisometropia.

    B. INCORRECT: Convex lenses are used for children who have hyperopia.

    C. **CORRECT:** Placing a patch over the strong eye to increase visual stimulation to the affected eye is used when treating strabismus.

    D. INCORRECT: Special lenses are used for children who have astigmatism and anisometropia.

    (N) NCLEX® Connection: Reduction of Risk Potential, Therapeutic Procedures

3. A. **CORRECT:** Headaches are a clinical manifestation of myopia.

    B. INCORRECT: Photophobia is a clinical manifestation of strabismus.

    C. **CORRECT:** Difficulty reading is a clinical manifestation of myopia.

    D. INCORRECT: Difficulty focusing on close objects is a clinical manifestation of hyperopia.

    E. **CORRECT:** Poor school performance is a clinical manifestation of myopia.

    (N) NCLEX® Connection: Basic Care and Comfort, Assistive Devices

4.   A. INCORRECT: Monotone speech is a clinical manifestation of a hearing impairment.

     B. **CORRECT:** Speaking loudly is a clinical manifestation of a hearing impairment.

     C. INCORRECT: Repeating sentences is an expected developmental task for a toddler.

     D. **CORRECT:** Shyness or withdrawn behavior are clinical manifestations of a hearing impairment.

     E. INCORRECT: Inattentiveness to surroundings is a clinical manifestation of a hearing impairment.

     Ⓝ NCLEX® Connection: Basic Care and Comfort, Assistive Devices

5.   A. **CORRECT:** Epiphora is a clinical manifestation of glaucoma.

     B. INCORRECT: Absent red reflex is a clinical manifestation of a cataract.

     C. INCORRECT: Strabismus is a clinical manifestation of a cataract.

     D. **CORRECT:** Blepharospasm is a clinical manifestation of glaucoma.

     E. **CORRECT:** Report of pain is a clinical manifestation of glaucoma.

     Ⓝ NCLEX® Connection: Basic Care and Comfort, Assistive Devices

6.   *Using the ATI Active Learning Template: Nursing Skill*

     A. Nursing Actions
         • Choose appropriate chart: Snellen Letter, tumbling E, or picture chart.
         • Place child 10 feet from the chart with heels on the 10-foot mark.
         • Screen child wearing glasses, if appropriate.
         • Child keeps both eyes open and covers one eye.
         • Have the child start at the bottom and read each line, continuing up until the child can pass a line.
         • Have the child start at the top and move down until the child can no longer pass a line.
         • To pass, the child needs to identify four of the six characters correctly.
         • Repeat the procedure with the other eye.

     B. Client Outcomes
         • Partial visual impairment is classified as visual acuity of 20/70 to 20/200.
         • Legal blindness is classified as visual acuity of 20/200 or worse.

     Ⓝ NCLEX® Connection: Health Promotion and Maintenance, Health Screening

UNIT 2 **Nursing Care of Children with System Disorders**

SECTION: RESPIRATORY DISORDERS

› Oxygen and Inhalation Therapy
› Acute and Infectious Respiratory Illnesses
› Asthma
› Cystic Fibrosis

NCLEX® CONNECTIONS

When reviewing the chapters in this unit, keep in mind the relevant sections of the NCLEX® outline, in particular:

Client Needs: Safety and Infection Control	Client Needs: Reduction of Risk Potential	Client Needs: Physiological Adaptation
› Relevant topics/tasks include: » Standard Precautions/ Transmission-Based Precautions/Surgical Asepsis › Understand communicable diseases and the modes of organism transmission.	› Relevant topics/tasks include: » Diagnostic Tests › Monitor the results of diagnostic testing and intervene as needed. » Laboratory Values › Identify laboratory values for ABGs, BUN, cholesterol, glucose, hematocrit, hemoglobin, glycosylated hemoglobin, platelets, potassium, sodium, WBC, creatinine, PT, PTT and APTT, INR. » Potential for Alterations in Body Systems › Identify the client's potential for aspiration.	› Relevant topics/tasks include: » Alterations in Body Systems › Provide pulmonary hygiene. » Illness Management › Manage the care of a client with impaired ventilation/ oxygenation. » Pathophysiology › Identify pathophysiology related to an acute or chronic condition.

chapter 16

CHAPTER 16　Oxygen and Inhalation Therapy

Overview

- Oxygen is used to maintain adequate cellular oxygenation. It is used in the treatment of many acute and chronic respiratory problems (hypoxemia, cystic fibrosis, asthma). Supplemental oxygen may be delivered using a variety of methods, depending on individual circumstances.

- Pulse oximetry is used to monitor the effectiveness of inhalation therapies.

- Common treatment methods for children with respiratory issues (acute or chronic)

  o Nebulized aerosol therapy

  o Metered-dose inhaler (MDI) or dry powder inhaler (DPI)

  o Chest physiotherapy (CPT)

  o Oxygen therapy

  o Suctioning

  o Artificial airway

Pulse Oximetry

- A noninvasive measurement of the oxygen saturation (SaO_2) of arterial blood.

- A pulse oximeter is a device that is operated by battery or electricity and has a sensor probe that is attached securely to the child's fingertip, toe, earlobe, or around the foot with a clip or band.

- Indications – Pulse oximetry is used for a variety of situations in which quick assessments of a child's respiratory status are needed.

- Interpretation of Findings

  o The expected reference range for SaO_2 is 95% to 100%. Acceptable levels may range from 91% to 100%. Some illnesses may allow for an SaO_2 of 85% to 89%.

  o Results less than 91% require nursing intervention to assist the child to regain acceptable SaO_2 levels. An SaO_2 of less than 86% is a life-threatening emergency. The lower the SaO_2 level, the less accurate the value.

- Preprocedure

  o Nursing Actions

    ▪ Find an appropriate probe site. The probe site must be dry and have adequate circulation. Remove polish from nails or remove earring if using the earlobe.

    ▪ Be sure the child is in a comfortable position and that the arm is supported if a finger is used as a probe site.

- Intraprocedure
  - Nursing Actions
    - Note the pulse reading and compare it with the child's radial pulse. Any discrepancy warrants further assessment.
    - If continuous monitoring is required, make sure the alarms are set for a low and a high limit, the alarms are functioning, and the sound is audible. Move the probe every 4 hr or per facility policy.
- Postprocedure
  - Nursing Actions – Report unexpected findings to the provider.
    - If a child's SaO_2 is less than prescribed range (usually 90 to 92%)
      - Confirm that the sensor probe is properly placed.
      - Confirm that the oxygen delivery system is functioning and that the child is receiving the prescribed oxygen flow rate. Increase oxygen rate as needed.
      - Place the child in a semi-Fowler's or Fowler's position to maximize ventilation.
      - Encourage deep breathing.
      - Report significant findings to the health care provider.
      - Remain with the child and provide emotional support to decrease anxiety.

Nebulized Aerosol Therapy

- The process of nebulization breaks up medications into minute particles that are then dispersed throughout the respiratory tract. These droplets are much finer than those created by inhalers.
- Indications – Respiratory conditions that necessitate bronchodilators, corticosteroids, mucolytics, or antibiotics.
- Nursing Actions
  - Preparation of the Client
    - Instruct the child and family that the treatment may take 10 to 15 min.
    - Determine if the child should use a mouthpiece, mask, or blow-by.
    - Perform a preprocedure assessment, including vital signs and oxygen saturation.
    - Pour the medication into the small container and attach the device to an air or oxygen source.
  - Ongoing Care
    - Encourage the child to take slow, deep breaths by mouth.
    - Monitor the child during the treatment.
    - Assess vital signs, oxygen saturation, and lung sounds at the completion of treatment.
    - Assist the family with obtaining a nebulizer for home use if needed.
    - Enforce recommendations for aerosolized medications.
    - Monitor for adverse reactions to medications.
- Client Education
  - Teach the family how to operate a home nebulizer.
  - Teach the family about adverse affects of the prescribed medications.

Metered-Dose Inhaler (MDI) or Dry Powder Inhaler (DPI)

- These are handheld devices that allow children to self-administer medications on an intermittent basis.
- Indications – respiratory conditions that necessitate bronchodilators or corticosteroids
- Nursing Actions
  - Provide instructions to the child and parents for use of an MDI.

 View Animation: Metered-Dose Inhaler

  - Remove the cap from the inhaler.
  - Shake the inhaler five to six times.
  - Attach the spacer. (A spacer should be encouraged for children to facilitate proper inhalation of the medication.)
  - Hold the inhaler with the mouthpiece at the bottom.
  - Hold the inhaler with the thumb near the mouthpiece, and the index and middle fingers at the top.
  - Instruct the child on an MDI placement technique.
    - Open-mouth method: Hold the inhaler approximately 2 to 4 cm (0.8 to 1.6 in) away from the front of the mouth.
    - Closed-mouth method: Place the inhaler between the lips and instruct the child to form a seal around the MDI.
  - Take a deep breath and then exhale.
  - Tilt the head back slightly, and press the inhaler. While pressing the inhaler, begin a slow, deep breath that lasts for 3 to 5 seconds to facilitate delivery to the air passages.
  - Hold the breath for approximately 10 seconds to allow the medication to deposit in the airways.
  - Take the inhaler out of the mouth and slowly exhale through the nose.
  - Resume normal breathing.
  - Provide instructions to the child and parents for the use of a DPI.
    - Do not shake the device.
    - Take the cover off the mouthpiece.
    - Follow the directions of the manufacturer, such as turning the wheel of the inhaler, for preparing the medication.
    - Exhale completely.
    - Place the mouthpiece between the lips and take a deep breath through the mouth.
    - Hold breath for 5 to 10 seconds.
    - Take the inhaler out of the mouth and slowly exhale through pursed lips.
    - Resume normal breathing.
  - If more than one puff is prescribed, instruct the child to wait the length of time directed before administering the second puff.
  - Instruct the child to remove the canister and rinse the inhaler, cap, and spacer once a day with warm running water. Instruct the child to dry the inhaler before reuse.

- Complications
  - Improper medication dosage related to improper use
    - Inhalation is too rapid.
    - Inability to coordinate inhalation with spray.
    - Not holding breath for adequate period.
    - Nursing Actions – Ensure the child uses the inhaler with proper technique.
    - Client Education – Reinforce proper technique with client and family.
  - Fungal infections
    - Fungal infections of the oral cavity may occur with corticosteroid use.
    - Nursing Actions
      - Assess mouth for signs of infections.
      - Assist the child with rinsing his mouth after administration.
    - Client Education – Instruct the child and parents to clean the MDI and spacer after each use and to have the child rinse his mouth and expectorate.

Chest Physiotherapy (CPT)

- Chest physiotherapy is a set of techniques that include percussion, vibration, and postural drainage. Gravity and positioning loosen respiratory secretions and move them into the central airways, where they can be eliminated by coughing or suctioning to rid excessive secretions from specific areas of the lungs.
- Indications
  - Client Presentation
    - Thick secretions with an inability to clear the airway
    - Contraindication – decreased cardiac reserves, pulmonary embolism, or increased intracranial pressure
- Preprocedure
  - Nursing Actions
    - Schedule treatments 1 hr before or 2 hr after meals and at bedtime to decrease the likelihood of vomiting or aspirating.
    - Administer a bronchodilator medication or nebulizer treatment prior to postural drainage if prescribed.
    - Offer an emesis basin and facial tissues.
- Intraprocedure
  - Nursing Actions
    - Perform hand hygiene, provide privacy, and explain the procedure to the child and parents.
    - Ensure proper positioning to promote drainage of specific areas of the lungs.
      - Apical sections of the upper lobes – Fowler's position
      - Posterior sections of the upper lobes – side-lying position
      - Right lobe – on the left side with a pillow under the chest wall
      - Left lobe – Trendelenburg position

- Apply manual percussion by using cupped hand or a special device to clap rhythmically on the chest wall to break up secretions.

- Electronic percussion is applied by a vest device worn by the child.

- Have the child remain in each postural drainage position for 10 to 15 min to allow time for percussion, vibration, and postural drainage.

- Discontinue the procedure if the child reports faintness or dizziness.

- Postprocedure
  - Nursing Actions
    - Perform lung auscultation and assess the amount, color, and character of the expectorated secretions.
    - Document interventions and repeat the procedure as prescribed (typically two to four times per day).

- Complications
  - Hypoxia (decrease in SaO_2)
    - Nursing Actions
      - Monitor respiratory status during the procedure.
      - Discontinue the procedure if dyspnea occurs.

Oxygen Therapy

- Oxygen therapy increases the oxygen concentration of the air that is being breathed.

- Oxygen can be delivered via nasal cannula, face mask, hood, or ventilator.
  - Humidification of oxygen moistens the airways, which promotes loosening and mobilization of pulmonary secretions and prevents drying and injury of respiratory structures.

- Indications
  - Diagnoses
    - Hypoxemia
      - Hypoxemia develops when there is an inadequate level of oxygen in the blood. Hypovolemia, hypoventilation, and interruption of arterial flow can lead to hypoxemia.

EARLY SIGNS	LATE SIGNS
› Tachypnea	› Confusion and stupor
› Tachycardia	› Cyanosis of skin and mucous membranes
› Restlessness	› Bradypnea
› Pallor of the skin and mucous membranes	› Bradycardia
› Evidence of respiratory distress (use of accessory muscles, nasal flaring, tracheal tugging, adventitious lung sounds)	› Hypotension or hypertension

- Nursing Actions
  - Preparation of the Client
    - Warm oxygen to prevent hypothermia.
    - Use a calm, nonthreatening approach.
    - Explain all procedures to the child and parents.
    - Place in semi-Fowler's or Fowler's position to facilitate breathing and to promote chest expansion.
    - Ensure that equipment is working properly.
  - Ongoing Care
    - Provide oxygen therapy at the lowest liter flow that corrects hypoxemia.
    - Assess/monitor lung sounds and respiratory rate, rhythm, and effort to determine the need for supplemental oxygen.
    - Do not allow oxygen to blow directly onto the faces of infants.
    - Change linens and clothing frequently.
    - Monitor temperature for hypothermia.
    - Assess/monitor oxygenation status with pulse oximetry and ABGs.
    - Apply the oxygen delivery device prescribed.
    - Provide oral hygiene as needed.
    - Promote turning, coughing, deep breathing, and use of incentive spirometry and suctioning.
    - Promote rest and decrease environmental stimuli.
    - Provide emotional support for children who appear anxious.
    - Assess nutritional status and provide supplements as prescribed.
    - Assess/monitor skin integrity. Provide moisture and pressure-relief devices as indicated.
    - Assess/monitor and document response to oxygen therapy.
    - Titrate oxygen to maintain the prescribed oxygen saturation.
    - Discontinue oxygen gradually.

DELIVERY SYSTEM	NURSING IMPLICATIONS
› Oxygen hood – small plastic hood that fits over the infant's head	› Use a minimum flow rate of 4 to 5 L/min to prevent carbon dioxide buildup. › Ensure that neck, chin, or shoulders do not rub against the hood. › Secure a pulse oximeter for continuous SaO_2 monitoring.
› Nasal cannula – disposable plastic tube with two prongs for insertion into the nostrils that delivers an oxygen concentrations of 24% to 40% FiO_2 at a flow rate of 1 to 6 L/min	› Nasal cannulas are safe, easy to apply, and well tolerated. › The child is able to eat, talk, and ambulate while wearing a cannula. › Cannulas may be used by infants and older children who are cooperative. › Assess the patency of the nares. › Ensure that the prongs fit in the nares properly. › A nasal cannula may cause skin breakdown and dry mucous membranes. › Supply the child with a water-soluble gel if the nares are dry. › Provide humidification for flow rates greater than 4 L/min. › Prongs can become dislodged easily; therefore, monitor the child frequently.
› Pediatric face mask – pediatric-size mask that covers the nose and mouth	› Face masks require a snug fit and may not be tolerated. › Used for supplying high oxygen flow rate or for children who are mouth breathers.

- Complications
  - Combustion – Oxygen is combustible.
    - Nursing Actions
      - Place "No Smoking" or "Oxygen in Use" signs to alert others of the combustion hazard.
      - Know where the closest fire extinguisher is located.
      - Have the child wear a cotton gown, because synthetics or wools may create sparks of static electricity.
      - Ensure that all electric machinery (monitors, suction machines) are grounded.
      - Avoid toys that may induce a spark.
      - Do not use volatile, flammable materials (alcohol, acetone) near children who are receiving oxygen.
    - Client Education – Educate the child and others about the fire hazards of smoking with oxygen use.
  - Oxygen toxicity
    - Oxygen toxicity may result from high concentrations of oxygen, long duration of oxygen therapy, and the child's degree of lung disease.
      - Hypoventilation and increased $PaCO_2$ levels allow for rapid progression into unconscious state.
    - Nursing Actions
      - Use the lowest level of oxygen necessary to maintain an adequate SaO_2.
      - Monitor ABGs and notify the health care provider if $PaCO_2$ levels rise outside of the expected reference range.
      - Use of an oxygen mask with continuous positive airway pressure (CPAP), bilevel positive airway pressure (BiPAP), or positive end-expiratory pressure (PEEP) while a child is on a mechanical ventilator may decrease the amount of oxygen needed.
      - Decrease the oxygen flow rate gradually.

Suctioning

- Suctioning can be accomplished orally, nasally, endotracheally, or through a tracheostomy tube.
- Indications – to remove mucus plugs and excessive secretions
  - Client Presentation
    - Early signs of hypoxemia (restlessness, tachypnea, tachycardia, decreased SaO_2 levels, adventitious breath sounds, visualization of secretions, cyanosis, absence of spontaneous cough)
- Nasal suctioning
  - Use clean technique.
  - Use a mushroom tip catheter.
- Oral suctioning
  - Use clean technique.
  - Use a hard catheter tip.
  - Insert in sides of mouth.

- Endotracheal and tracheal suctioning
  - Preprocedure
    - Nursing Actions
      - Perform hand hygiene, provide privacy, and explain the procedure to the child.
      - Don the required personal protective equipment. Assist the child to a high-Fowler's or Fowler's position for suctioning if possible.
      - Perform through a tracheostomy or an endotracheal tube. Obtain a suction catheter with an outer diameter of no more than 1 cm (0.4 in) of the internal diameter of the tube.
      - Ask for assistance if necessary.
      - Hyperoxygenate the child using a bag-valve-mask (BVM) resuscitator or specialized ventilator function with an FiO_2 of 100%.
      - Obtain baseline breath sounds and vital signs, including oxygen saturation (SaO_2) by pulse oximeter. Oxygen saturation may be monitored continually during the procedure.
  - Intraprocedure
    - Nursing Actions
      - Use correct surgical aseptic technique as identified in appropriate resources.
      - Maintain ongoing assessments of oxygen status while performing the procedure.
  - Postprocedure
    - Nursing Actions – Document the child's response.
- Complications
  - Hypoxia
    - Nursing Actions
      - Stop the procedure.
      - Hyperoxygenate the child.

Artificial Airways

- A tracheotomy is a sterile surgical incision into the trachea through the skin and muscles for the purpose of establishing an airway.
- A tracheotomy can be performed as an emergency procedure or as a scheduled surgical procedure.
- A tracheostomy is the stoma/opening that results from a tracheotomy to provide and secure a patent airway. A tracheostomy can be permanent or temporary.
- Artificial airways can be placed orotracheally, nasotracheally, or through a tracheostomy to assist with respiration.
  - Pediatric tracheostomy tubes made of plastic have a more acute angle than adult tubes. Pediatric tracheostomy tubes soften with body temperature to shape to the contour of the child's trachea. No inner cannula is necessary, because this material resists the accumulation of dried secretions.
- Indications
  - Client Presentation – obstruction of the upper airway requiring the use of artificial ventilation

- Nursing Actions
  - Assess/monitor:
    - Oxygenation, ventilation (respiratory rate, effort, SaO_2), and vital signs hourly.
    - Thickness, quantity, odor, and color of mucous secretions.
    - The stoma and the skin surrounding the stoma for signs of inflammation or infection (redness, swelling, or drainage).
  - Provide adequate humidification and hydration to thin secretions and decrease the risk of mucus plugging.
  - Do not suction routinely. This may cause mucosal damage, bleeding, and bronchospasm.
  - Assess/monitor the need for suctioning. Suction on a PRN basis when assessment findings indicate the need to do so (audible/noisy secretions, crackles, restlessness, tachypnea, tachycardia, and mucus in the airway).
  - Maintain surgical aseptic technique when suctioning to prevent infection.
  - Provide emotional support to the child and parents.
  - Provide oral hygiene, usually every 2 hr.
  - For cuffed tubes, keep the pressure below 20 mm Hg to reduce the risk of tracheal necrosis due to prolonged compression of tracheal capillaries.
  - Provide tracheostomy care every 8 hr.
  - Change nondisposable tracheostomy tubes every 6 to 8 weeks or per protocol.
  - Reposition the client every 2 hr to prevent atelectasis and pneumonia.
  - Keep an emergency tracheostomy tube (one size smaller) at the bedside.
  - Client Education
    - Provide discharge teaching regarding the following:
      - Tracheostomy care
      - Findings that the family should immediately report to the health care provider (signs of infection or copious secretions)
      - Ways to promote improved nutrition
- Complications
  - Accidental decannulation
    - Accidental decannulation in the first 72 hr after surgery is an emergency because the tracheostomy tract has not matured and replacement may be difficult.
    - Nursing Actions – Always have an additional staff member present when moving the tube or during any situation in which decannulation may occur.
    - Client Education
      - When caring for the tube at home, have a second tube available in the event of dislodgement.
      - Have scissors available to cut the old strings in an emergency.
  - Occlusion
    - Occlusion is a situation in which the tube is clogged with secretions and prevents adequate air exchange.
    - Nursing Actions – Maintain a patent airway with suctioning.
    - Client Education – Instruct the parents about the need to suction to prevent occlusion.

APPLICATION EXERCISES

1. A nurse is teaching an adolescent to self-administer a corticosteroid medication per dry powder inhaler (DPI). Which of the following should be included in the teaching? (Select all that apply.)

_____ A. Shake the device prior to use.

_____ B. Rinse and expectorate after administration.

_____ C. Inhale with medication administration.

_____ D. Exhale quickly after medication administered.

_____ E. Attach a spacer to the device prior to use.

2. A nurse caring for a child who is receiving oxygen therapy and is on a continuous oxygen saturation monitor that is reading 89%. Which of the following is the priority action for the nurse to take?

A. Increase the oxygen flow rate.

B. Encourage the child to take deep breaths.

C. Ensure proper placement of the sensor probe.

D. Place the child in the Fowler's position.

3. A nurse is assessing a child. Which of the following is an early indication of hypoxemia?

A. Nonproductive cough

B. Hypoventilation

C. Nasal flaring

D. Nasal stuffiness

4. A nurse is caring for a child who is receiving oxygen. Which of the following is a clinical manifestations of oxygen toxicity?

A. Increased blood pressure

B. Hyperventilation

C. Decreased $PaCO_2$

D. Unconsciousness

5. A nurse is caring for a child who is receiving a bronchodilator medication by nebulized aerosol therapy. Which of the following are appropriate actions for the nurse to take? (Select all that apply.)

_____ A. Instruct the child that the treatment will last 30 min.

_____ B. Obtain vital signs prior to the procedure.

_____ C. Tell the child to take slow deep breaths.

_____ D. Determine if the child should use a mask.

_____ E. Attach the device to an air source.

6. A nurse is teaching a child how to use a metered-dose inhaler. What information should be included in the teaching? Use the ATI Active Learning Template: Nursing Skill to complete this item.

APPLICATION EXERCISES KEY

1. A. INCORRECT: A DPI is a powder medication and should not be shaken prior to administration.

    B. **CORRECT:** Corticosteroids can cause an oral fungal infection. The client should rinse and expectorate following medication administration.

    C. **CORRECT:** The client should take a quick, deep inhalation from the device to administer the medication into the lungs.

    D. INCORRECT: After inhalation of the medication, the client should hold his breath for 5 to 10 seconds.

    E. INCORRECT: A spacer is not used with a DPI device.

    Ⓝ NCLEX® Connection: Pharmacological and Parenteral Therapies, Medication Administration

2. A. INCORRECT: Increasing the oxygen flow rate for a child who has an oxygen saturation of 89% is important, but this is not the priority action.

    B. INCORRECT: Encouraging the child to take deep breaths to increase oxygenation is important, but this is not the priority action.

    C. **CORRECT:** The first action the nurse should take using the nursing process approach is to assess. Ensuring the sensor probe is properly placed is the priority action.

    D. INCORRECT: Placing the child in Fowler's position to increase oxygenation is important, but this is not the priority action.

    Ⓝ NCLEX® Connection: Physiological Adaptations, Illness Management

3. A. INCORRECT: Nonproductive cough is a clinical manifestation of a respiratory infection.

    B. INCORRECT: Hypoventilation is a clinical manifestation of oxygen toxicity.

    C. **CORRECT:** Early signs of hypoxemia include indications of respiratory distress, such as nasal flaring.

    D. INCORRECT: Nasal stuffiness is a clinical manifestation of a respiratory infection.

    Ⓝ NCLEX® Connection: Physiological Adaptations, Illness Management

4. A. INCORRECT: Increased blood pressure is not a clinical manifestation of oxygen toxicity.

    B. INCORRECT: Hypoventilation is a clinical manifestation of oxygen toxicity.

    C. INCORRECT: An increased $PaCO_2$ is a clinical manifestation of oxygen toxicity.

    D. **CORRECT:** Children who exhibit oxygen toxicity progress into an unconscious state rapidly.

    Ⓝ NCLEX® Connection: Pharmacological and Parenteral Therapies, Expected Actions/Outcomes

5.   A. INCORRECT: Nebulized medications take approximately 10 to 15 min to deliver.

     B. **CORRECT:** Baseline vital signs should be obtain prior to a nebulized medication for purposes of comparison with how the client tolerates the medication.

     C. **CORRECT:** The client should take slow, deep breaths to inhale the medication deeply into the respiratory tract.

     D. **CORRECT:** Nebulized medications can be delivered by mask, mouthpiece, or blow-by. The nurse should determine the best method of delivery.

     E. **CORRECT:** Nebulized medications need to have an air source to break the medication into small particles for inhalation.

     Ⓝ NCLEX® Connection: Reduction of Risk Potential, Potential for Complications from Surgical Procedures and Health Alterations

6.   *Using the ATI Active Learning Template: Nursing Skill*
     • Remove the cap from the inhaler
     • Shake the inhaler five to six times.
     • Attach the spacer. (A spacer should be encouraged for children to facilitate proper inhalation of the medication.)
     • Hold the inhaler with the mouthpiece at the bottom.
     • Hold the inhaler with the thumb near the mouthpiece and the index and middle fingers at the top.
       ○ Open-mouth technique: Hold the inhaler approximately 2 to 4 cm (0.8 to 1.6 in) away from the front of the mouth.
       ○ Closed-mouth method: Place the inhaler between the lips and instruct the child to form a seal around the inhaler.
     • Take a deep breath and then exhale.
     • Tilt the head back slightly, and press the inhaler. While pressing the inhaler, begin a slow, deep breath that lasts for 3 to 5 seconds to facilitate delivery to the air passages.
     • Hold the breath for approximately 10 seconds to allow the medication to deposit in the airways.
     • Take the inhaler out of the mouth and slowly exhale through the nose.
     • Resume normal breathing.

     Ⓝ NCLEX® Connection: Pharmacological and Parenteral Therapies, Medication Administration

chapter 17

Overview

- Acute and infectious respiratory illnesses prevalent in children include tonsillitis, nasopharyngitis, pharyngitis, croup syndromes, bacterial tracheitis, bronchitis, bronchiolitis, allergic rhinitis, and pneumonia.

TONSILLITIS AND TONSILLECTOMY

Overview

- Tonsils are masses of lymph-type tissue found in the pharyngeal area. They filter pathogenic organisms (viral and bacterial), which helps to protect the respiratory and gastrointestinal tracts. In addition, they contribute to antibody formation.

- Palatine tonsils are located on both sides of the oropharynx. These are the tonsils removed during a tonsillectomy.

- Other tonsils are the pharyngeal tonsils, also known as the adenoids. These are removed during an adenoidectomy.

- Tonsils are highly vascular, which helps them to protect against infection because foreign materials, such as viral or bacterial organisms, enter the body through the mouth.

- In some instances, enlarged tonsils can block the nose and throat. This can interfere with breathing, nasal and sinus drainage, sleeping, swallowing, and speaking.

- Enlarged tonsils also can disrupt the function of the eustachian tube, which can impede hearing.

- Acute tonsillitis occurs when the tonsils become inflamed and reddened. Small patches of yellowish pus also may become visible. Acute tonsillitis may become chronic.

Assessment

- Risk Factors
  - Exposure to a viral or bacterial agent
  - Immature immune systems (younger children)
- Subjective Data
  - Report of sore throat with difficulty swallowing
  - History of otitis media and hearing difficulties

- Objective Data
  - Physical Assessment Findings
    - Mouth odor
    - Mouth breathing
    - Snoring
    - Nasal qualities in the voice
    - Fever
    - Tonsil inflammation with redness and edema
  - Laboratory Tests
    - Throat culture for group A β-hemolytic streptococci (GABHS)

Patient-Centered Care

- Nursing Care
  - Tonsillitis
    - Provide symptomatic treatment for viral tonsillitis (rest, cool fluids, warm salt-water gargles).
    - Administer antibiotic therapy as prescribed for bacterial tonsillitis.
- Medications
  - Antipyretics – acetaminophen (Tylenol) or ibuprofen (Advil)
    - Antipyretics decrease fever and manage pain.
    - Nursing Considerations – Be aware of allergies.
    - Client Education – Teach appropriate dosing for acetaminophen and ibuprofen.
  - Antibiotics – IM penicillin G, erythromycin, azithromycin, cephalosporins, amoxicillin
    - Nursing Considerations – Be aware of allergies.
    - Client Education – Teach parents to administer antibiotics for the full course of treatment.
- Therapeutic Procedures
  - Tonsillectomy
    - Nursing Actions
      - Preoperative
        - ▸ Maintain NPO status.
      - Postoperative

NURSING CONSIDERATION	NURSING ACTIONS
Positioning	› Place in side-lying position or on abdomen to facilitate drainage.
	› Elevate head of bed when child is fully awake.
Assessment	› Assess for evidence of bleeding, which includes frequent swallowing, clearing the throat, restlessness, bright red emesis, tachycardia, and/or pallor.
	› Assess the airway and vital signs.
	› Monitor for difficulty breathing related to oral secretions, edema, and/or bleeding.

NURSING CONSIDERATION	NURSING ACTIONS
Comfort measures	› Administer analgesics (acetaminophen and codeine) as prescribed. › Provide an ice collar. › Offer ice chips or sips of water to keep throat moist. › Administer pain medication on a regular schedule.
Diet	› Encourage clear liquids and fluids after a return of the gag reflex, avoiding red-colored liquids, citrus juice, and milk-based foods initially. › Advance the diet with soft, bland foods.
Instruction	› Discourage coughing, throat clearing, and nose blowing in order to protect the surgical site. › Refrain from placing pointed objects in the back of the mouth. › Alert parents that there may be clots or blood-tinged mucus in vomitus.

- Client Education
  - Instruct the family to notify the provider if bright red bleeding occurs.
  - Encourage the child to rest.
- Care After Discharge
  - Client Education
    - Instruct the parents to contact the provider if the child experiences difficulty breathing, lack of oral intake, increase in pain, and/or indications of infection.
    - Tell the parents to ensure that the child does not put anything sharp (ice-cream stick, straw, pointed object) in the mouth.
    - Teach the parents to administer pain medications for discomfort.
    - Encourage fluid intake and diet advancement to a soft diet with no spicy foods or hard, sharp foods like corn chips until full recovery.
    - Instruct the child and family to limit strenuous activity and physical play with no swimming for 2 weeks as prescribed.
    - Instruct the child and family that full recovery usually occurs in approximately 14 days.
    - Teach the family of clinical manifestations of hemorrhage, dehydration, and infection, and when to notify the provider.

Complications

- Hemorrhage
  - Nursing Actions
    - Use a good light source and possibly a tongue depressor to directly observe the throat.
    - Assess for findings of bleeding (tachycardia, repeated swallowing and clearing of throat, hemoptysis). Hypotension is a late sign of shock.
    - Contact the provider immediately if there is any indication of bleeding.
  - Client Education
    - Instruct the family to report indications of bleeding (frequent swallowing, clearing the throat, restlessness, bright red emesis, tachycardia, pallor).

- Dehydration
  - ○ Nursing Actions
    - ▪ Encourage oral fluids.
    - ▪ Monitor I&O.
  - ○ Client Education
    - ▪ Instruct the family to encourage oral fluids.
    - ▪ Teach the family about clinical manifestations of dehydration.
- Chronic infection
  - ○ Chronically infected tonsils with group A β-hemolytic streptococci may pose a potential threat to other parts of the body. Some children who frequently have tonsillitis may develop other diseases, such as rheumatic fever and kidney infection.
  - ○ Client Education – Instruct the family to seek medical attention when the child presents with manifestations of tonsillitis.

COMMON RESPIRATORY ILLNESSES

Overview

- Disorders can affect both the upper (nasopharynx, pharynx, larynx, and upper part of the trachea) and lower (lower trachea, mainstem bronchi, segmental bronchi, subsegmental bronchioles, terminal bronchioles, and alveoli) respiratory tracts.
- Infections of the respiratory tract may affect more than one area.

Assessment

- Risk Factors
  - ○ Age
    - ▪ Infants between 3 and 6 months of age are at an increased risk due to the decrease of maternal antibodies acquired at birth and the lack of antibody protection.
    - ▪ Viral infections are more common in toddlers and preschoolers. The incidence of these infections decreases by age 5.
    - ▪ Certain viral agents can cause serious illness during infancy, but only cause a mild illness in older children.
  - ○ Anatomy
    - ▪ A short, narrow airway can become easily obstructed with mucus or edema.
    - ▪ A short respiratory tract allows infections to travel quickly to the lower airways.
    - ▪ Infants and young children have small surface areas for gas exchange.
    - ▪ Infectious agents have easy access to the middle ear through the short and open eustachian tubes of infants and young children.

- o Decreased resistance
  - Compromised immune system
  - Anemia
  - Nutritional deficiencies
  - Allergies
  - Chronic medical conditions (asthma, cystic fibrosis, congenital heart disease)
  - Exposure to second-hand smoke
- o Seasonal variables
  - Children with asthma have a greater incidence of respiratory infections during cold weather.
  - Respiratory syncytial virus (RSV) and other common respiratory infections are more common during the winter and spring.
  - Infections caused by *Mycoplasma pneumoniae* are more frequent during autumn and early winter.
- Subjective Data
  - o Nursing history that includes recent infections, medications taken, immunization status, and family coping
  - o Reports of sore throat, decreased activity level, chest pain, fatigue, difficulty breathing, shortness of breath, cough, and decreased appetite
- Objective Data
  - o Physical Assessment Findings

RESPIRATORY ILLNESS	CLINICAL MANIFESTATIONS
› Nasopharyngitis (common cold) » Self-limiting virus that persists for 7 to 10 days	› Nasal inflammation, rhinorrhea, cough, dry throat, sneezing, and nasal qualities in voice › Fever, decreased appetite, and irritability
› Bacterial tracheitis » Infection of the lining of the trachea	› Thick, purulent drainage from the trachea that can obstruct the airway and cause respiratory distress › Fever, croupy cough, stridor
› Bronchitis (tracheobronchitis) » Associated with an upper respiratory infection (URI) and inflammation of large airways » Self-limiting and requires symptomatic relief	› Persistent cough as a result of inflammation › Resolves in 5 to 10 days
› Bronchiolitis » Mostly caused by RSV » Primarily affects the bronchi and bronchioles » Occurs at the bronchiolar level	› Rhinorrhea – intermittent fever, cough, and wheezing › Coughing that progresses toward wheezing, increased respiratory rate, nasal flaring, retractions, and cyanosis › Possible posttussive vomiting due to coughing

RESPIRATORY ILLNESS	CLINICAL MANIFESTATIONS
› Allergic rhinitis » Caused by seasonal reaction to allergens most often in the autumn or spring	› Watery rhinorrhea; nasal congestion; itchiness of the nose, eyes, and pharynx; itchy, watery eyes; nasal quality of the voice; dry, scratchy throat; snoring; poor sleep leading to poor performance in school; and fatigue
› Pneumonia (RSV, *Streptococcus pneumoniae, Haemophilus influenzae, Mycoplasma pneumoniae*)	› High fever › Cough that may be unproductive or productive of white sputum › Retractions and nasal flaring › Rapid, shallow respirations › Report of chest pain › Adventitious breath sounds (rhonchi, crackles) › Pale color that progresses to cyanosis › Irritability, anxiety, agitation, and fatigue › Abdominal pain, diarrhea, lack of appetite, and vomiting › Sudden onset, usually following a viral infection (bacterial pneumonia)
Croup Syndromes	
› Bacterial epiglottitis (acute supraglottitis) » Medical emergency » Caused by *Haemophilus influenzae*	› Predictive signs – absence of cough, drooling, and agitation › Sitting with chin pointing out, mouth opened, and tongue protruding › Dysphonia (hoarseness or difficulty speaking) › Dysphagia (difficulty swallowing) › Inspiratory stridor (noisy inspirations) › Sore throat, high fever, and restlessness
› Acute laryngotracheobronchitis » Causative agents include RSV, influenza A and B, and *Mycoplasma pneumoniae*	› Low-grade fever, restlessness, hoarseness, barky cough, dyspnea, inspiratory stridor, and retractions
› Acute spasmodic laryngitis » Self-limiting illness that may result from allergens	› Barky cough, restlessness, difficulty breathing, hoarseness, and nighttime episodes of laryngeal obstruction
› Influenza A and B » Mild, moderate, or severe	› Sudden onset of fever and chills › Dry throat and nasal mucosa › Dry cough › Flushed face › Photophobia › Myalgia › Fatigue

- ○ Laboratory Tests
  - ▪ Blood samples
    - □ Elevated serum antistreptolysin-O (ASO) titer
    - □ Elevated C-reactive protein (CRP) or sedimentation rate in response to an inflammatory reaction
    - □ CBC to assess for anemia and infection
  - ▪ Sputum culture and sensitivity to detect infection
- ○ Diagnostic Procedures
  - ▪ Collection of direct aspiration of nasal secretions
    - □ The secretions are collected for immunofluorescence analysis to detect RSV. Instill 1 to 3 mL of 0.9% sodium chloride into one of the child's nostrils. The fluid is then aspirated for evaluation.
    - □ Nursing Actions
      - ▸ Place the child in a supine position.
      - ▸ Use a sterile syringe without a needle.
    - □ Client Education – Caregivers should be educated about the potential need for isolation, dependent on the results of laboratory tests.
  - ▪ Chest x-ray
    - □ Identifies infiltration in pneumonia
    - □ Nursing Actions – Ensure the child is positioned correctly to avoid the need for a repeat x-ray.
    - □ Client Education – Inform adolescents of childbearing age of the need for confirmation of nonpregnant status.

Patient-Centered Care

- • Nursing Care
  - ○ Closely monitor progression of illness and ensuing respiratory distress. Observe for increased heart and respiratory rate, retractions, nasal flaring, and restlessness.
  - ○ Make emergency equipment for intubation readily accessible.
  - ○ Position the child to have optimal ventilation without increasing distress that would contribute to increasing respiratory distress.
  - ○ Implement isolation precautions if indicated.
- • Nasopharyngitis – Instruct parents about home management.
  - ○ Give antipyretic for fever.
  - ○ Rest.
  - ○ Provide vaporized air (cool mist).
  - ○ Give decongestants for children older than 1 year.
  - ○ Give cough suppressants with caution (avoid oversedation).
  - ○ Antihistamines are not recommended.
  - ○ Antibiotics are not indicated.

- Bacterial tracheitis
  - Administer oxygen as prescribed.
  - Monitor continuous oximetry.
  - Administer antipyretics for fever.
  - Administer IV antibiotics as prescribed.
- Bronchitis – Instruct parents about home management.
  - Give antipyretics for fever.
  - Give a cough suppressant.
  - Provide increased humidity (cool mist vaporizer).
- Bronchiolitis
  - Provide humidified oxygen as prescribed.
  - Monitor continuous oximetry.
  - Encourage fluid intake if tolerated.
  - Administer IV fluids if oral intake not tolerated.
  - Suction nasopharynx as needed.
  - Administer nebulized bronchodilator.
  - Corticosteroids and antihistamines are not recommended.
  - Antibiotics are not recommended for RSV.
  - Chest percussion and postural drainage is not recommended.
  - Ribavirin administration is controversial.
- Allergic rhinitis – Instruct parents about home management.
  - Avoid allergens.
  - Give antihistamines.
  - Give nasal corticosteroids.
- Pneumonia
  - Viral (symptom management)
    - Administer oxygen with cool mist as prescribed.
    - Monitor continuous oximetry.
    - Administer antipyretics for fever.
    - Monitor intake and output.
  - Bacterial
    - Encourage rest.
    - Promote increased oral intake.
    - Monitor I&O.
    - Administer antipyretics for fever.
    - Chest percussion and postural drainage is controversial.

- Administer IV fluids as prescribed.
- Administer oxygen as prescribed.
- Monitor continuous oximetry.
- Administer IV antibiotics as prescribed.
- Bacterial epiglottitis
  - Protect airway.
    - Avoid throat culture or using a tongue blade.
  - Prepare for intubation.
  - Provide humidified oxygen.
  - Monitor continuous oximetry.
  - Administer racemic epinephrine, corticosteroids, and IV fluids as prescribed.
  - Administer antibiotic therapy (ceftriaxone sodium or cephalosporin), starting with IV, then transition to oral to complete a 10-day course, as prescribed.
- Acute laryngotracheobronchitis and acute spasmodic laryngitis
  - Provide humidity with cool mist.
  - Administer oxygen if needed.
  - Monitor continuous oximetry.
  - Administer nebulized racemic epinephrine as prescribed.
  - Administer corticosteroids: oral (prednisone), IM (dexamethasone), or nebulized (budesonide).
  - Encourage oral intake if tolerated.
  - Administer IV fluids as prescribed.
- Influenza – Instruct parents about home management.
  - Promote increased fluid intake.
  - Rest.
  - Give medications, as prescribed.
    - Amantadine (Symmetrel) – for type A
      - Shortens the length of the illness.
      - Administer within 24 to 48 hr of onset of symptoms.
    - Rimantadine (Flumadine) – for type A
      - Treats manifestations.
      - Give orally two times per day for 7 days for children older than 1 year.
    - Zanamivir (Relenza) – for type A and B
      - Treatment of influenza for children 7 and older or for prophylaxis for children 5 and older.
      - Start within 48 hr of manifestations.
      - Inhaled two times per day for 5 days.

- Oseltamivir (Tamiflu) – for type A and B
  - Decreases manifestations.
  - Give orally for 5 days for children older than 1 year.
  - Start within 48 hr of manifestations.
- Influenza vaccine – prevention
  - Recommended for children 6 months and older.
  - Live vaccination should not be used in children who are immunocompromised, have respiratory conditions, are pregnant, or have a history of Guillain-Barre syndrome.
- Antipyretic (pain or fever)

- Care After Discharge
  - Use a cool-air vaporizer to provide humidity.
  - Rest during febrile illness.
  - Maintain adequate fluid intake. Infants may be given commercially prepared oral rehydration solutions, and older children may be given sports drinks.
  - Apply ice or warm pack to the neck to decrease pain from enlarged cervical nodes.
  - Administer medications using accurate dosages and appropriate time intervals.
  - Develop strategies to decrease the spread of infection. Strategies include performing good hand hygiene; covering the nose and mouth with tissues when sneezing and coughing; properly disposing of tissues; not sharing cups, eating utensils, and towels; and keeping infected children from contact with children who are well.
  - Seek further medical attention for the child if symptoms worsen or respiratory distress occurs.

Complications

- Pneumothorax – accumulation of air in the pleural space
  - Clinical Manifestations – dyspnea, chest pain, back pain, labored respirations, decreased oxygen saturations, and tachycardia
  - Nursing Interventions
    - Prepare client for an emergent needle aspiration with insertion of chest tube to closed drainage.
    - Provide for chest tube management.
    - Assess respiratory status.
    - Administer oxygen as prescribed.
- Pleural effusion – accumulation of fluid in the pleural space
  - Clinical manifestations – dyspnea, chest pain, back pain, labored respirations, decreased oxygen saturations, and tachycardia
  - Nursing Interventions
    - Prepare the client for an emergent needle aspiration with insertion of chest tube to closed drainage.
    - Provide for chest tube management.
    - Assess respiratory status.
    - Administer oxygen as prescribed.

APPLICATION EXERCISES

1. A nurse is caring for a child who has bronchiolitis. Which of the following are appropriate actions for the nurse to take? (Select all that apply.)

_____ A. Administer oral prednisone.

_____ B. Initiate chest percussion and postural drainage.

_____ C. Administer humidified oxygen.

_____ D. Suction the nasopharynx as needed.

_____ E. Administer oral penicillin.

2. A nurse is teaching a group of parents about influenza. Which of the following should be included in the teaching?

A. "Amantadine will prevent the illness."

B. "Rimantadine is administered intramuscularly."

C. "Zanamivir can be given to children 1 year and older."

D. "Oseltamivir should be given within 48 hours of onset of symptoms."

3. A nurse is caring for a child who is in the postoperative period following a tonsillectomy. Which of the following is a clinical finding of postoperative bleeding?

A. Hgb of 11.6 and Hct of 37%

B. Inflamed and reddened throat

C. Frequent swallowing and clearing of the throat

D. Blood-tinged mucus

4. A nurse is caring for a child in the postoperative period following a tonsillectomy. Which of the following is an appropriate action for the nurse to take?

A. Encourage the child to blow her nose gently.

B. Administer analgesics on a schedule.

C. Offer orange juice.

D. Position the child supine.

5. A nurse is assessing a child. Which of the following are clinical manifestations of epiglottitis? (Select all that apply.)

_____ A. Hoarseness and difficulty speaking

_____ B. Difficulty swallowing

_____ C. Low-grade fever

_____ D. Drooling

_____ E. Dry, barking cough

_____ F. Stridor

6. A nurse is teaching a parent of a child who has an infectious respiratory illness. What should be included in the teaching? Use the ATI Active Learning Template: Basic Concept to complete this item to include Related Content: Identify at least three strategies to decrease the spread of infection.

APPLICATION EXERCISES KEY

1. A. INCORRECT: Corticosteroids are not indicated for a client who has bronchiolitis.

    B. INCORRECT: Chest percussion and postural drainage are not indicated for a client who has bronchiolitis.

    C. **CORRECT:** Humidified oxygen provides moisture to the airway and is an appropriate action for the nurse to take.

    D. **CORRECT:** Suctioning the nasopharynx will assist the client to clear secretions and is an appropriate action for the nurse to take.

    E. INCORRECT: Antibiotics are not indicated for a client who has bronchiolitis.

    Ⓝ NCLEX® Connection: Physiological Adaptations, Alterations in Body Systems

2. A. INCORRECT: Amantadine can shorten the length of the illness.

    B. INCORRECT: Rimantadine is administered orally two times per day for 7 days.

    C. INCORRECT: Zanamivir is approved for children over the age of 5 years.

    D. **CORRECT:** Oseltamivir decrease flu manifestations in clients who have findings for less than 48 hr.

    Ⓝ NCLEX® Connection: Physiological Adaptations, Alterations in Body Systems

3. A. INCORRECT: A Hgb of 11.6 and Hct of 37% are within the expected reference range.

    B. INCORRECT: Inflamed and reddened throat is an expected finding following a tonsillectomy.

    C. **CORRECT:** Frequent swallowing and clearing of the throat indicates that there is an increased amount of fluid in the back of the throat, which is a clinical finding in the client who is experiencing postoperative bleeding.

    D. INCORRECT: Blood-tinged mucus is an expected finding following a tonsillectomy.

    Ⓝ NCLEX® Connection: Physiological Adaptations, Unexpected Response to Therapies

4. A. INCORRECT: Blowing the nose causes pressure and could increase the risk of bleeding.

    B. **CORRECT:** Analgesics should be administered on a scheduled basis to provide pain relief.

    C. INCORRECT: Citrus juices such as orange juice can cause discomfort and should be avoided postoperatively.

    D. INCORRECT: The client should be positioned on the abdomen or side-lying following a tonsillectomy.

    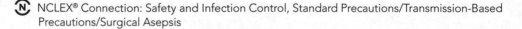 NCLEX® Connection: Physiological Adaptations, Alterations in Body Systems

5. A. **CORRECT:** Hoarseness and difficulty speaking is a clinical manifestation of epiglottitis.

    B. **CORRECT:** Difficulty swallowing is a clinical manifestation of epiglottitis.

    C. INCORRECT: A high fever is a clinical manifestation of epiglottitis.

    D. **CORRECT:** Drooling is a clinical manifestation of epiglottitis.

    E. INCORRECT: Dry, barking cough is a clinical manifestation of croup.

    F. **CORRECT:** Stridor is a clinical manifestation of epiglottitis.

    NCLEX® Connection: Physiological Adaptations, Medical Emergencies

6. *Using the ATI Active Learning Template: Basic Concept*
    - Related Content
      ○ Perform appropriate hand hygiene.
      ○ Cover the nose and mouth with tissues when sneezing and coughing.
      ○ Dispose of tissues properly.
      ○ Do not share cups, eating utensils, or towels.
      ○ Keep infected children from contact with children who are well.

    NCLEX® Connection: Safety and Infection Control, Standard Precautions/Transmission-Based Precautions/Surgical Asepsis

chapter 18

Overview

- Asthma is a chronic inflammatory disorder of the airways that results in intermittent and reversible airflow obstruction of the bronchioles.

- The obstruction occurs either by inflammation or airway hyper-responsiveness.

  View Video: Asthma

- Asthma diagnoses are based on symptoms and classified into one of four categories.

  - Intermittent – Symptoms occur two or fewer times per week, nighttime symptoms two or fewer per month, no interference with normal activity, uses short-acting ß-agonist less than two times per week.

  - Mild persistent – Symptoms occur more than twice a week, but not daily. Nighttime symptoms one to two times per month for 0- to 4-year-old and three to four times per month for 5- to 11-year-old. Minor limitations with activity, use of short-acting ß-agonist more than two days per week but not daily.

  - Moderate persistent – Daily symptoms. Nighttime symptoms three to four times a month for 0- to 4-year-old and more than one time per week, but not daily for 5- to 11-year-old. Some limitation in activity. Uses short-acting ß-agonist daily.

  - Severe persistent – Symptoms occur continually, nighttime symptoms more than one time per week for 0- to 4-year-old and nightly for 5- to 11-year-old. Limited activity. Use short-acting ß-agonist several times per day.

Assessment

- Risk Factors
  - Family history of asthma
  - Family history of allergies
  - Allergies
- Triggers to asthma
  - Allergens
    - Indoor: mold, cockroach, house dust mites
    - Outdoor: grass, pollen, trees, shrubs, molds, spores, air pollution
  - Exercise/Activity
  - Cold air or changes in weather

- ○ Tobacco smoke
- ○ Infections/colds
- ○ Animal hair or dander
- ○ Medications
- ○ Strong odors
- ○ Emotions
- ○ Gastroesophageal reflux
- ○ Food allergies or additives
- Subjective Data
  - ○ Chest tightness
  - ○ History regarding current and previous asthma exacerbations
    - ▪ Onset and duration
    - ▪ Precipitating factors
    - ▪ Changes in medication regimen
    - ▪ Medications that relieve symptoms
    - ▪ Other medications
    - ▪ Self-care methods used to relieve symptoms
- Objective Data
  - ○ Physical Assessment Findings
    - ▪ Dyspnea
    - ▪ Cough
    - ▪ Audible wheezing
    - ▪ Coarse lung sounds, wheezing throughout possible crackles
    - ▪ Mucus production
    - ▪ Restlessness
    - ▪ Anxiety
    - ▪ Red ears, dark red lips
    - ▪ Sweating
    - ▪ Use of accessory muscles
    - ▪ Decreased oxygen saturation (low SaO_2)
  - ○ Laboratory Tests – CBC
  - ○ Diagnostic Procedures
    - ▪ Pulmonary function tests (PFTs) are the most accurate tests for diagnosing asthma and its severity.
      - ▫ Baseline test at time of diagnosis
      - ▫ After treatment is initiated and child is stabilized
      - ▫ Yearly testing

- Peak expiratory flow rates
    - Measures the amount of air that can be forcefully exhaled in 1 second
    - Each child needs to establish personal best
- Bronchoprovocation testing
    - Exposure to methacholine, cold air, or histamine
    - Exercise challenge
- Skin prick testing (SPT)
    - Identify allergens that trigger asthma
- Chest x-ray showing hyperexpansion and infiltrates

Patient-Centered Care

- Nursing Care
    - Assess airway patency, respiratory rate, symmetry, effort, and use of accessory muscles.
    - Assess breath sounds in all lung fields.
    - Monitor for shortness of breath, dyspnea, and audible wheezing. An absence of wheezing may indicate severe constriction of the alveoli.
    - Monitor vital signs and oxygen saturation.
    - Check CBC and chest x-ray results, possible ABGs.
    - Position the child to maximize ventilation.
    - Administer oxygen therapy as prescribed.
    - Initiate and maintain IV access as prescribed.
    - Maintain a calm and reassuring demeanor.
    - Encourage appropriate vaccinations and prompt medical attention for infections.
    - Administer medications as prescribed.
    - Antibiotics are not used to treat asthma, only if a bacterial infection is confirmed.
- Medications
    - Bronchodilators (inhalers)
        - Short-acting beta$_2$ agonists (albuterol [Proventil], levalbuterol [Xopenex], terbutaline [Brethine])
            - Used for acute exacerbations
            - Prevention of exercised-induced asthma
        - Cholinergic antagonists (anticholinergic medications), such as ipratropium (Atrovent), block the parasympathetic nervous system, providing relief of acute bronchospasms.
        - Nursing Considerations
            - Instruct the child and family in the proper use of MDI, DPI, or nebulizer.
            - Watch the child for tremors and tachycardia when taking albuterol.
            - Observe the child for dry mouth when taking ipratropium.

- Client Education
  - Encourage older children who are taking ipratropium to suck on hard candies to help with dry mouth.
  - Teach children to administer prior to exercise or activity.
- ○ Anti-inflammatory agents
  - Anti-inflammatory agents decrease airway inflammation.
  - Corticosteroids
    - Methylprednisolone (Solu-Medrol)
      - ▶ IV or oral
      - ▶ Children less than 12 years: 1 to 2 mg/kg/day divided every 12 hr for 3 to 10 days
      - ▶ Children older than 12 years: 40 to 60 mg/day divided every 12 hr for 3 to 10 days
    - Prednisone
      - ▶ Oral
      - ▶ Dosing by age
        - ▷ Younger than 1 year: 10 mg every 12 hr
        - ▷ 1 to 4 years: 20 mg every 12 hr
        - ▷ 5 to 13 years: 30 mg every 12 hr
        - ▷ 13 years and older: 40 mg every 12 hr
      - ▶ Administer for 3 to 5 days
  - Leukotriene modifiers (montelukast [Singulair]), mast cell stabilizers (cromolyn sodium [Intal]), and monoclonal antibodies (omalizumab [Xolair])
  - Combination medications
    - Fluticasone/salmeterol (Advair)
    - Inhaled corticosteroid/long-acting beta$_2$ agonist)
  - Nursing Considerations
    - Observe the child's oral mucosa for infection secondary to use of inhaled medication.
    - Assess the child's weight, blood pressure, electrolytes, glucose, and growth with oral corticosteroid use.
  - Client Education
    - Encourage the child to drink plenty of fluids to promote hydration.
    - Encourage the child to take a oral corticosteroids with food.
    - Instruct the child to rinse her mouth after the use of a corticosteroid inhaler.
    - Instruct the child and family to watch for redness, sores, or white patches in the mouth, and report them to the provider.
    - Teach the family to follow prescription for medication administration (dosage, tapering off medication, length of time to take).

- Teamwork and Collaboration
  - Consult respiratory services for inhalers and breathing treatments.
  - Contact nutritional services for weight loss or gain related to medications or diagnosis.
  - Consult rehabilitation if the child has prolonged weakness and needs assistance with increasing level of activity.
- Care After Discharge
  - Client Education
    - Instruct the family and the child to identify personal triggering agents.
    - Assist the child in avoiding triggering agents.
    - Provide the family and child with an asthma action plan.
    - Teach the child how to use a peak flow meter. (Use same time each day.)
      - Ensure the marker is zeroed.
      - Have the child stand up straight.
      - Close lips tightly around the mouthpiece (ensure the tongue is not occluding).
      - Blow out as hard and as quickly as possible.
      - Read the number on the meter.
      - Repeat two more times (wait at least 30 seconds between attempts).
      - Record highest number.
    - Teach the family and child how to recognize an asthma exacerbation.
    - Teach the family and the child about when to use each of the prescribed medications (rescue medications vs. maintenance medications).
    - Instruct the child how to properly self-administer medications (nebulizers, inhalers, and spacer).
    - Educate the child and family regarding infection prevention techniques.
      - Promote good nutrition.
      - Reinforce importance of good hand hygiene.
    - Encourage prompt medical attention for infections.
    - Stress the importance of keeping immunizations, including seasonal influenza and pneumonia vaccines, up to date.
    - Encourage regular exercise as part of asthma therapy.
      - Promotes ventilation and perfusion
      - Maintains cardiac health
      - Enhances skeletal muscle strength
    - Children may require medication before exercise.

Complications

- Status asthmaticus
  - A life-threatening episode of airway obstruction that is often unresponsive to common treatment
  - Manifestations include wheezing, labored breathing, nasal flaring, lack of air movement in lungs, use of accessory muscles, distended neck veins, and risk for cardiac and/or respiratory arrest.
  - Nursing Actions
    - Monitor oxygen saturations continuously.
    - Place on continuous cardiorespiratory monitoring.
    - Position the child sitting upright, standing, or leaning slightly forward.
    - Administer humidified oxygen.
    - Administer three nebulizer treatments of a beta$_2$-agonist, 20 to 30 min apart or continuously. Ipratropium bromide may be added to the nebulizer to increase bronchodilation.
    - Obtain IV access.
    - Monitor ABGs and serum electrolytes.
    - Administer corticosteroid.
    - Prepare for emergency intubation.
- Respiratory failure
  - Persistent hypoxemia related to asthma can lead to respiratory failure.
  - Nursing Actions
    - Monitor oxygenation levels and acid-base balance.
    - Prepare for intubation and mechanical ventilation as indicated.

APPLICATION EXERCISES

1. A nurse is assessing a child who has asthma. Which of the following are indications of deterioration in the child's respiratory status? (Select all that apply.)

_____ A. Oxygen saturation 95%

_____ B. Wheezing

_____ C. Retraction of sternal muscles

_____ D. Warm extremities

_____ E. Nasal flaring

2. A nurse is teaching an adolescent about the appropriate use of his asthma medications. Which of the following should the client be instructed to take as needed before exercise?

A. Fluticasone/salmeterol (Advair)

B. Montelukast (Singulair)

C. Prednisone (Deltasone)

D. Albuterol (Proventil)

3. A nurse is planning caring for a child who has asthma. Which of the following interventions should be included in the plan of care? (Select all that apply.)

_____ A. Perform chest percussion.

_____ B. Place the child in an upright position.

_____ C. Monitor oxygen saturation.

_____ D. Administer bronchodilators.

_____ E. Administer dornase alfa (Pulmozyme) daily.

4. A nurse is teaching a child who has asthma how to use a peak flow meter. Which of the following should be included in the teaching? (Select all that apply.)

_____ A. Zero the meter before each use.

_____ B. Record the average of the attempts.

_____ C. Perform three attempts.

_____ D. Deliver a long, slow breath into the meter.

_____ E. Sit in a chair with feet on the floor.

5. A nurse is preparing to administer methylprednisolone (Solu-Medrol) IV 2 mg/kg/day divided in two equal doses to a child who weighs 50 kg. How many mg per dose should the nurse administer? (Round the answer to the nearest tenth.)

6. A nurse is teaching a child about triggers to asthma. What should be included in the teaching? Use the ATI Active Learning Template: Systems Disorder to complete this item to include Client Education: List at least eight possible triggers to asthma.

APPLICATION EXERCISES KEY

1. A. INCORRECT: Oxygen saturation of 95% is within the expected reference range for a child.

    B. **CORRECT:** Wheezing is an indication of bronchoconstriction and of deterioration in a child's respiratory status.

    C. **CORRECT:** Retractions of sternal muscles are an indication of increased work of breathing and of deterioration in a child's respiratory status.

    D. INCORRECT: Warm extremities is an expected finding in a child.

    E. **CORRECT:** Nasal flaring is an indication of increased work of breathing and of deterioration in a child's respiratory status.

    Ⓝ NCLEX® Connection: Physiological Adaptations, Alterations in Body Systems

2. A. INCORRECT: Fluticasone/salmeterol (Advair) is a combination medication used for maintenance control of asthma.

    B. INCORRECT: Montelukast (Singulair) is a medication used for maintenance control of asthma.

    C. INCORRECT: Prednisone (Deltasone) is a medication used for exacerbations of asthma.

    D. **CORRECT:** Albuterol is a beta$_2$-agonist used for bronchodilation and should be administered prior to exercise.

    Ⓝ NCLEX® Connection: Pharmacological and Parenteral Therapies, Medication Administration

3. A. INCORRECT: Chest percussion promotes movement of mucus plugs and is commended for children who have cystic fibrosis.

    B. **CORRECT:** Children who are experiencing an asthma exacerbation have decreased oxygenation. Placing them in an upright position is an appropriate intervention.

    C. **CORRECT:** Children who are experiencing an asthma exacerbation have decreased oxygenation. Monitoring oxygen saturation is an appropriate intervention.

    D. **CORRECT:** Children who are experiencing an asthma exacerbation experience bronchoconstriction. Administering bronchodilators is an appropriate intervention.

    E. INCORRECT: Dornase alfa is a mucolytic and is recommended for children who have cystic fibrosis.

    Ⓝ NCLEX® Connection: Physiological Adaptations, Alterations in Body Systems

4. A. **CORRECT:** The monitor should be zeroed each time it is used to achieve accurate results.

   B. INCORRECT: The highest number achieved is recorded.

   C. **CORRECT:** Three attempts should be performed to achieve accurate results.

   D. INCORRECT: A hard, fast breath should be used for the peak flow meter.

   E. INCORRECT: The child should be standing upright when using a peak flow meter.

   Ⓝ NCLEX® Connection: Reduction of Risk Potential, Diagnostic Tests

5. **50** mg

Using Ratio and Proportion, Desired Over Have, and Dimensional Analysis

STEP 1: *What is the unit of measurement to calculate?*
mg

STEP 2: *Set up an equation and solve for X.*
mg x kg/day = X
2 mg x 50 kg = 100 mg

STEP 3: *Round if necessary.*

STEP 4: *Reassess to determine whether the amount makes sense.*
If the prescribed amount is 2 mg/kg/day and the client weighs 50 kg, it makes sense to give 100 mg/day or 50 mg/dose.

Ⓝ NCLEX® Connection: Pharmacological and Parenteral Therapies, Dosage Calculation

6. *Using the ATI Active Learning Template: Systems Disorder*
   • Client Education
     ○ Allergens
       ▪ Indoor: mold, cockroaches, house dust mites
       ▪ Outdoor: grass, pollen, trees, shrubs, molds, spores, air pollution
     ○ Exercise/activity
     ○ Cold air or changes in weather
     ○ Tobacco smoke
     ○ Infections/colds
     ○ Animal hair or dander
     ○ Medications
     ○ Strong odors
     ○ Emotions
     ○ Gastroesophageal reflux
     ○ Food allergies or additives

   Ⓝ NCLEX® Connection: Physiological Adaptations, Alterations in Body Systems

chapter 19

Overview

- Cystic fibrosis is a respiratory disorder that results from inheriting a mutated gene. It is characterized by:
  - Mucus glands that secrete an increase in the quantity of thick, tenacious mucus, which leads to mechanical obstruction of organs (pancreas, lungs, liver, small intestine, and reproductive system).
  - An increase in organic and enzymatic constituents in the saliva.
  - An increase in the sodium and chloride content of sweat.
  - Central nervous system abnormalities.

Assessment

- Risk Factors
  - Both biological parents carry the recessive trait for cystic fibrosis.
- Subjective Data
  - Family history of cystic fibrosis
  - Past medical history, including respiratory infections, failure to thrive
- Objective Data
  - Physical Assessment Findings
    - Meconium ileus at birth manifested as distention of the abdomen, vomiting, and inability to pass stool
    - Respiratory findings
      - Early signs
        - Wheezing
        - Dry, nonproductive cough
      - Increased involvement
        - Dyspnea
        - Paroxysmal cough
        - Mucus plugs and atelectasis on x-ray
      - Advanced involvement
        - Cyanosis
        - Barrel-shaped chest
        - Clubbing of fingers and toes
        - Multiple episodes of bronchitis or bronchopneumonia

- Gastrointestinal findings
  - Large, loose, fatty, sticky, foul-smelling stools
  - Voracious appetite (early), loss of appetite (late)
  - Failure to gain weight or weight loss
  - Delayed growth patterns
  - Distended abdomen
  - Thin arms and legs
  - Deficiency of fat-soluble vitamins
  - Anemia
- Integumentary findings
  - Sweat, tears, and saliva are abnormally salty
- Endocrine and reproductive system findings
  - Viscous cervical mucus
  - Decreased or absent sperm
- Laboratory Tests
  - Blood specimen
    - CBC, CRP, nutritional panel, blood glucose, complete metabolic panel, ABGs
  - Sputum culture for detection of infection
    - *Pseudomonas aeruginosa, Haemophilus influenzae, Burkholderia cepacia, S. aureus, Escherichia coli,* or *Klebsiella pneumoniae*
  - Stool analysis
    - For presence of fat and enzymes
    - 72 hr sample with documented food intake
- Diagnostic Procedures
  - To diagnose cystic fibrosis
    - Sweat chloride test
      - ▶ A special device stimulates sweat production
      - ▶ Collection of sweat from two different sites for adequate sample
      - ▶ Expected reference range is the presence of chloride less than 40 mEq/L
      - ▶ Diagnostic confirmation of cystic fibrosis: chloride greater than 60 mEq/L for infants less than 3 months of age and greater then 40 mEq/L for all others
  - DNA testing to isolate the mutation
  - Pulmonary Function Tests (PFTs)
  - Chest x-ray
    - ▶ May indicate diffuse atelectasis and obstructive emphysema
  - Abdominal x-ray
    - Detect meconium ileus

Patient-Centered Care

- Nursing Care
  - Assess lung sounds and respiratory status.
  - Vital signs with oxygen saturation.
  - Obtain IV access (peripherally inserted central catheter [PICC]).
  - Obtain sputum for culture and sensitivity.
  - Contact isolation for *B. cepacia* and *P. aeruginosa*.
  - Provide support to the child and family.
  - Provide pulmonary management.
    - Perform chest physiotherapy (CPT) with postural drainage as prescribed (traditional or vest). Avoid CPT before and after meals.
    - Perform airway clearance therapy (flutter mucus clearance device) twice daily.
    - Administer aerosol therapy as prescribed (bronchodilator, human deoxyribonuclease).
    - Administer IV antibiotics as prescribed (tobramycin, ticarcillin, or gentamicin).
    - Administer IV antifungal medications as prescribed.
    - Encourage physical exercise (stationary bicycle).
    - Provide oxygen as prescribed (assess for carbon dioxide retention).
  - Gastrointestinal management
    - Provide a well-balanced diet that's high in protein and calories.
    - Give three meals a day with snacks.
    - Encourage oral fluid intake.
    - Administer pancreatic enzymes as prescribed 30 min within eating.
    - Administer vitamin supplements as prescribed: multivitamin; vitamins A, D, E, and K.
    - Administer polyethylene-glycol electrolyte solution (GoLYTELY) via nasogastric tube for constipation as prescribed.
    - Administer histamine-receptor antagonist and motility medications for GERD as prescribed.
    - Administer possible formula supplements via gastric tube.
    - Consult dietitian.
  - Endocrine management
    - Monitor blood glucose.
    - Administer insulin as prescribed.
- Medications
  - Respiratory Medications
    - Short-acting beta$_2$- agonists, such as albuterol (Proventil)
    - Cholinergic antagonists (anticholinergics), such as ipratropium bromide (Atrovent)
    - Fluticasone propionate/salmeterol (Advair)

- Dornase alfa (Pulmozyme)
  - Decreases the viscosity of mucus and improves lung function
  - Nursing Considerations
    - Monitor sputum thickness and ability of client to expectorate.
    - Monitor the child for improvement in PFTs.
  - Client Education
    - Instruct the child how to use a nebulizer.
    - Instruct the child to administer once a day.
- Nursing Considerations
  - Instruct the child and family about how to properly use an MDI, DPI, or nebulizer.
  - Monitor the child for tremors and tachycardia when he is taking albuterol.
  - Observe the child for dry mouth when taking ipratropium.
- Client Education
  - Wait 5 min between ipratropium bromide and other inhaled medications.
  - Rinse mouth after fluticasone propionate/salmeterol.

- Antibiotics
  - Administer through IV or aerosol.
  - Specific to treat pulmonary infection – common medications include tobramycin, ticarcillin, or gentamicin.
  - Nursing Considerations
    - Assess for allergies.
    - High doses may be prescribed. Collect blood specimens before and after some IV antibiotics to maintain therapeutic levels.
    - Implement special precautions for aerosol antibiotics.

- Pancreatic enzymes – pancrelipase (Pancrease)
  - Treats pancreatic insufficiency associated with cystic fibrosis
  - Nursing Considerations
    - Monitor stools for adequate dosing (increase dose if loose, fatty stools present; decrease dose if constipation present).
    - Administer capsules with all meals and snacks.
    - Client can swallow or sprinkle capsules on food.

- Vitamins
  - Daily multivitamin and vitamins A, E, D, and K

- Teamwork and Collaboration
  - Respiratory and physical therapy, social services, pulmonologist, pharmacist, pediatrician, infectious disease specialists, and dieticians may be involved in the care of the child who has cystic fibrosis.
  - Transplantation of heart, lung, pancreas, and liver for clients with advanced disease may be a consideration.
- Care After Discharge
  - Ensure that the family has information regarding access to medical equipment and medications.
  - Provide teaching about equipment and medications prior to discharge.
  - Instruct the family about ways to provide CPT and breathing exercises.
  - Promote regular provider visits.
  - Emphasize the need for up-to-date immunizations and a yearly influenza vaccine.
  - Teach about diet and ways to increase calorie intake.
  - Teach signs and symptoms of infection and when to call the provider.
  - Teach parents about ways to manage chronic illness in children.
  - Promote regular physical activity.
  - Encourage the family to participate in a support group and use community resources.

Complications

- Respiratory Complications
  - Respiratory infections, respiratory colonizations, bronchial cysts, emphysema, pneumothorax, nasal polyps
- Gastrointestinal complications
  - Meconium ileus, prolapse of the rectum, distal intestinal obstruction syndrome, GERD
- Endocrine complications
  - Diabetes mellitus

APPLICATION EXERCISES

1. A nurse is preparing to administer tobramycin 100 mg via intermittent IV bolus. Available is tobramycin 100 mg in 0.9% sodium chloride 100 mL. The nurse is planning to administer the medication over 30 min. The nurse should set the pump to deliver how many milliliters per hour? (Round the answer to the nearest whole number.)

2. A nurse is caring for a child who is suspected of having cystic fibrosis. Which of the following tests should the nurse prepare to administer to confirm this diagnosis?

    A. Sweat chloride

    B. Pulmonary function test

    C. Arterial blood gases

    D. Chest percussion

3. A nurse is admitting a child who has cystic fibrosis. Which of the following medications should the nurse anticipate including in the plan of care? (Select all that apply.)

    _____ A. Tobramycin

    _____ B. Solu-medrol

    _____ C. Fat-soluble vitamins

    _____ D. Albuterol

    _____ E. Dornase alfa

4. A nurse is caring for a child who has cystic fibrosis. Which of the following are expected findings? (Select all that apply.)

    _____ A. Wheezing

    _____ B. Clubbing of fingers and toes

    _____ C. Barrel-shaped chest

    _____ D. Thin, watery mucus

    _____ E. Rapid growth spurts

5. A nurse is planning care for a child who has cystic fibrosis. Which of the following interventions should she include in the plan of care?

    A. Provide a low-calorie, low-protein diet.

    B. Administer pancreatic enzymes with meals and snacks.

    C. Promote an increase in fluids after 1800.

    D. Restrict physical activity.

6. A nurse is caring for a child who has cystic fibrosis. What nursing interventions should the nurse anticipate providing? Use the Systems Disorder ATI Active Learning Template to complete this item to include:

    A. Nursing Care:
- Describe at least three general nursing actions.
- Describe three nursing actions related to the management of pulmonary function.
- Describe two nursing actions related to gastrointestinal system management.
- Describe two nursing actions related to endocrine system management.

APPLICATION EXERCISES KEY

1. **200** mL/hr

Using Ratio and Proportion, Desired Over Have, and Dimensional Analysis

STEP 1: *What is the unit of measurement to calculate?*
mL/hr

STEP 2: *What is the volume needed? Volume needed = Volume*
100 mL

STEP 3: *What is the total infusion time? Time available = Time*
30 min

STEP 4: *Should the nurse convert the units of measurement?*
Yes (min ≠ hr)

$$\frac{1\,hr}{60\,min} = \frac{X\,hr}{30\,min}$$

X = 0.5

STEP 5: *Set up an equation and solve for X.*

$$\frac{Volume\,(mL)}{Time\,(hr)} = X$$

$$\frac{100\,mL}{0.5\,hr} = X\,mL/hr$$

200 = X

STEP 6: *Round if necessary.*

STEP 7: *Reassess to determine whether the IV flow rate makes sense.*
If the amount prescribed is 100 mL to infuse over 30 min (0.5 hr), it makes sense to administer 200 mL/hr. The nurse should set the IV pump to deliver 100 mg in 0.9% sodium chloride 100 mL at 200 mL/hr.

Ⓝ NCLEX® Connection: Pharmacological and Parenteral Therapies, Parenteral/Intravenous Therapies

2. A. **CORRECT:** Children who have cystic fibrosis excrete an abnormal amount of sodium and chloride in their sweat. Therefore, a sweat chloride test is diagnostic of cystic fibrosis and should be performed.

    B. INCORRECT: Pulmonary function tests evaluate lung function and are used for children who have cystic fibrosis. However, they are not diagnostic of the disease.

    C. INCORRECT: Arterial blood gases are used for children who have cystic fibrosis to determine oxygenation status. However, they are not diagnostic of the disease.

    D. INCORRECT: Chest percussion is used for children who have cystic fibrosis to assist with expectoration of mucus from their lungs, but it is not diagnostic of the disease.

Ⓝ NCLEX® Connection: Reduction of Risk Potential, Diagnostic Tests

3.   A. **CORRECT:** Children who have cystic fibrosis have pulmonary infections. Therefore, administering antibiotics should be part of the plan of care.

    B. INCORRECT: Corticosteroid use has been associated with short stature, glucose intolerance, and cataracts, and should not be part of the plan of care.

    C. **CORRECT:** Children who have cystic fibrosis have difficulty absorbing fat. Therefore, supplementation of the fat-soluble vitamins should be part of the plan of care.

    D. **CORRECT:** Children who have cystic fibrosis have mucus plugs. Therefore, administering a bronchodilator should be part of the plan of care.

    E. **CORRECT:** Children who have cystic fibrosis have mucus plugs. Therefore, administering dornase alfa, which decreases the viscosity of the mucus, should be part of the plan of care.

    (N) NCLEX® Connection: Pharmacological and Parenteral Therapies, Expected Actions/Outcomes

4.   A. **CORRECT:** Wheezing is a manifestations of cystic fibrosis.

    B. **CORRECT:** Clubbing of fingers and toes is a late manifestation of cystic fibrosis.

    C. **CORRECT:** A barrel-shaped chest is a late manifestation of cystic fibrosis.

    D. INCORRECT: Thick, viscous mucus is a manifestation of cystic fibrosis.

    E. INCORRECT: Delayed growth is a manifestation of cystic fibrosis.

    (N) NCLEX® Connection: Physiological Adaptations, Pathophysiology

5.   A. INCORRECT: Children who have cystic fibrosis should eat a high-calorie, high-protein diet to allow for proper growth.

    B. **CORRECT:** Children who have cystic fibrosis have pancreatic insufficiency. Therefore, administering pancreatic enzymes with meals and snacks should be part of the plan of care.

    C. INCORRECT: Children who have cystic fibrosis should increase fluids throughout the day to assist in thinning thick mucus.

    D. INCORRECT: Children who have cystic fibrosis should engage in daily activity to assist with lung expansion and stimulate mucus excretion.

    (N) NCLEX® Connection: Physiological Adaptations, Alterations in Body Systems

6. *Using the Systems Disorder ATI Active Learning Template*

    A. Nursing Care
       • General Nursing Actions
          ○ Assess lung sounds and respiratory status.
          ○ Assess vital signs with oxygen saturation.
          ○ Obtain IV access (peripherally inserted central catheter [PICC]).
          ○ Obtain sputum for culture and sensitivity.
          ○ Contact isolation for *B. cepacia* and *P. aeruginosa*.
          ○ Provide support to the child and family.
       • Pulmonary Management
          ○ Perform chest physiotherapy (CPT) with postural drainage as prescribed (traditional or vest). Avoid immediately before and after meals.
          ○ Perform airway clearance therapy (flutter mucus clearance device) twice daily.
          ○ Administer aerosol therapy, as prescribed (bronchodilator, human deoxyribonuclease).
          ○ Administer IV antibiotics, as prescribed (tobramycin, ticarcillin, or gentamicin).
          ○ Administer IV antifungals as prescribed.
          ○ Encourage physical exercise (stationary bicycle).
          ○ Provide oxygen as prescribed (assess for carbon dioxide retention).
       • Gastrointestinal Management
          ○ Consume a well-balanced diet that's high in protein and calories.
          ○ Eat three meals a day with snacks.
          ○ Encourage oral fluid intake.
          ○ Administer pancreatic enzymes as prescribed 30 min within eating.
          ○ Take vitamin supplements: multivitamin, vitamins A, D, E, and K.
          ○ Administer polyethylene-glycol electrolyte solution (GoLYTELY) via nasogastric tube for constipation as prescribed.
          ○ Administer histamine-receptor antagonist and motility medications for GERD as prescribed.
          ○ Administer possible formula supplements via a gastric tube.
          ○ Consult a dietitian.
       • Endocrine Management
          ○ Monitor blood glucose.
          ○ Administer insulin as prescribed.

    (N) NCLEX® Connection: Physiological Adaptations, Illness Management

UNIT 2   Nursing Care of Children with System Disorders

SECTION: CARDIOVASCULAR AND HEMATOLOGIC DISORDERS

› Cardiovascular Disorders
› Hematologic Disorders

NCLEX® CONNECTIONS

When reviewing the chapters in this unit, keep in mind the relevant sections of the NCLEX® outline, in particular:

Client Needs: Pharmacological and Parenteral Therapies

› Relevant topics/tasks include:
  » Adverse Effects/ Contraindications/Side Effects/Interactions
    › Monitor for anticipated interactions among the client's prescribed medications and fluids.
  » Dosage Calculation
    › Use clinical decision making/critical thinking when calculating dosages.
  » Medication Administration
    › Review pertinent data prior to medication administration.

Client Needs: Reduction of Risk Potential

› Relevant topics/tasks include:
  » Changes/Abnormalities in Vital Signs
    › Apply knowledge of client pathophysiology when measuring vital signs.
  » Potential for Complications of Diagnostic Tests/ Treatments/Procedures
    › Monitor the client for signs of bleeding.
  » System Specific Assessment
    › Assess the client for abnormal peripheral pulses after a procedure or treatment.

Client Needs: Physiological Adaptation

› Relevant topics/tasks include:
  » Alterations in Body Systems
    › Evaluate achievement of the client treatment goals.
  » Hemodynamics
    › Provide the client with strategies to manage decreased cardiac output.
  » Illness Management
    › Apply knowledge of client pathophysiology to illness management.

chapter 20

Overview

- Heart disease may be congenital or acquired.

- Anatomic abnormalities present at birth can lead to congenital heart disease (CHD). These abnormalities result primarily in heart failure and hypoxemia. Congenital disorders that result primarily in heart failure and hypoxemia to be discussed in this chapter include:

  - Ventricular defect (VSD)

  - Atrial septal defect (ASD)

  - Patent ductus arteriosus (PDA)

  - Pulmonary stenosis

  - Aortic stenosis

  - Tetralogy of Fallot

  - Coarctation of the aorta

  - Transposition of the great arteries

  - Tricuspid atresia

  - Truncus arteriosus

  - Hypoplastic left heart syndrome

- Acquired cardiovascular disorder

  - Rheumatic fever

  - Hyperlipidemia

- Vascular dysfunction

  - Kawasaki disease

- Heart failure occurs when the heart is unable to pump adequate blood to meet the metabolic and physical demands of the body.

- Due to changing lifestyles and socioeconomic conditions, the incidence of hyperlipidemia is on the rise in children. The result is obesity in childhood and leads to heart disease during adulthood.

CONGENITAL HEART DISEASE (CHD)

Overview

- Anatomic defects of the heart prevent normal blood flow to the pulmonary and/or systemic system. Defects are categorized by blood flow patterns in the heart.
  - Increased pulmonary blood flow (ASD, VSD, PDA)
  - Decreased pulmonary blood flow (Tetralogy of Fallot, tricuspid atresia)
  - Obstruction to blood flow (coarctation of the aorta, pulmonary stenosis, aortic stenosis)
  - Mixed blood flow (transposition of the great arteries, truncus arteriosus, hypoplastic left heart syndrome)

Assessment

- Risk Factors
  - Maternal factors
    - Infection
    - Alcohol and/or other substance abuse during pregnancy
    - Diabetes mellitus
  - Genetic factors
    - History of congenital heart disease in other family members
    - Certain syndromes such as Trisomy 21 (Down syndrome)
    - Presence of other congenital anomalies or chromosomal abnormalities
- Subjective and Objective Data

> **View Images**
> › Ventricular Septal Defect
> › Pulmonary Stenosis
> › Coarctation of the Aorta
> › Tetralogy of Fallot

CONGENITAL HEART DEFECT	MANIFESTATIONS
› Ventricular septal defect (VSD) – a hole in the septum between the right and left ventricle that results in increased pulmonary blood flow (left-to-right shunt)	› Loud, harsh murmur auscultated at the left sternal border › Heart failure › Many VSDs close spontaneously
› Atrial septal defect (ASD) – a hole in the septum between the right and left atria that results in increased pulmonary blood flow (left-to-right shunt)	› Loud, harsh murmur with a fixed split second heart sound › Heart failure › Asymptomatic (possibly)

CONGENITAL HEART DEFECT	MANIFESTATIONS
› Patent ductus arteriosus (PDA) – a condition in which the normal fetal circulation conduit between the pulmonary artery and the aorta fails to close and results in increased pulmonary blood flow (left-to-right shunt)	› Murmur (machine hum) › Wide pulse pressure › Bounding pulses › Asymptomatic (possibly) › Heart failure
› Pulmonary stenosis – a narrowing of the pulmonary valve or pulmonary artery that results in obstruction of blood flow from the ventricles	› Systolic ejection murmur › Asymptomatic (possibly) › Cyanosis varies with defect, worse with severe narrowing › Cardiomegaly › Heart failure
› Aortic stenosis – a narrowing of the aortic valve	› Infants » Faint pulses » Hypotension » Tachycardia » Poor feeding tolerance › Children » Intolerance to exercise » Dizziness » Chest pain » Possible ejection murmur
› Coarctation of the aorta – a narrowing of the lumen of the aorta, usually at or near the ductus arteriosus, that results in obstruction of blood flow from the ventricle	› Elevated blood pressure in the arms › Bounding pulses in the upper extremities › Decreased blood pressure in the lower extremities › Cool skin of lower extremities › Weak or absent femoral pulses › Heart failure in infants › Dizziness, headaches, fainting, or nosebleeds in older children
› Transposition of the great arteries – a condition in which the aorta is connected to the right ventricle instead of the left, and the pulmonary artery is connected to the left ventricle instead of the right a septal defect or a PDA must exist in order to oxygenate the blood	› Murmur depending on presence of associated defects › Severe to less cyanosis depending on the size of the associated defect › Cardiomegaly › Heart failure
› Tricuspid atresia – A complete closure of the tricuspid valve that results in mixed blood flow. An atrial septal opening needs to be present to allow blood to enter the left atrium.	› Infants – cyanosis, dyspnea, tachycardia › Older children – hypoxemia, clubbing of fingers

CONGENITAL HEART DEFECT	MANIFESTATIONS
› Tetralogy of Fallot – four defects that result in mixed blood flow » Pulmonary stenosis » Ventricular septal defect » Overriding aorta » Right ventricular hypertrophy	› Cyanosis at birth – progressive cyanosis over the first year of life › Systolic murmur › Episodes of acute cyanosis and hypoxia (blue spells)
› Truncus arteriosus – failure of septum formation, resulting in a single vessel that comes off of the ventricles	› Heart failure › Murmur › Variable cyanosis › Delayed growth › Lethargy › Fatigue › Poor feeding habits
› Hypoplastic left heart syndrome – Left side of the heart is underdeveloped. An ASD or patent foramen ovale allows for oxygenation of the blood.	› Mild cyanosis › Heart failure › Lethargy › Cold hands and feet › Once PDA closes, progression of cyanosis and decreased cardiac output result in eventual cardiac collapse

- Manifestations of heart failure (HF)
  - Impaired myocardial function
    - Sweating, tachycardia, fatigue, pallor, cool extremities with weak pulses, hypotension, gallop rhythm, cardiomegaly
  - Pulmonary congestion
    - Tachypnea, dyspnea, retractions, nasal flaring, grunting, wheezing, cyanosis, cough, orthopnea, exercise intolerance
  - Systemic venous congestion
    - Hepatomegaly, peripheral edema, ascites, neck vein distention, periorbital edema, weight gain
- Manifestations of hypoxemia
  - Cyanosis, poor weight gain, tachypnea, dyspnea, clubbing, polycythemia

 View Image: Clubbed Fingers

  - Hypercyanotic spells (blue, or "Tet," spells) manifest as acute cyanosis and hyperpnea.
- Laboratory Tests
  - Hemoglobin (Hgb), hematocrit (Hct), and serum electrolytes

○ Diagnostic Procedures

- ECG monitoring to identify cardiac dysrhythmias

  □ Nursing Actions

  ▸ Assist with the application of electrodes.

  ▸ Assist with maintaining the child in a quiet position.

  □ Client Education – Tell the child that the test will not be painful.

- Radiography (chest x-ray) to determine heart size and blood flow

  □ Nursing Actions – Assist with positioning the client.

- Echocardiography to determine cardiac defects and heart function

  □ Nursing Actions – Assist with positioning the child.

- Cardiac catheterization

  □ Cardiac catheterization is an invasive test used for diagnosing, repairing some defects, and evaluating dysrhythmias. A radiopaque catheter is peripherally inserted and threaded into the heart with the use of fluoroscopy. A contrast medium (may be iodine-based) is injected, and images of the blood vessels and heart are taken as the medium is diluted and circulated throughout the body.

  □ Nursing Actions

  ▸ Preprocedure

  ▷ Perform a nursing history and physical exam. Evidence of infection, such as a severe diaper rash, may necessitate canceling the procedure if femoral access is required.

  ▷ Check for allergies to iodine and shellfish.

  ▷ Provide age-appropriate teaching.

  ▷ Describe how long the procedure will take, how the child will feel, and what care will be required after the procedure.

  ▷ Provide for NPO status 4 to 6 hr prior to the procedure. (If the procedure is performed as outpatient, be sure the child and family are given instructions in advance.)

  ▷ Obtain baseline vital signs including oxygen saturation.

  ▷ Locate and mark the dorsalis pedis and posterior tibial pulses on both extremities.

  ▷ Administer presedation as prescribed based on the child's age, height, weight, condition, and type of procedure being performed.

  ▸ Postprocedure

  ▷ Provide for continuous cardiac monitoring and oxygen saturation to assess for bradycardia, dysrhythmias, hypotension, and hypoxemia.

  ▷ Assess heart and respiratory rate for one full minute.

  ▷ Assess pulses for equality and symmetry.

  ▷ Assess temperature and color. A cool extremity with skin that blanches may indicate arterial obstruction.

  ▷ Assess insertion site (femoral or antecubital area) for bleeding and/or hematoma.

  ▷ Maintain clean dressing.

▷ Prevent bleeding by maintaining the affected extremity in a straight position for 4 to 8 hr.

▷ Monitor I&O to assess for adequate urine output, hypovolemia, or dehydration.

▷ Monitor for hypoglycemia. IV fluids with dextrose may be necessary.

▷ Encourage oral intake, starting with clear liquids.

▷ Encourage the child to void to promote excretion of the contrast medium.

◻ Client Education

▸ Encourage fluid intake to help with the removal of the dye from the body.

▸ Advise the parents and child to monitor the site for infection.

Patient-Centered Care

- Nursing Care
  - General Interventions
    - Remain calm when providing care.
    - Keep the child well-hydrated.
    - Conserve the child's energy by providing frequent rest periods; clustering care; providing small, frequent meals; bathing PRN; and keeping crying to a minimum in cyanotic children.
    - Perform daily weight and I&O to monitor fluid status and nutritional status.
    - Monitor heart rate, blood pressure, serum electrolytes, and renal function to assess for complications.
    - Provide support and resources for parents to promote developmental growth in the child.
    - Monitor family coping and provide support.
    - Administer prescribed medications.
    - Maintain fluid and electrolyte balance.
      - ◻ Administer potassium supplements if prescribed. These may not be indicated if the child is concurrently taking an ACE inhibitor.
      - ◻ Maintain sodium and fluid restrictions if prescribed.
    - Decrease workload of the heart.
      - ◻ Maintain bedrest.
      - ◻ Position the infant in a car seat or hold at a 45° angle. Keep safety restraints low and loose on the abdomen.
      - ◻ Allow the child to sleep with several pillows and encourage a semi-Fowler's or Fowler's position while awake.
    - Provide for adequate nutrition.
      - ◻ Plan to feed the infant using a feeding schedule of every 3 hr. The infant should be rested, which occurs soon after awakening.
      - ◻ Use a soft preemie nipple or a regular nipple with a slit to provide an enlarged opening.
      - ◻ Hold the infant in a semi-upright position.
      - ◻ Allow the infant to rest during feedings, taking approximately 30 min to complete the feeding.

- □ Gavage feed the infant if he is unable to consume enough formula or breast milk.
- □ Increase caloric density of formula gradually from 20 kcal/oz to 30 kcal/oz.
- □ Encourage mothers who are breastfeeding to alternate feedings with high-density formula or fortified breast milk.
  - ▪ Increase tissue oxygenation.
    - □ Provide cool, humidified oxygen via an oxygen hood (or tent), mask, or nasal cannula.
    - □ Suction the airway as indicated.
    - □ Monitor oxygen saturation every 2 to 4 hr.
- Medications
  - ○ Digoxin (Lanoxin) – improves myocardial contractility
    - ▪ Nursing Actions
      - □ Monitor the pulse and withhold the medication as ordered. Generally, if an infant's pulse is less than 90/min, the medication should be withheld. In children, the medication should be withheld if the pulse is less than 70/min.
      - □ Monitor for toxicity as evidenced by bradycardia, dysrhythmias, nausea, vomiting, or anorexia.
      - □ Monitor serum digoxin levels.
  - ○ Captopril (Capoten) or enalapril (Vasotec)
    - ▪ Angiotensin-converting enzyme (ACE) inhibitors reduce afterload by causing vasodilation, resulting in decreased pulmonary and systemic vascular resistance.
    - ▪ Nursing Considerations
      - □ Monitor blood pressure before and after the medication is administered.
      - □ Monitor for evidence of hyperkalemia.
    - ▪ Client Education – Instruct parents to monitor blood pressure frequently.
  - ○ Metoprolol or carvedilol (Coreg) – beta-blockers, which decrease heart rate and blood pressure, and promote vasodilation
    - ▪ Nursing Considerations
      - □ Monitor blood pressure and pulse prior to administration.
      - □ Monitor for adverse effects such as dizziness, hypotension, and headache.
  - ○ Furosemide (Lasix) or chlorothiazide (Diuril) – Potassium-wasting diuretics rid the body of excess fluid and sodium.
    - ▪ Nursing Considerations
      - □ Encourage a diet high in potassium.
      - □ Monitor I&O.
      - □ Monitor for adverse affects such as hypokalemia, nausea, vomiting, and dizziness.
      - □ Monitor weight daily.

- Nonsurgical and Surgical Intervention
  - VSD
    - Closure during cardiac catheterization
    - Surgical procedures such as:
      - Pulmonary artery banding
      - Complete repair with patch
  - ASD
    - Closure during cardiac catheterization
    - Surgical procedure: patch closure
  - PDA
    - Administration of indomethacin
    - Insertion of coils to occlude PDA during cardiac catheterization
    - Surgical procedure: thoracoscopic repair
  - Pulmonary stenosis
    - Balloon angioplasty with cardiac catheterization
    - Surgical procedures
      - Infants: Brock procedure
      - Children: pulmonary valvotomy
  - Aortic stenosis
    - Balloon dilation with cardiac catheterization
    - Surgery
      - Norwood procedure
      - Aortic valvotomy
  - Coarctation of the aorta
    - Infants and children: balloon angioplasty
    - Adolescents: placement of stents
    - Surgery: repair of defect recommended for infants less than 6 months of age
  - Transposition of the great arteries
    - Surgery to switch the arteries within the first 2 weeks of life
  - Tricuspid atresia
    - Surgery in 3 stages: shunt placement, Glenn procedure, modified Fontan procedure
  - Tetralogy of Fallot
    - Shunt placement until able to undergo primary repair
    - Complete repair within the first year of life

○ Truncus arteriosus

▪ Surgical repair within the first month of life

○ Hypoplastic left heart syndrome

▪ Surgery in three stages starting shortly after birth: Norwood procedure, Glenn shunt, and Fontan procedure

• Teamwork and Collaboration

○ Dieticians should be consulted to assist the family with appropriate food choices.

• Care After Discharge

○ Client Education

▪ Cardiac catheterization

□ Teach the family to monitor for possible complications (bleeding, infection, thrombosis).

□ Limit activity for 24 hr.

□ Encourage fluids.

▪ Digoxin administration

□ Take pulse prior to medication administration. Notify provider if pulse is lower than specified rate.

□ Administer digoxin every 12 hr.

□ Direct oral elixir toward the side and back of mouth when administering.

□ Give water following administration to prevent tooth decay if the child has teeth.

□ If a dose is missed, do not give an extra dose or increase the next dose.

□ If the child vomits, do not readminister the dose.

□ Observe for signs of digoxin toxicity (decreased heart rate, decreased appetite, nausea, and/or vomiting). Notify the provider if these occur.

□ Keep the medication in a locked cabinet.

▪ Diuretic administration

□ Mix the oral elixir in a small amount of juice to disguise the bitter taste and prevent intestinal irritation.

□ Observe for adverse effects of diuretics, which may include nausea, vomiting, and diarrhea.

□ Observe for manifestations of serum potassium level imbalances (muscle weakness, irritability, excessive drowsiness, and increased or decreased heart rate).

□ Encourage the child to eat foods high in potassium, such as bran cereals, potatoes, tomatoes, bananas, melons, oranges, and orange juice.

□ Teach the family to monitor weight daily.

▪ Instruct the family to report evidence of worsening heart failure, such as increased sweating and decreased urinary output (fewer wet diapers or less frequent toileting).

Complications

- Cardiac catheterization (potential)
  - ○ Nausea, vomiting
  - ○ Low-grade fever
  - ○ Loss of pulse in the catheterized extremity
  - ○ Transient dysrhythmias
  - ○ Acute hemorrhage from entry site
  - ○ Nursing Actions
    - ▪ Apply direct continuous pressure at 2.5 cm (1 in) above the catheter entry site to localize pressure over the location of the vessel puncture.
    - ▪ Position the child flat to reduce the gravitational effect on the rate of bleeding.
    - ▪ Notify the provider immediately.
    - ▪ Prepare for the possible administration of replacement fluids and/or medication to control emesis.
  - ○ Client Education
    - ▪ Monitor for infection.
    - ▪ Monitor for bleeding.
- Hypoxemia
  - ○ A hypercyanotic spell can result in severe hypoxemia, which leads to cerebral hypoxemia, and should be treated as an emergency.
  - ○ Nursing Actions – Immediately place the child in the knee-chest position, attempt to calm the child, and call for help.
- Bacterial endocarditis or subacute bacterial endocarditis
  - ○ Children with congenital or acquired heart disease are at increased risk for infection of the valves or lining of the heart.
  - ○ The client should follow the American Heart Association's recommendations for bacterial endocarditis prophylaxis. These include receiving prophylactic antibiotic therapy prior to dental and surgical procedures (dental extractions, endodontic surgery, surgical procedures that involve the respiratory or gastrointestinal mucosa).
  - ○ Causative organisms include *Streptococcus viridans* and *Staphylococcus aureus*.
  - ○ Nursing Actions – Administer antibiotics parenterally for an extended length of time usually via a peripherally inserted central catheter.
  - ○ Client Education
    - ▪ Counsel the family about the need for prophylactic antibiotics prior to dental and surgical procedures.
    - ▪ Teach the family clinical manifestations of endocarditis (low-grade fever, malaise, decreased appetite with weight loss).

- Heart failure requiring transplant
  - Cardiomyopathy and congenital heart disease are causes of heart failure.
  - Nursing Actions
    - Maintain pharmacological support as ordered (oxygen, diuretics, digoxin, afterload reducers such as ACE inhibitors).
    - Provide family and child support.
  - Client Education
    - Teach the importance of adhering to the medication regimen.
    - Inform the child and family about infection control precautions.

RHEUMATIC FEVER

Overview

- Rheumatic fever is an inflammatory disease that occurs as a reaction to Group A β-hemolytic streptococcus (GABHS) infection of the throat.

Assessment

- Risk Factors
  - Rheumatic fever usually occurs within 2 to 6 weeks following an untreated or partially treated upper respiratory infection (strep throat) with GABHS.
- Subjective and Objective Data
  - History of recent upper respiratory infection
  - Fever
  - Tachycardia, cardiomegaly, prolonged PR interval, new or changed heart murmur, muffled heart sounds, pericardial friction rub, and report of chest pain, which may indicate carditis
  - Nontender, subcutaneous nodules over bony prominence

  - Large joints (knees, elbows, ankles, wrists, shoulders) with painful swelling, indicating polyarthritis
    - Findings may be present for a few days and then disappear without treatment, frequently returning in another joint.
  - Pink, nonpruritic macular rash on the trunk and inner surfaces of extremities that appears and disappears rapidly, indicating erythema marginatum
  - CNS involvement (chorea) including involuntary, purposeless muscle movements; muscle weakness; involuntary facial movements; difficulty performing fine motor activities; labile emotions; and random, uncoordinated movements of the extremities
  - Irritability, poor concentration, and behavioral problems

- ○ Laboratory Tests
  - ▪ Throat culture for GABHS
  - ▪ Serum antistreptolysin-O (ASO) titer – elevated or rising titer, most reliable diagnostic test
  - ▪ C-reactive protein (CRP) – elevated in response to an inflammatory reaction
  - ▪ Erythrocyte sedimentation rate – elevated in response to an inflammatory reaction
- ○ Diagnostic Procedures
  - ▪ Cardiac function
    - □ ECG to reveal the presence of conduction disturbances and to evaluate the function of the heart and valves.
    - □ Nursing Actions – Position the child correctly for the procedure.
    - □ Client Education – Explain the need for decreased movement during the procedure.
  - ▪ The diagnosis of rheumatic fever is made on the basis of modified Jones criteria. The child should demonstrate the presence of two major criteria or the presence of one major and two minor criteria following an acute infection with GABHS infection.
    - □ Major criteria
      - ▸ Carditis
      - ▸ Subcutaneous nodules
      - ▸ Polyarthritis
      - ▸ Rash (erythema marginatum)
      - ▸ Chorea
    - ⊓ Minor criteria
      - ▸ Fever
      - ▸ Arthralgia

Patient-Centered Care

- • Nursing Care
  - ○ Encourage bed rest during the acute illness.
  - ○ Administer antibiotic as prescribed.
  - ○ Encourage nutritionally balanced meals.
  - ○ Assess for chorea.
- • Medications
  - ○ Antibiotic prophylaxis
    - ▪ Follow the prescribed prophylactic treatment regimen, which can include one of the following: two daily oral doses of 200,000 units of penicillin, a monthly IM injection of 1.2 million units of penicillin G, or a daily oral dose of 1 g sulfadiazine (Microsulfon). The length of treatment varies according to residual heart disease, ranging from 5 years to indefinitely.
    - ▪ Nursing Considerations
      - □ Assess for an allergic response (anaphylaxis, hives, rashes).
      - □ Assess for nausea, vomiting, or diarrhea.
    - ▪ Client Education
      - □ Encourage compliance with medication regimen.

- Care After Discharge
  - Client Education
    - Promote rest during the acute phase.
    - Provide information and reassurance related to the development of chorea and its self-limiting nature.
    - Encourage well-balanced meals.
    - Seek medical care if infection recurrence is suspected.

Complications

- Carditis and heart disease

HYPERLIPIDEMIA

Overview

- Hyperlipidemia is excess lipids (fat) in circulating blood.
- Cholesterol is part of the lipoprotein complex in blood.
- Triglycerides come from two sources: naturally made in the body from carbohydrates, and the end product of fat ingestion.
- Total cholesterol – the sum of all forms of cholesterol.
- High density lipoprotein (HDL) cholesterol – "good" cholesterol, having low level of cholesterol and triglycerides and high level of protein.
- Low density lipoprotein (LDL) cholesterol – "bad" cholesterol, having a high level of cholesterol, low level of triglycerides, and moderate levels of protein.

Assessment

- Risk Factors
  - Genetic
  - Obesity
  - Lack of exercise
  - History of health condition: diabetes, kidney disease, hypothyroidism
  - Medications: birth control pills, diuretics, beta-blockers
- Subjective and Objective Data
  - Clients who have risk factors should be evaluated.
  - Laboratory Tests
    - Lipid profile – fasting for 12 hr prior to test
    - Fasting blood glucose

- Patient-Centered Care
  - Nursing Care/Client Education
    - Assist in screening clients at risk.
    - Teach the client to keep a diet history for review by the dietician.
    - Assess the client for febrile illness 3 weeks prior to screening (illness will alter results).
    - Teach diet to lower cholesterol: low fat, whole grains, fruit and vegetables.
    - Encourage use of olive oil and canola oil.
    - Assist with an exercise program (60 min per day for 5 days per week of aerobic exercise).
- Medication
  - Cholestyramine (Questran) and colestipol (Colestid)
    - Used in clients who fail conventional treatment
    - Used in children 8 years and older who have a LDL of 190 mg/dL or higher or 160 mg/dL in clients who have risk factors
    - Nursing Considerations
      - Powdered medication mixed in 4 to 6 oz of water or juice, then administered immediately.
      - Monitor for adverse effects: constipation, abdominal pain, flatulence, nausea and abdominal bloating.
      - Monitor laboratory findings: liver function tests, CBC, creatinine kinase and fasting lipid profile at 4 and 8 week intervals and with any dosage change.
  - Client Education
    - Teach the client and family how to administer medications.
    - Teach the client about adverse effects of medications.
    - Teach the client to discontinue medication if he exhibits dark urine or muscle aches, and to notify the provider.
- Teamwork and Collaboration
  - Dietary counseling

Complications

- Atherosclerosis and coronary heart disease
  - Nursing Considerations
    - Identify clients who are at risk and promote early screening.
    - Teach health eating to families and client.

KAWASAKI DISEASE

Overview

- Acute systemic vasculitis

Assessment

- Risk Factors – etiology unknown
- Subjective and Objective Data
  - Acute phase: onset of high fever that is unresponsive to antipyretics, with development of other clinical manifestations
    - Fever greater than 38.9° C (102° F) lasting 5 days to 2 weeks and unresponsive to antipyretics
    - Irritability
    - Red eyes without drainage
    - Bright red, chapped lips
    - Strawberry tongue with white coating or red bumps on the posterior aspect
    - Red oral mucous membranes
    - Swelling of hand and feet with red palms and soles
    - Nonblistering rash
    - Bilateral joint pain
    - Enlarged lymph nodes
  - Subacute phase: resolution of the fever and gradual subsiding of other clinical manifestations
    - Irritability
    - Peeling skin around the nails, on the palms and soles
  - Convalescent: no clinical manifestations seen except altered laboratory findings. Resolution in about 6 to 8 weeks from onset.
  - Laboratory Tests
    - CBC, CRP, ESR, serum albumin
  - Diagnostic Procedures
    - Chest x-ray
    - Echocardiogram and/or ECG to indicate myocarditis, pericarditis, arthritis, meningitis, inflammation

Patient-Centered Care

- Nursing Care
  - Monitor vital signs and cardiac status. Maintain cardiac monitoring.
  - Assess client for heart failure (decreased urine output, gallop heart rhythm, tachycardia, respiratory distress).
  - Monitor I&O. Obtain daily weight.
  - Administer IV fluids to prevent dehydration. Offer clear liquids and soft foods.
  - Administer IV gamma globulin according to facility policy.
  - Administer aspirin as prescribed.
  - Provide care to promote comfort due to clinical findings.
    - Oral hygiene.
    - Apply cool cloths to skin.
    - Apply skin lotions to maintain hydration.
    - Provide for a calm, quiet environment.
    - Promote rest by clustering care.
- Medication
  - Gamma globulin (IVGG)
    - Nursing Consideration
      - Administer via IV infusion.
      - High dosage: 2 g/kg over 10 to 12 hr.
      - Ideally administer within the first 7 days of illness.
      - Repeat for clients who remain febrile.
      - Monitor vital signs.
      - Assess for allergic reaction.
  - Aspirin
    - High dose: 80 to 100 mg/kg/day divided every 6 hr.
    - Once afebrile: 3 to 5 mg/kg/day to continue until platelet count returns to expected range which may be approximately 6 to 8 weeks.
    - If coronary abnormalities develop, continue aspirin therapy indefinitely.
- Care after discharge
  - Teach the family about disease progression.
  - Encourage the family to maintain follow-up appointments.
  - Teach the family that the irritability may last 2 months.
  - Teach the family that arthritic symptoms may last several weeks.
  - Teach the family that the skin manifestations are painless but the skin could be tender.

- ○ Encourage passive ROM exercises in the bathtub.
- ○ Avoid live immunizations for 11 months.
- ○ Notify the provider of any fever.
- Ongoing Care
  - ○ Avoid smoking.
  - ○ Maintain a heart healthy diet.
  - ○ Screen for heart disease as child age.
    - ▪ Serum cholesterol testing
    - ▪ Blood pressure monitoring
    - ▪ Periodic imaging of the heart

Complications

- Coronary artery dilation or aneurysm formation
  - ○ Most common in the subacute phase
  - ○ Echocardiogram to monitor for changes
  - ○ Administer anticoagulation medications as prescribed (enoxaparin [Lovenox])

APPLICATION EXERCISES

1. A nurse is caring for an infant. Which of the following are clinical manifestations of coarctation of the aorta? (Select all that apply.)

_____ A. Weak femoral pulses

_____ B. Cool skin of lower extremities

_____ C. Severe cyanosis

_____ D. Clubbing of the fingers

_____ E. Heart failure

2. A nurse is assessing an infant. Which of the following should the nurse recognize as clinical manifestations of heart failure? (Select all that apply.)

_____ A. Bradycardia

_____ B. Cool extremities

_____ C. Peripheral edema

_____ D. Increased urinary output

_____ E. Nasal flaring

3. A nurse is providing teaching to the mother of an infant who is to start taking digoxin (Lanoxin). Which of the following instructions should the nurse include?

A. "Do not offer your baby fluids after giving the medication."

B. "Digoxin increases your baby's heart rate."

C. "Give the correct dose of medication at regularly scheduled times."

D. "If your baby vomits a dose, you should repeat the dose to ensure that he gets the correct amount."

4. A nurse is caring for a 2-year-old child who is cyanotic and is in the hospital for a cardiac catheterization to repair cardiac defects. The child will be transferred to the pediatric ICU following the procedure. Which of the following is an appropriate nursing action when providing care to this child?

A. Place on NPO status for 12 hr prior to the procedure.

B. Check for iodine or shellfish allergies prior to the procedure.

C. Elevate the affected extremity following the procedure.

D. Limit fluid intake following the procedure

5. A nurse is caring for a child who is suspected of having rheumatic fever. Which of the following manifestations support this diagnosis? (Select all that apply.)

_____ A. Erythema marginatum (rash)

_____ B. Continuous joint pain of the digits

_____ C. Tender, subcutaneous nodules

_____ D. Decreased erythrocyte sedimentation rate

_____ E. Elevated C-reactive protein

6. A nurse is discussing care of a child who has Kawasaki disease with a newly hired nurse. What should be included in this discussion? Use the ATI Active Learning Template: Systems Disorder to complete this item to include:

A. Clinical Manifestations: Identify for the acute, subacute, and convalescent phase.

B. Nursing Care: List seven for this client.

APPLICATION EXERCISES KEY

1. A. **CORRECT:** Narrowing of the lumen of the aorta results in obstruction of blood flow from the ventricle, resulting in weak or absent femoral pulses.

    B. **CORRECT:** Narrowing of the lumen of the aorta results in obstruction of blood flow from the ventricle, resulting in cool skin of the lower extremities.

    C. INCORRECT: A client who has coarctation of the aorta exhibits adequate oxygenation of blood. Therefore, severe cyanosis is not present.

    D. INCORRECT: Clubbing of the fingers is a clinical manifestation of chronic hypoxemia and will not be observed in an infant who has coarctation of the aorta.

    E. **CORRECT:** Heart failure occurs when the heart is unable to meet the body's demands, and is a clinical manifestation of coarctation of the aorta.

    Ⓝ NCLEX® Connection: Physiological Adaptations, Pathophysiology

2. A. INCORRECT: A client who has heart failure will exhibit tachycardia as the heart attempts to meet the body's demands.

    B. **CORRECT:** A client who has heart failure will exhibit cool extremities as the heart is unable to adequately circulate oxygenated blood.

    C. **CORRECT:** A client who has heart failure will exhibit peripheral edema as the heart is unable to adequately circulate blood through the body and back to the heart.

    D. INCORRECT: With heart failure, the heart is unable to keep up with the body's demands. A decrease in urinary output is a clinical manifestation of heart failure.

    E. **CORRECT:** A client who has heart failure will exhibit nasal flaring due to inadequate oxygenation of blood.

    Ⓝ NCLEX® Connection: Physiological Adaptations, Pathophysiology

3.   A. INCORRECT: Digoxin can be given without regard to food or fluids.

    B. INCORRECT: Digoxin slows the heart rate by increasing contractility of the heart.

    C. **CORRECT:** The correct amount of digoxin should be administered at regularly scheduled times to maintain therapeutic blood levels.

    D. INCORRECT: It is not recommended to repeat digoxin following an emesis because it is impossible to determine how much medication was lost.

    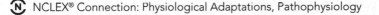 NCLEX® Connection: Pharmacological and Parenteral Therapies, Medication Administration

4.   A. INCORRECT: The child should remain NPO 4 to 6 hr prior to the procedure.

    B. **CORRECT:** Iodine-based dyes may be used in this procedure, so the child is assessed for allergies to iodine or shellfish which could lead to anaphylaxis.

    C. INCORRECT: The affected extremity should be maintained in a straight position following the procedure.

    D. INCORRECT: Fluids should be encouraged after the procedure to maintain adequate urine output and promote excretion of the dye.

    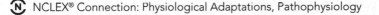 NCLEX® Connection: Reduction of Risk Potential, Diagnostic Tests

5.   A. **CORRECT:** Rheumatic fever is caused by Group A β-hemolytic streptococcus. An erythema marginatum (rash) is a clinical manifestation.

    B. INCORRECT: A client who has rheumatic fever exhibits migratory joint pain of the large joints.

    C. INCORRECT: A client who has rheumatic fever exhibits nontender subcutaneous nodules of bony prominences.

    D. INCORRECT: Rheumatic fever is caused by Group A β-hemolytic streptococcus, which results in an elevated erythrocyte sedimentation rate.

    E. **CORRECT:** Rheumatic fever is caused by Group A β-hemolytic streptococcus. An increase in C-reactive protein is a clinical manifestation.

    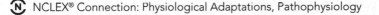 NCLEX® Connection: Physiological Adaptations, Pathophysiology

6. *Using the ATI Active Learning Template: Systems Disorder*

A. Clinical Manifestations

- Acute phase: onset of high fever that is unresponsive to antipyretics, with development of other manifestations
  - Fever greater than 38.9° C (102° F) lasting 5 days to 2 weeks and unresponsive to antipyretics
  - Irritability
  - Red eyes without drainage
  - Bright red, chapped lips
  - Strawberry tongue with white coating or red bumps on the posterior aspect
  - Red oral mucous membranes
  - Swelling of hands and feet with red palms and soles
  - Non-blistering rash
  - Bilateral joint pain
  - Enlarged lymph nodes
- Subacute phase: resolution of the fever and gradual subsiding of other manifestations
  - Irritability
  - Peeling skin around the nails, on the palms and soles
- Convalescent phase: no clinical manifestations seen except altered laboratory findings. Resolution in about 6 to 8 weeks from onset.

B. Nursing Care

- Monitor vital signs, ECG, and cardiac status.
- Assess client for heart failure (decreased urine output, gallop heart rhythm, tachycardia, respiratory distress).
- Monitor I&O. Obtain daily weight.
- Administer IV fluids. Offer clear liquids and soft foods.
- Administer IV gamma globulin according to facility policy.
- Administer aspirin as prescribed.
- Provide care to include oral hygiene, cool cloths to extremities, application of skin lotion; providing for a quiet environment to promote rest; cluster nursing care.

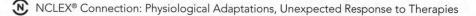 NCLEX® Connection: Physiological Adaptations, Unexpected Response to Therapies

chapter 21

Overview

- Blood disorders that may affect children include:
  - Epistaxis
  - Iron deficiency anemia
  - Sickle cell anemia
  - Hemophilia

EPISTAXIS

Overview

- Short, isolated occurrences of epistaxis are common in childhood.
- Although epistaxis is rarely an emergency, it causes the child and the child's caregivers anxiety.

Assessment

- Risk Factors
  - Trauma, such as picking or rubbing the nose, can cause mucous membranes in the nose, which are vascular and fragile, to tear and bleed.
  - Low humidity, allergic rhinitis, upper respiratory infection, blunt injury, or a foreign body in the nose can all precipitate a nosebleed.
  - Medications that affect clotting factors can increase bleeding.
  - Epistaxis may be the result of underlying diseases (von Willebrand disease, hemophilia, idiopathic thrombocytopenia purpura [ITP], leukemia).
- Subjective Data
  - History of bleeding gums or blood in body fluids and/or stool
  - History of trauma, illness, allergies, or placing foreign bodies in the nose
- Objective Data
  - Physical Assessment Findings
    - Active bleeding from nose
    - Restlessness and agitation

Patient-Centered Care

- Nursing Care
  - Maintain a calm demeanor with the child and family.
  - Have the child sit up with the head tilted slightly forward to prevent aspiration of blood.
  - Apply pressure to the lower nose with the thumb and forefinger for at least 10 min.
  - If needed, cotton or tissue can be packed into the side of the nose that is bleeding.
  - Encourage the child to breathe through her mouth while her nose is bleeding.
  - Apply ice across the bridge of the nose if bleeding continues.
  - Water-soluble jelly or petroleum can be inserted after a nose bleed to prevent crusting of the blood and possible recurrence of bleeding episode.
- Care After Discharge
  - Client Education
    - Keep fingernails short.
    - Use a cool-mist humidifier during the dry winter months.
    - For recurrences, remind the child to sit up and slightly forward so blood does not flow down the throat and cause coughing.
    - Inform the family that bleeding usually stops within 10 min.

Complications

- Hemorrhage
  - Nursing Actions
    - Provide support to the child during cauterization or packing.
  - Client Education
    - Instruct the child and family to seek medical care if bleeding lasts longer than 30 min, and that repeated episodes require further evaluation for bleeding disorders.

IRON DEFICIENCY ANEMIA

Overview

- Iron deficiency anemia is the most common anemia in the United States.
- Children ages 12 to 36 months are at risk due to consuming a diet high in cow's milk without adequate intake of foods high in iron.
- Adolescents are at risk due to poor diets, menses, and obesity.
- The production of Hgb requires iron. Iron deficiency will result in decreased Hgb levels.
- Iron deficiency anemia usually results from an inadequate dietary supply of iron, and is the most preventable mineral disturbance.

Assessment

- Risk Factors
  - Premature birth resulting in decreased iron stores
  - Excessive intake of cows' milk in toddlers
    - Milk is not a good source of iron.
    - Milk takes the place of iron-rich solid foods.
  - Malabsorption disorders due to prolonged diarrhea
  - Poor dietary intake of iron
  - Increased iron requirements (blood loss)
  - Chronic disorders (folate deficiency, sickle cell anemia, hemophilia)
- Subjective and Objective Data
  - Shortness of breath
  - Pallor
  - Brittle, spoon-shaped fingernails
  - Fatigue, irritability, and muscle weakness
  - Systolic heart murmur, enlarged heart, and/or heart failure
  - Laboratory Tests

EXPECTED REFERENCE RANGES		
AGE	HGB	HCT
2 months	9.0 to 14.0 g/dL	28% to 42%
6 to 12 years	11.5 to 15.5 g/dL	35% to 45%
12 to 18 years	13.0 to 16.0 g/dL (male)	37% to 49% (male)
	12.0 to 16.0 g/dL (female)	36% to 46% (female)

  - CBC – decreased RBC count, Hgb, and Hct
  - RBC indices – decreased, indicating microcytic/hypochromic RBCs
    - Mean corpuscular volume (MVC) – average size of RBC
    - Mean corpuscular Hgb (MCH) – average weight of RBC
    - Mean corpuscular hemoglobin concentration (MCHC) – amount of Hgb relative to size of cell
  - Reticulocyte count – may be decreased (indicates bone marrow production of RBCs)
  - Decreased serum ferritin level (indicator of iron stores)

Patient-Centered Care

- Nursing Care
  - Provide iron supplements for preterm and low-birth-weight infants by the age of 2 months.
  - Provide iron supplements to infants who are exclusively breastfed by the age of 4 months.
  - Recommend iron-fortified formula for infants who are not being breastfed.
  - Modify the infant's diet to include high iron, vitamin C, and protein content.
  - Monitor milk intake in toddlers.
    - Limit milk intake to 32 oz (950 mL) per day.
    - Delay giving milk until after a meal.
    - Do not allow toddlers to carry bottles or cups of milk.
  - Allow frequent rest periods.
  - If packed RBCs are required, follow protocols for administration.
- Medications
  - Iron Supplements
    - Nursing Considerations
      - Give 1 hr before or 2 hr after milk or antacid to prevent decreased absorption.
      - Gastrointestinal upset (diarrhea, constipation, nausea) is common at the start of therapy. These will decrease over time.
      - If tolerated, administer iron supplements on an empty stomach. Give with meals and start with reduced dose and gradually increase if GI distress occurs.
      - Give with vitamin C to increase absorption.
      - Use a straw with liquid preparation to prevent staining of teeth.
      - Use a Z-track into deep muscle for parenteral injections. Do not massage after injection.
    - Client Education
      - Educate the child and family to expect stools to turn a tarry green color if dose is adequate.
      - Instruct child to brush teeth after oral dose to minimize or prevent staining.
- Care After Discharge
  - Client Education
    - Advise the family that diarrhea, constipation, or nausea may occur at the start of therapy, but these adverse effects are usually self-limiting.
    - Provide information regarding appropriate iron administration.
    - Increase fiber and fluids if constipation develops.
    - Dietary sources of iron
      - Infants – iron-fortified cereals and formula
      - Older children – dried beans and lentils; peanut butter; green, leafy vegetables; iron-fortified breads and flour; poultry; and red meat

- To prevent overdose store no more than a month's supply in a child-proof bottle, and out of reach of children.
- Encourage parents to allow the child to rest.
- Inform parents that the length of treatment will be determined by the child's response to the treatment. If Hgb levels aren't increased after one month of therapy further evaluation is warranted.
- Instruct parents to return for follow-up laboratory tests to determine the effectiveness of treatment.

Complications

- Heart failure
  - Heart failure can develop due to the increased demand on the heart to deliver oxygen to tissues.
  - Nursing Actions
    - Treat anemia.
    - Monitor cardiac rhythm.
    - Give cardiac medications as prescribed.
  - Client Education
    - Educate the child and family on the manifestations of heart failure.
    - Teach the family how to monitor pulse rates.
- Developmental delay
  - Nursing Actions
    - Assess level of functioning.
    - Improve nutritional intake.
    - Refer to appropriate developmental services.
  - Client Education
    - Provide support to the family.

SICKLE CELL ANEMIA

Overview

- Sickle cell disease (SCD) is a group of diseases in which abnormal sickle hemoglobin S (HbS) replaces normal adult hemoglobin (Hgb A).
- Sickle cell anemia (SCA) is the homozygous and most common form of SCD.
- Manifestations and complications of SCA are the result of RBC sickling, which leads to increased blood viscosity, obstruction of blood flow, and tissue hypoxia.
  - Manifestations of SCA are not usually apparent until later in infancy due to the presence of fetal Hgb.
- Tissue hypoxia causes tissue ischemia, which results in pain.
- Increased destruction of RBCs occurs.
- Sickle cell crisis is the exacerbation of SCA.

Assessment

- Risk Factors
  - SCD is an autosomal recessive genetic disorder.
  - SCA primarily affects African-Americans. Other forms of SCD may affect individuals of Mediterranean, Indian, or Middle Eastern descent.
  - Children with sickle cell trait do not manifest the disease but can pass the trait to their offspring.
- Subjective and Objective Data
  - Family history of sickle cell anemia or sickle cell trait
  - Reports of pain
  - Shortness of breath/fatigue
  - Pallor/pale mucous membranes
  - Jaundice
  - Hands and feet cool to touch
  - Dizziness
  - Headache

CRISIS	MANIFESTATIONS
Vaso-occlusive (painful episode) › Usually lasts 4 to 6 days	› Acute » Severe pain, usually in bones, joints, and abdomen » Swollen joints, hands, and feet » Anorexia, vomiting, and fever » Hematuria » Obstructive jaundice » Visual disturbances › Chronic » Increased risk of respiratory infections and osteomyelitis » Retinal detachment and blindness » Systolic murmurs » Renal failure and enuresis » Liver cirrhosis; hepatomegaly » Seizures » Skeletal deformities; shoulder or hip avascular necrosis
Sequestration	› Excessive pooling of blood primarily in the spleen (splenomegaly), and sometimes in the liver (hepatomegaly) › Reduced circulating blood volume results in hypovolemia and can progress to shock › Hypovolemic shock: irritability, tachycardia, pallor, decreased urinary output, tachypnea, cool extremities, thready pulse, hypotension
Aplastic	› Extreme anemia as a result of decreased RBC production › Typically triggered by an infection
Hyperhemolytic	› Increased rate of RBC destruction leading to anemia, jaundice, and/or reticulocytosis

- ○ Laboratory Tests
  - ▪ Screening for SCA in newborns is mandatory in most states.
  - ▪ CBC to detect anemia
  - ▪ Sickledex (sickle-turbidity) – a screening tool that detects the presence of HbS but will not differentiate the trait from the disease
  - ▪ Hemoglobin electrophoresis – separates the various forms of Hgb and is the definitive diagnosis of sickle cell anemia
  - ▪ Sickle-cell crisis
    - □ Hgb is decreased
    - □ WBC count is elevated
    - □ Bilirubin and reticulocyte levels are elevated
    - □ Peripheral blood smear reveals sickled cells
- ○ Diagnostic Procedures

  - ▪ Transcranial Doppler (TCD) test
    - □ Used to assess intracranial vascular flow and detect the risk for cerebrovascular accident (CVA).
    - □ A TCD is performed annually on children ages 2 to 16 years who have SCD.

Patient-Centered Care

- • Nursing Care
  - ○ Promote rest to decrease oxygen consumption.
  - ○ Administer oxygen as prescribed if hypoxia is present.
  - ○ Maintain fluid and electrolyte balance.
    - ▪ Monitor I&O.
    - ▪ Give oral fluids.
    - ▪ Administer IV fluids with electrolyte replacement.
  - ○ Pain Management
    - ▪ Use an interprofessional approach.
    - ▪ Treat mild to moderate pain with acetaminophen (Tylenol) or ibuprofen (Advil). Manage severe pain with opioid analgesics.
    - ▪ Apply comfort measures, such as warm packs to painful joints.
    - ▪ Schedule analgesics to prevent pain.
  - ○ Administer blood products, usually packed RBCs, and exchange transfusions per facility protocol. Observe for manifestations of hypervolemia and transfusion reaction.
  - ○ Treat and prevent infection.
    - ▪ Administer antibiotics.
    - ▪ Perform frequent hand hygiene.

    - ▪ Give oral prophylactic penicillin.
    - ▪ Administer pneumococcal conjugate vaccine (PCV), meningococcal vaccine (MCV4), and yearly seasonal influenza vaccine.
  - ○ Monitor and report laboratory results

 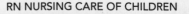

- Medications
  - Opioids – codeine, morphine sulfate, oxycodone, hydrocodone (Dilaudid), and methadone (Dolophine)
    - Opioids provide analgesia for pain management.
    - Nursing Considerations
      - Administer orally (immediate or sustained release) or IV.
      - Administer on a regular schedule to maintain control, or prevent pain if possible.
      - Use patient-controlled analgesia if appropriate.
    - Client Education
      - Educate the child and family about the need to avoid activities that require mental alertness.
      - Provide reassurance that analgesics may be necessary in high doses, and that addiction is rare.
- Care After Discharge
  - Client Education
    - Provide emotional support, and refer to social services if appropriate.
    - Teach child and family about manifestations of crisis and infection.
    - Advise the family of the importance of promoting rest and providing adequate nutrition for the child.
    - Encourage the child and family to maintain good hand hygiene and avoid individuals with colds/infection/viruses.
    - Give specific directions regarding fluid intake requirements, such as how many bottles or glasses of fluid should be consumed daily.
    - Provide information about genetic counseling.
    - Encourage maintenance of up-to-date immunizations.
    - Advise the child to wear a medical identification wristband or medical identification tags.

Complications

- CVA
  - Nursing Actions
    - Assess and report manifestations, which include:
      - Seizures
      - Abnormal behavior
      - Weakness of, or inability to move an extremity
      - Slurred speech
      - Visual changes
      - Vomiting
      - Severe headache
  - Client Education
    - Blood transfusions are usually performed every 3 to 4 weeks to prevent a repeat CVA.

- Acute chest syndrome
  - Can be life-threatening
  - Nursing Actions
    - Assess and report manifestations, which include:
      - Chest, back, or abdominal pain
      - Fever of 38.5° C (101.3° F) or higher
      - Cough
      - Tachypnea
      - Dyspnea
      - Retractions
      - Decreased oxygen saturations

HEMOPHILIA

Overview

- Hemophilia is a group of disorders characterized by difficulty controlling bleeding.
- Bleeding time is extended due to lack of a factor required for blood to clot. Bleeding is internal or external.
- Bleeding tendencies are sometimes recognized during infancy following circumcision, but may not become apparent until the infant becomes more active and prone to injuries during the toddler years.
- Hemophilia varies in severity based on the percentage of clotting factor a child's body contains. For example, a child with mild hemophilia may have up to 49% of the normal factor VIII in his body, while a child with severe hemophilia has very little factor VIII.
- Both hemophilia A and B are X-linked recessive disorders.

TYPES OF HEMOPHILIA	
Hemophilia A	Hemophilia B
› Deficiency of factor VIII	› Deficiency of factor IX
› Referred to as classic hemophilia	› Referred to as Christmas disease
› Accounts for 80% of cases	

Assessment

- Subjective Data
  - Episodes of bleeding, excessive bleeding, reports of joint pain and stiffness, impaired mobility, easy bruising, and activity intolerance
- Objective Data
  - Physical Assessment Findings
    - Active bleeding, which includes bleeding gums, epistaxis, hematuria, and/or tarry stools
    - Hematomas and/or bruising, even with minor injuries
    - Hemarthrosis as evidenced by joint pain, stiffness, warmth, swelling, redness, loss of range of motion, and deformities
    - Headache, slurred speech, and a decreased level of consciousness
  - Laboratory Tests
    - Prolonged partial thromboplastin time (aPTT)
    - Factor-specific assays to determine deficiency
    - Platelets and prothrombin time are within expected reference ranges
    - Whole blood clotting time is within expected range or prolonged
  - Diagnostic Procedures
    - DNA testing – detects classic hemophilia trait in females

Patient-Centered Care

- Nursing Care
  - Management of bleeding in the hospital
    - Avoid taking temperature rectally.
    - Avoid unnecessary skin punctures and use surgical aseptic technique.
    - Apply pressure for 5 min after injections, venipuncture, or needle sticks.
    - Monitor urine, stool, and nasogastric fluid for occult blood.
    - Control localized bleeding.
      - Administer factor replacement.
      - Observe for adverse effects, which include headache, flushing, low sodium, and alterations in heart rate and blood pressure.
      - Encourage the child to rest and immobilize the affected joints.
      - Elevate and apply ice to the affected joints.

- Medications
  - 1-deamino-8-d-arginine vasopressin (DDAVP) is a synthetic form of vasopressin that increases plasma factor VIII (antihemophilic factor [AHF])
    - Effective for mild, but not severe, hemophilia
    - Not effective for hemophilia B, which involves a factor IX deficiency
    - Nursing Considerations – can be given prior to dental or surgical procedures
  - Factor VIII, products that contain factor VIII, pooled plasma, and recombinant products
    - Used to prevent and treat hemorrhage
    - Nursing Considerations – Administer by IV infusion.
    - Client Education
      - Instruct the child and family that treatment can require numerous doses.
      - Periodic administration has proven effective for preventing bleeding complications.
  - Corticosteroids
    - Used to treat hematuria, acute episodes of hemarthrosis, and chronic synovitis
    - Nursing Considerations – Monitor for infection and bleeding.
    - Client Education
      - Encourage the client and family to maintain good hand hygiene and avoid individuals with colds/infection/viruses.
  - Nonsteroidal anti-inflammatory agents
    - Used to treat chronic synovitis
    - Nursing considerations – Monitor for infection.
    - Client Education
      - Administer cautiously due to potential inhibition of platelet function.
      - Encourage the client to take the medication with food.
- Teamwork and Collaboration
  - An interprofessional approach includes the pediatrician, hematologist, orthopedist, nurse, physical therapist, and social worker.
- Care After Discharge
  - Client Education
    - Teach parents to prevent bleeding at home.
      - Place the infant or child in a padded crib.
      - Provide a safe home and a play environment that is free of clutter. Place padding on corners of furniture.
      - Dress toddlers in extra layers of clothing to provide additional padding.
      - Set activity restrictions to avoid injury. Acceptable activities include low-contact sports (tennis, swimming, golf). While participating in these activities, children should wear protective equipment.
      - Encourage the use of soft-bristled toothbrushes.

- Encourage regular exercise and physical therapy after active bleeding is controlled.

- Encourage the family to maintain up-to-date immunizations.

- Teach the importance of wearing a medical identification wristband or medical identification tags.

- Teach manifestations of internal bleeding and hemarthrosis.

- Teach to control bleeding episodes using the RICE (rest, ice, compression, elevation) method.

- Encourage the family to participate in a support group.

Complications

- Uncontrolled bleeding (intracranial hemorrhage, airway obstruction from bleeding in mouth, neck, or chest)
  - Nursing Actions
    - Monitor vital signs for evidence of impending shock.
    - Take measures to control bleeding.
    - Administer appropriate factor replacement during bleeding episodes to treat excessive bleeding or hemarthrosis.
    - Administer a blood transfusion as prescribed.
    - Conduct a neurologic assessment for evidence of intracranial bleed.
    - Provide prophylaxis treatment. Regimens include infusion of factor VIII concentrate:
      - Prior to joint bleed
      - Three times a week after the first joint bleed
  - Client Education – Tell the client to report signs of bleeding.
- Joint deformity (most often elbows, knees, and ankles)
  - Repeated episodes of hemarthrosis (bleeding into joint spaces) lead to impaired range of motion, pain, tenderness, and swelling, which can develop into joint deformities.
  - Nursing Actions
    - Take appropriate measures to rest, immobilize, elevate, and apply ice to the affected joints during active bleeding.
    - Encourage active range of motion after active bleeding is controlled.
    - Encourage maintenance of ideal weight to minimize stress on joints.
    - Encourage maintenance of regular exercise and physical therapy.

APPLICATION EXERCISES

1. A nurse is providing teaching about the management of epistaxis to a child and his family. Which of the following positions should the nurse instruct the child to take when experiencing a nosebleed?

    A. Sit up and lean forward.

    B. Sit up and tilt the head up.

    C. Lie in a supine position.

    D. Lie in a prone position.

2. A nurse is providing teaching about epistaxis to the parent of a school-age child. Which of the following should the nurse include as an appropriate action to take when managing an episode of epistaxis? (Select all that apply.)

    _____ A. Press the nares together at least 10 min.

    _____ B. Breathe through the nose until bleeding stops.

    _____ C. Pack cotton or tissue into the naris that is bleeding.

    _____ D. Apply a warm cloth across the bridge of the nose.

    _____ E. Insert petroleum into the naris after the bleeding stops.

3. A nurse is providing teaching to the parent of a child who has a new prescription for liquid oral iron supplements. Which of the following statements by the parent indicates an understanding of the teaching?

    A. "I should take my child to the emergency department if his stools become dark."

    B. "My child should avoid eating citrus fruits while taking the supplements."

    C. "I should give the iron with milk to help prevent an upset stomach."

    D. "My child should take the supplement through a straw."

4. A nurse is preparing to administer iron dextran (Proferdex) IM to a school-age child who has iron deficiency anemia. Which of the following actions by the nurse is appropriate?

    A. Administer the dose in the deltoid muscle.

    B. Use the Z-track method when administering the dose.

    C. Avoid injecting more than 2 mL with each dose.

    D. Massage the injection site for 1 min after administering the dose.

5. A nurse is caring for an infant whose screening test reveals that he may have sickle cell disease. Which of the following tests should be performed to distinguish if the infant has the trait or the disease?

    A. Sickle solubility test (Sickledex)

    B. Hemoglobin electrophoresis

    C. Complete blood count

    D. Transcranial Doppler

6. A nurse is caring for a child who is newly diagnosed with hemophilia A. Use the ATI Active Learning Template: Systems Disorder to complete this item to include the following:

    A. Objective and Subjective Data: List two physical assessment findings associated with hemophilia.

    B. Client Education: List three concepts to include in the teaching with the family and child.

APPLICATION EXERCISES KEY

1. A. **CORRECT:** The nurse should instruct the child to sit up and lean to prevent aspiration when experiencing a nosebleed.

   B. INCORRECT: Sitting up and tilting the head up could cause aspiration of blood, and is not an appropriate position when experiencing a nosebleed.

   C. INCORRECT: Lying in a supine position could cause aspiration of blood, and is not an appropriate position when experiencing a nosebleed.

   D. INCORRECT: Lying in a prone position could cause aspiration of blood, and is not an appropriate position when experiencing a nosebleed.

   Ⓝ NCLEX® Connection: Reduction of Risk Potential, Therapeutic Procedures

2. A. **CORRECT:** Pressing the nares together for at least 10 min is an appropriate action to take when managing an episode of epistaxis.

   B. INCORRECT: The child should breathe through the mouth until the bleeding stops.

   C. **CORRECT:** Packing cotton or tissue into the naris that is bleeding is an appropriate action when managing an episode of epistaxis.

   D. INCORRECT: Applying an ice pack across the bridge of the nose is an appropriate action when managing an episode of epistaxis.

   E. **CORRECT:** Inserting petroleum into the naris after the bleeding stops is an appropriate action when managing an episode of epistaxis.

   Ⓝ NCLEX® Connection: Reduction of Risk Potential, Therapeutic Procedures

3. A. INCORRECT: The child's stools will become a tarry-green color if the iron supplement dose is adequate.

   B. INCORRECT: Vitamin C increases absorption of the iron and should be encouraged while taking the supplement.

   C. INCORRECT: Milk prevents absorption of the iron. The supplement should be given 1 hr before or 2 hr after consuming milk.

   D. **CORRECT:** The child should take the supplement through a straw to prevent or minimize staining of the teeth.

   Ⓝ NCLEX® Connection: Pharmacological and Parenteral Therapies, Medication Administration

4. A. INCORRECT: The nurse should administer the dose in to a large muscle mass.

    B. **CORRECT:** The nurse should use the Z-track method when administering the dose.

    C. INCORRECT: The nurse should avoid injecting more than 1 mL with each dose.

    D. INCORRECT: To reduce irritation and skin staining, the nurse should not massage the injection site after administering the dose.

     NCLEX® Connection: Pharmacological and Parenteral Therapies, Medication Administration

5. A. INCORRECT: The Sickle solubility test is a screening tool that detects the presence of abnormal hemoglobin, but does not distinguish between the trait and the disease.

    B. **CORRECT:** The hemoglobin electrophoresis test should be performed to distinguish if the infant has the trait or the disease.

    C. INCORRECT: A complete blood count tests for anemia, and tells the average size of the red blood cells, and the amount of hemoglobin in the red blood cells. It will not distinguish between sickle cell disease and sickle cell trait.

    D. INCORRECT: The transcranial Doppler is performed to assess intracranial vascular flow and detect the risk for cerebrovascular accident, and will not distinguish between sickle cell disease and sickle cell trait.

    NCLEX® Connection: Reduction of Risk Potential, Diagnostic Tests

6. *Using the ATI Active Learning Template: Systems Disorder*

    A. Objective and Subjective Data
       - Active bleeding (possibly from the gums, epistaxis, hematuria, and/or GI tract)
       - Hematomas and bruising occur easily even with minor injuries
       - Joint pain and stiffness, warmth, swelling, redness, loss of range of motion of the joints
       - Cerebral bleeding can cause headaches, slurred speech, and decreased level of consciousness

    B. Client Education
       - Prevent bleeding at home
         - Provide a safe home and a play environment that is free of clutter.
         - Place padding on corners of furniture.
         - Set activity restrictions to avoid injury. Stress importance of wearing protective equipment during activities.
         - Recommend the use of soft-bristled toothbrushes or disposable oral sponges.
       - Encourage regular exercise and physical therapy when not actively bleeding.
       - Encourage recommended immunizations remain up-to-date.
       - Teach the importance of wearing a medical identification wristband or medical identification tags.
       - Teach manifestations of internal bleeding and hemarthrosis
       - Inform of the RICE method (rest, ice, compression, elevation) to control active bleeding.

    NCLEX® Connection: Physiological Adaptations, Alterations in Body Systems

UNIT 2   Nursing Care of Children with System Disorders

SECTION: GASTROINTESTINAL DISORDERS

› Acute Infectious Gastrointestinal Disorders
› Gastrointestinal Structural and Inflammatory Disorders

NCLEX® CONNECTIONS

When reviewing the chapters in this unit, keep in mind the relevant sections of the NCLEX® outline, in particular:

Client Needs: Basic Care and Comfort	Client Needs: Reduction of Risk Potential	Client Needs: Physiological Adaptation

› Relevant topics/tasks include:
» Elimination
  › Assess and manage the client with an alteration in elimination.
» Nutrition and Oral Hydration
  › Monitor the client's hydration status.
	› Relevant topics/tasks include:
	» Potential for Alterations in Body Systems
	  › Monitor the client's output for changes from baseline.
	» System Specific Assessment
	  › Perform focused assessment.
	» Therapeutic Procedures
	  › Provide pre and/or postoperative education.
		› Relevant topics/tasks include:
		» Alterations in Body Systems
		  › Identify signs, symptoms, and incubation periods of infectious diseases.
		» Illness Management
		  › Implement interventions to manage the client recovering from an illness.
		» Pathophysiology
		  › Understand general principles of pathophysiology.

chapter 22

Overview

- Diarrhea may be mild to severe, and acute or chronic. It may result in mild to severe dehydration.
  - Acute diarrhea is a sudden increase in frequency and change in consistency of stool.
    - It is usually secondary to an infectious agent in the GI tract, upper respiratory infection, urinary tract infection, antibiotic use, or laxative use.
    - Self-resolution occurs in less than 14 days if dehydration does not occur.
  - Acute infectious diarrhea is caused by a variety of viral, bacterial, or parasitic pathogens.
  - Chronic diarrhea is an increase in frequency and change of consistency of stool(s) for more than 14 days.
    - It is caused by chronic conditions such as malabsorption syndrome, food allergies, or inflammatory bowel disease.
  - Chronic nonspecific diarrhea has no identified cause.
- Dehydration is a body fluid disturbance when the output exceeds intake. It results from many causes such as fluid losses through the skin, respiratory tract, urinary tract, or GI tract.

Assessment

- Risk Factors
  - Lack of clean water, poor hygiene, crowded living environments, poor sanitation, and nutritional deficiency.
- Subjective and Objective Data
  - Reports of fatigue, malaise, change in behavior, change in stool pattern, poor appetite, weight loss, and pain.
  - Assess for clinical manifestations of dehydration.

PATHOGEN	CLINICAL MANIFESTATIONS	TRANSMISSION/INCUBATION
Rotavirus – viral infection	› Most common cause of diarrhea in children younger than 5 years › Affects children of all ages › Fever › Onset of foul-smelling, watery stools, diarrhea for 5 to 7 days › Vomiting for approximately 2 days	› Transmission: fecal-oral › Incubation period: 48 hr
Yersinia enterocolitis – bacterial infection	› Mucoid, possibly bloody diarrhea › Abdominal pain, fever, and vomiting	› Transmission: pets and food › Incubation period: 1 to 3 weeks

PATHOGEN	CLINICAL MANIFESTATIONS	TRANSMISSION/INCUBATION
Escherichia coli (*E. coli*) – bacterial infection	› Watery diarrhea for 1 to 2 days, followed by abdominal cramping and bloody diarrhea › Could lead to hemolytic uremic syndrome (HUS)	› Transmission: depends on strain of *E. coli* › Incubation period: 3 to 4 days
Salmonella nontyphoidal groups – bacterial infection	› Mild to severe nausea, vomiting, abdominal cramping, bloody diarrhea, and fever (may be afebrile in infants) › Diarrhea may last as long as 2 to 3 weeks › Possible headache, confusion, drowsiness, and seizures › May lead to meningitis or septicemia	› Transmission: person to person, undercooked meats and poultry › Incubation period: 6 to 72 hr
Clostridium difficile (*C. difficile*) – bacterial infection	› Mild, watery diarrhea for a few days › Possible less severe symptoms in children than adults › Possible leukocytosis, hypoalbuminemia, and high fever in certain children › Possible pseudomembranous colitis	› Transmission: contact with colonized spores, commonly in health care settings › Incubation period: nonspecified
Clostridium botulinum (*C. botulinum*) – bacterial infection	› Symptoms depend on strain › Abdominal pain, cramping, and diarrhea › Possible respiratory or CNS problems	› Transmission: contaminated food products › Incubation period: 12 to 26 hr
Shigella groups Shigellosis – bacterial infection	› Sick appearance › Fever, fatigue, and anorexia › Cramping abdomen followed by watery or bloody diarrhea lasting 5 to 10 days	› Transmission: contaminated food or water › Incubation period: 1 to 7 days
Norwalk-like organisms Caliciviruses – viral infection	› Abdominal cramps, nausea and vomiting, malaise, watery diarrhea › Lasts 2 to 3 days	› Transmission: contaminated water › Incubation period: 12 to 48 hr
Staphylococcus – bacterial infection	› Diarrhea, nausea, and vomiting	› Transmission: inadequately cooked or refrigerated food › Incubation period: 1 to 8 hr
Enterobius vermicularis (pinworm) – helminthic infection	› Perianal itching, enuresis, sleeplessness, restlessness, and irritability due to itching	› Transmission: fecal-oral › Ingested or inhaled eggs hatch in the upper intestine, and mature. After mating, worms migrate out of the intestine and lay eggs. Eggs can survive for 2 to 3 weeks on surfaces.
Giardia lamblia – parasitic pathogen	› Children 5 years of age or younger » Diarrhea » Vomiting » Anorexia › Older children » Abdominal cramps » Intermittent loose, malodorous, pale, greasy stools	› Transmission: person to person, food, animals › The nonmotile stage of protozoa may survive in the environment for months.

- ○ Laboratory Tests
  - ▪ Perform a CBC with differential to determine anemia and/or infection.
  - ▪ Hct, Hgb, BUN, creatinine, and urine-specific gravity levels are usually elevated with dehydration.
  - ▪ Stool test for occult blood.
  - ▪ Perform a urinalysis.
- ○ Diagnostic Procedures
  - ▪ Tape test
    - □ A tape test should be performed to check for *Enterobius vermicularis*.
    - □ Client Education
      - ‣ Tell the parents to place transparent tape over the child's anus at night. The tape should be removed the following morning prior to the child toileting or bathing. If possible, have the parent apply the tape after the child has gone to sleep and remove it before the child awakens.
      - ‣ Inform the parents that the specimen should be brought to the laboratory for microscopic evaluation.
      - ‣ Teach the parents to use good hand hygiene during this procedure.
  - ▪ Infectious gastroenteritis
    - □ Rotavirus – Enzyme immunoassay (stool sample)
    - □ *E. coli* – Sorbitol-MacConkey agar (stool sample)
    - □ *Salmonella* – Gram-stained stool culture
    - □ *C. difficile* – Stool culture
    - □ *C. botulinum* – Blood and stool culture
    - □ *Staphylococcus* – Identification of organism in stool, blood, food, or aspirate
    - □ *G. lamblia* – Enzyme immunoassay (stool sample)
    - □ Shigellosis – Blood and stool culture
    - □ Caliciviruses – Enzyme immunoassay (stool sample)
    - □ Yersinia enterocolitis – Identification of organism in stool, blood, oral secretions, urine, or bile

Patient-Centered Care

- • Nursing Care
  - ○ Obtain baseline height and weight.
  - ○ Obtain daily weights at the same time each day.
  - ○ Avoid taking a rectal temperature.
  - ○ Assess and monitor I&O (urine and stool).
  - ○ Initiate IV fluids as ordered.
  - ○ Administer antibiotic as prescribed (*Shigella*, *C. difficile*, and *G. lamblia*).
  - ○ Avoid antibiotics (*C. botulinum*, *E. coli*, *Salmonella*).

- Avoid antimotility agents (*E. coli*, *Salmonella*, *Shigella*).
- Administer oral rehydration therapy (ORT).
    - Start replacement with an oral replacement solution (ORS) of 75 to 90 sodium mEq/L at 40 to 50 mL/kg over 4 hr.
    - Determine the need for further rehydration after initial replacement.
        - Initiate maintenance therapy with ORS of 40 to 60 sodium mEq/L and limit to 150 mL/kg/day.
            - Give ORS alternately with appropriate intake.
                - Give infants water, breast milk, or lactose-free formula if supplementary fluid is needed.
                - Older children may resume their regular diets for additional intake.
            - Replace each diarrheal stool with 10 mL/kg of ORS for ongoing diarrhea.
- Medications
    - Metronidazole (Flagyl) and tinidazole (Tindamax)
        - Indicated for *C. difficile* and *G. lamblia*
        - Nursing Considerations
            - Monitor for allergies.
            - Monitor for GI upset.
        - Client Education
            - Instruct the client to take the medication as prescribed and to report any GI disturbances.
    - Mebendazole, albendazole (Albenza), and pyrantel pamoate (Pin-X) – indicated for *Enterobius vermicularis*
        - Nursing Considerations
            - Administer in a single dose that may need to be repeated in 2 weeks.
            - Administer mebendazole for children older than 2 years of age.
        - Client Education
            - Entire family should be treated at the same time.
- Care After Discharge
    - Client Education
        - Have the parents inform the child's school or day care center of the infection/infestation. The child should stay home during the incubation period.
        - Teach the family to use commercially prepared ORS when the child experiences diarrhea. Foods and fluids to avoid include
            - Fruit juices, carbonated sodas, and gelatin, which all have high carbohydrate content, low electrolyte content, and a high osmolality
            - Caffeine, due to its mild diuretic effect
            - Chicken or beef broth, which has too much sodium and not enough carbohydrates
            - Bananas, rice, applesauce, and toast (BRAT diet)
                - This diet has low nutritional value, high carbohydrate content, and low electrolytes.

- Teach prevention measures, including immunization for rotavirus.
- Provide frequent skin care to prevent skin breakdown.
- Teach the family how to avoid the spread of infectious diseases.
    - Change bed linens and underwear daily for several days.
    - Cleanse toys and child care areas thoroughly to prevent further spread or reinfestation.
    - Keep toys separate and avoid shaking linens to prevent the spread of disease.
    - Shower frequently.
    - Avoid undercooked or under-refrigerated food.
    - Perform proper hand hygiene after toileting and after changing diapers.
    - Do not share dishes and utensils. Wash them in hot, soapy water or in the dishwasher.
    - Clip nails and discourage nail biting and thumb sucking.
    - Clean toilet areas.

Complications

- Dehydration

TYPE	MANIFESTATIONS
Isotonic	› Water and sodium are lost in nearly equal amounts. › Major loss of fluid from extracellular fluid leads to a reduced volume of circulating fluid. › Hypovolemic shock may result. › Serum sodium is within normal limits (130 to 150 mEq/L).
Hypotonic	› Electrolyte loss is greater than water loss. › Water changes from extracellular fluid to intracellular fluid. › Physical manifestations are more severe with smaller fluid loss. › Shock is likely. › Serum sodium is less than 130 mEq/L.
Hypertonic	› Water loss is greater than electrolyte loss. › Fluid shifts from intracellular to extracellular. › Shock is less likely. › Neurologic changes (change in level of consciousness, irritability, hyperreflexia) may occur. › Serum sodium concentration is greater than 150 mEq/L.

LEVEL	WEIGHT LOSS	MANIFESTATIONS
Mild	3% to 5% in infants 3% to 4% in children	› Behavior, mucous membranes, anterior fontanel, pulse, and blood pressure are all within normal limits. › Capillary refill is greater than 2 seconds. › Slight thirst may be experienced.
Moderate	6% to 9% in infants 6% to 8% in children	› Capillary refill is between 2 and 4 seconds. › Thirst and irritability may be experienced. › Pulse is slightly increased with normal to orthostatic blood pressure. › Mucous membranes are dry and tears and skin turgor are decreased. › Slight tachypnea. › Normal to sunken anterior fontanel on infants.
Severe	Greater than 10% in infants 10% in children	› Capillary refill is greater than 4 seconds. › Tachycardia is present and orthostatic blood pressure may progress to shock. › Extreme thirst is present. › Mucous membranes are very dry and skin is tented. › Hyperpnea. › No tearing with sunken eyeballs. › The anterior fontanel is sunken. › Oliguria or anuria is present.

- ○ Nursing Actions
  - Oral rehydration is attempted first for mild and moderate cases of dehydration.
    - □ Mild: 50 mL/kg rehydration fluid every 4 to 6 hr
    - □ Moderate: 100 mL/kg rehydration fluid every 4 to 6 hr
    - □ Replacement of diarrhea losses with 10 mL/kg each stool
  - Administer parenteral fluid therapy as prescribed.
    - □ Initiate when a child is unable to drink enough oral fluids to correct fluid losses, and those with severe dehydration or continued vomiting.
    - □ Isotonic solution at 20 mL/kg IV bolus with possible repeat for isotonic and hypotonic dehydration.
    - □ Hypertonic dehydration rapid fluid replacement is contradicted because of the risk of cerebral edema.
    - □ Administer maintenance IV fluids as prescribed.
    - □ Avoid potassium replacement until kidney function is verified.
  - Assess capillary refill.
  - Assess vital signs.
  - Monitor weight.
  - Maintain accurate I&O.
- ○ Client Education
  - Encourage oral fluids.
  - Resume normal diet as soon as possible.
  - Monitor how many times the child voids.

APPLICATION EXERCISES

1. A nurse is caring for a child who has had watery diarrhea for the past 3 days. Which of the following is an appropriate action for the nurse to take?

    A. Offer chicken broth.

    B. Initiate oral rehydration therapy.

    C. Start hypertonic IV solution.

    D. Keep NPO until the diarrhea subsides.

2. A nurse is caring for a child who is suspected to have *Enterobius vermicularis*. Which of the following is an appropriate action for the nurse to take?

    A. Perform a tape test.

    B. Collect stool specimen for culture.

    C. Test the stool for occult blood.

    D. Initiate IV fluids.

3. A nurse is assessing a child who has a rotavirus infection. Which of the following are expected findings? (Select all that apply.)

    _____ A. Fever

    _____ B. Vomiting

    _____ C. Watery stools

    _____ D. Bloody stools

    _____ E. Confusion

4. A nurse is teaching a group of parents about *Salmonella*. Which of the following should be included in the teaching? (Select all that apply.)

    _____ A. Incubation period is nonspecific.

    _____ B. It is a bacterial infection.

    _____ C. Bloody diarrhea is common.

    _____ D. Transmission can be from house pets.

    _____ E. Antibiotics are used for treatment.

5. A nurse is teaching a group of parents about *E. coli*. Which of the following should be included in the teaching? (Select all that apply.)

_____ A. Severe abdominal cramping occurs.

_____ B. Watery diarrhea is present for more than 5 days.

_____ C. It can lead to hemolytic uremic syndrome.

_____ D. It is a foodborne pathogen.

_____ E. Antibiotics are given for treatment.

6. A nurse is teaching a parent of a child who has an acute gastrointestinal infection. What should be included in the teaching? Use the ATI Active Learning Template: Systems Disorder to complete this item to include Client Education: Describe at least 10 points to review regarding care after discharge.

APPLICATION EXERCISES KEY

1. A. INCORRECT: Chicken broth is avoided for children who have diarrhea because of increased sodium and inadequate carbohydrates.

    B. **CORRECT:** Oral rehydration therapy is recommended to replace lost electrolytes for children who have diarrhea.

    C. INCORRECT: Isotonic IV solutions are recommended for children who experience severe dehydration.

    D. INCORRECT: Children who experience diarrhea are at risk for dehydration. Therefore, keeping them NPO is contraindicated.

    Ⓝ NCLEX® Connection: Physiological Adaptations, Fluid and Electrolyte Imbalances

2. A. **CORRECT:** A tape test is used when diagnosing *Enterobius vermicularis*.

    B. INCORRECT: Stool cultures are obtained to diagnose *Salmonella* or *C. difficile*.

    C. INCORRECT: A clinical manifestation of *E. coli* is bloody stools.

    D. INCORRECT: IV fluids are initiated for children who are dehydrated.

    Ⓝ NCLEX® Connection: Reduction of Risk Potential, Diagnostic Tests

3. A. **CORRECT:** Fever is a clinical manifestation of rotavirus infection.

    B. **CORRECT:** Vomiting for approximately 2 days is a clinical manifestation of rotavirus infection.

    C. **CORRECT:** Foul-smelling, watery stools is a clinical manifestation of rotavirus infection.

    D. INCORRECT: Bloody stools is a clinical manifestation of *E. coli*.

    E. INCORRECT: Confusion is a clinical manifestation of *Salmonella*.

    Ⓝ NCLEX® Connection: Physiological Adaptations, Alterations in Body Systems

4. A. INCORRECT: The incubation period of *Salmonella* is 6 to 72 hr.

    B. **CORRECT:** *Salmonella* is classified as a bacterial infection.

    C. **CORRECT:** *Salmonella* clinical manifestations include bloody diarrhea, nausea, vomiting, and abdominal cramping.

    D. **CORRECT:** *Salmonella* can be transmitted to children from household pets such as cats, dogs, hamsters, and turtles.

    E. INCORRECT: *Salmonella* is a bacterial infection. However, antibiotics are not recommended for treatment.

    Ⓝ NCLEX® Connection: Physiological Adaptations, Illness Management

5.   A. **CORRECT:** Severe abdominal cramping is a clinical manifestation of *E. coli.*

B. INCORRECT: Watery diarrhea lasts 1 to 2 days, then advances to bloody diarrhea.

C. **CORRECT:** *E. coli* can lead to hemolytic uremic syndrome.

D. **CORRECT:** *E. coli* is a foodborne pathogen.

E. INCORRECT: Antibiotics can worsen an *E. coli* infection. Therefore, they are not recommended.

(N) NCLEX® Connection: Physiological Adaptations, Illness Management

6.   *Using the ATI Active Learning Template: Systems Disorder*
   • Client Education
      ○ Have the parents inform the child's school or day care center of the infection/infestation. The child should stay home during the incubation period.
      ○ Teach the family to use commercially prepared oral rehydration therapy when the child experiences diarrhea. Foods and fluids to avoid include
         ▪ Fruit juices, carbonated sodas, and gelatin, which all have high carbohydrate content, low electrolyte content, and a high osmolality
         ▪ Caffeine, due to its mild diuretic effect
         ▪ Chicken or beef broth, which has high sodium content and inadequate carbohydrates
         ▪ Bananas, rice, applesauce, and toast (BRAT diet) due to low nutritional value, high carbohydrate content, and low electrolytes
      ○ Teach prevention measures including immunization for rotavirus.
      ○ Provide frequent skin care to prevent skin breakdown.
      ○ Teach the family how to avoid the spread of infectious diseases.
      ○ Change bed linens and underwear daily for several days.
      ○ Cleanse toys and child care areas thoroughly to prevent further spread or reinfestation.
      ○ Keep toys separate, and avoid shaking linens to prevent the spread of disease.
      ○ Shower frequently.
      ○ Avoid undercooked or under-refrigerated food.
      ○ Perform proper hand hygiene after toileting and after changing diapers.
      ○ Do not share dishes and utensils. Wash them in hot, soapy water or in the dishwasher.
      ○ Clip nails, and discourage nail-biting and thumb-sucking.
      ○ Clean toilet areas.

(N) NCLEX® Connection: Physiological Adaptations, Illness Management

chapter 23

Overview

- Gastrointestinal structural disorders
    - Cleft lip and palate
    - Gastroesophageal reflux disease (GERD)
    - Hypertrophic pyloric stenosis
    - Hirschsprung's disease
    - Intussusception
- Inflammatory disorders
    - Appendicitis
    - Meckel's diverticulum

CLEFT LIP AND PALATE

Overview

- Cleft lip (CL) results from the incomplete fusion of the oral cavity during intrauterine life. Cleft palate (CP) results from the incomplete fusion of the palatine plates during intrauterine life.

  View Image: Cleft Palate

- Although a cleft lip and palate may occur together, either defect may appear alone. The defects can be unilateral (one-sided) or bilateral (two-sided)

Assessment

- Risk Factors
    - Other syndromes
    - Combination of maternal and environmental factors
        - Family history of cleft lip or palate
        - Exposure to alcohol, cigarette smoke, anticonvulsants, or steroids during pregnancy
        - Folate deficiency during pregnancy

- Objective Data
  - Physical Assessment Findings
    - Cleft lip is a visible separation from the upper lip toward the nose.
    - Cleft palate is a visible or palpable opening of the palate connecting the mouth and the nasal cavity.

Patient-Centered Care

- Nursing Care
  - Support and encourage parents in the general care of their child.
  - Promote parent-infant bonding.
  - Promote healthy self-esteem throughout the child's development.
- Teamwork and Collaboration
  - Care of the child with CL and CP requires care from members of various disciplines (plastic surgeon, orthodontist, ENT specialist, speech and language therapist, occupational therapist, dietitian, social services worker).
- Surgical Interventions
  - Cleft Lip
    - Repair is typically done between 2 to 3 months
    - Infant should be at least 10 weeks old, weigh 10 lb, and Hgb 10 g/dL.
    - Revisions are usually required in severe defects.
  - Cleft Palate
    - Repair is typically done between 6 to 12 months.
    - Majority require a second surgery.
  - Nursing Actions
    - Preoperative
      - Cleft lip and cleft palate repair
        - Inspect the infant's lip and palate using a gloved finger to palpate the infant's palate.
        - Assess the infant's ability to suck.
        - Obtain the infant's baseline weight.
        - Observe interaction between the family and infant.
        - Determine family coping and support.
        - Refer parents to appropriate support groups.
        - Consult with social services to provide needed services (financial, insurance) for the family and infant.
        - Instruct the parents about proper feeding and cares.
        - Assess ability to feed.

- Initiate strategies for successful feeding.
  - For isolated CL
    - Encourage breast feeding.
    - Use a wide-based nipple for bottle feeding.
    - Squeeze the infant's cheeks together during feeding to decrease the gap.
  - For CP or CL/CP
    - Position the infant upright while cradling the head during feeding.
    - Use a specialized bottle with a one-way valve and a specially cut nipple.
    - Burp the infant frequently.
    - Syringe feeding may be necessary for the infant who is unsuccessful with other methods.
  - Postoperative
    - Cleft lip and cleft palate repair
      - Perform standard postoperative care, including assessment of vital signs and pain management using an age-appropriate tool.
      - Keep the infant pain-free to decrease crying and stress on repair.
      - Administer analgesics as prescribed.
      - Assess the operative sites for signs of crusting and infection.
      - Avoid sucking on nipple or pacifier.
      - Avoid hard toys that the infant may bring to their mouth to protect the incision site.
      - Monitor I&O and weigh daily.
      - Observe the family's interaction with the infant.
      - Assess family coping and support.
    - Cleft lip repair
      - Monitor the integrity of the postoperative protective device to ensure proper positioning.
      - Position the infant on her back and upright or on her side during the immediate postoperative period to maintain the integrity of the repair. Apply elbow restraints to keep the infant from injuring the repair site.
      - Restraints should be removed periodically to assess skin, allow limb movement, and provide for comfort.
      - Use saline on a sterile swab to clean the incision site. Apply antibiotic ointment if prescribed.
      - Gently aspirate secretions of mouth and nasopharynx to prevent respiratory complications.
    - Cleft palate repair
      - Change the infant's position frequently to facilitate breathing. The infant may be placed on the abdomen in the immediate postoperative period.
      - Maintain intravenous fluids until the infant is able to eat and drink.
      - Monitor packing, which is usually removed in 2 to 3 days.
      - Avoid placing objects (tongue depressor, pacifier) in the infant's mouth after cleft palate repair.
      - Elbow restraints may needed to be used to prevent the infant from injuring the repair

- Client Education
  - Inform the parents that the infant may require elbow restraints for 4 to 6 weeks. Instruct the parents in the proper use of the restraints.
  - Instruct the parents on the postoperative diet and feeding techniques.
  - Instruct parents in proper care of operative site.

Complications

- Ear infections and hearing loss
  - Related to altered structure and recurrent infections
  - Nursing Actions
    - Feed the infant in an upright position. Monitor temperature.
  - Client Education
    - Teach parents manifestations of ear infections.
    - Encourage early intervention.
- Speech and language impairment
  - More common with cleft palate
  - Client Education
    - Refer to early intervention.
    - Refer parents to a speech therapist for care.
- Dental problems
  - Teeth may not erupt normally, and orthodontia is usually necessary later in life.
  - Client Education
    - Instruct the parents and child to promote healthy dental hygiene.
    - Encourage parents to seek early dental care.

GASTROINTESTINAL REFLUX DISEASE (GERD)

Overview

- Gastroesophageal reflux (GER) occurs when the gastric contents reflux back up into the esophagus, making esophageal mucosa vulnerable to injury from gastric acid and resulting in gastroesophageal reflux disease (GERD).
- Gastroesophageal reflux disease (GERD) is tissue damage from GER.
- GER is self-limiting and usually resolves by 1 year of age.

Assessment

- Risk Factors
  - GER – prematurity, bronchopulmonary dysplasia, neurological impairments, asthma, cystic fibrosis, cerebral palsy, scoliosis
  - GERD – neurologic impairments, hiatal hernia, esophageal atresia, morbid obesity
- Subjective and Objective Data
  - Infants
    - Excessive spitting up or forceful vomiting, irritability, excessive crying, blood in stool or vomitus, arching of back, stiffening
    - Respiratory problems
    - Failure to thrive
    - Apnea
  - Children
    - Heartburn, abdominal pain, difficulty swallowing, chronic cough, chest pain
- Diagnostic Procedures
  - Upper GI to detect GI structural abnormalities
  - 24-hr intraesophageal pH study to measures the amount of gastric acid reflux into the esophagus
  - Endoscopy with biopsy to detect esophagitis and strictures
  - Scintigraphy to identify the cause of gastric content aspiration

Patient-Centered Care

- Nursing Care
  - GER
    - Depends on the severity of the symptoms.
    - Offer small, frequent meals.
    - Thicken infants formula with 1 tsp to 1 tbsp rice cereal per 1 oz formula.
    - Avoid foods that cause reflux (caffeine, citrus, peppermint, spicy or fried foods).
    - Assist with weight control.
    - Position the child with the head elevated at 30° for 1 hr after meals.
  - GERD
    - Initiate interventions for GER plus.
    - Administer a proton pump inhibitor such as omeprazole (Prilosec), or an H_2-receptor antagonist such as ranitidine (Zantac).
- Therapeutic Procedures
  - Nissen fundoplication
    - Laparoscopic surgical procedure that wraps the fundus of the stomach around the distal esophagus to decrease reflux.
    - Used for clients who have severe cases of GERD

Complications

- Recurrent pneumonia, weight loss, and failure to thrive

  - Repeated reflux of stomach contents can lead to erosion of the esophagus or pneumonia if stomach contents are aspirated. Esophageal damage can lead to the inability to eat.

  - Nursing Actions

    - Evaluate the prescribed treatment plan.

    - Monitor for clinical manifestations of pneumonia and failure to thrive.

  - Client Education

    - Reinforce the plan of care with the family.

    - Teach the parents about clinical manifestations for pneumonia.

HYPERTROPHIC PYLORIC STENOSIS

Overview

- Hypertrophic pyloric stenosis is the thickening of the pyloric sphincter, which creates an obstruction.
- Usually occurs the first 5 weeks of life.

Assessment

- Risk Factors – genetic predisposition
- Subjective and Objective Data

  - Vomiting that often occurs following a feeding, but can occur up to several hours following a feeding and becomes projectile as obstruction worsens

  - Blood-tinged vomit

  - Constant hunger

  - Olive-shaped mass in the right upper quadrant of the abdomen and possible peristaltic wave that moves from left to right when lying supine

  - Failure to gain weight and signs of dehydration, such as skin that is dry and/or pale, cool lips, dry mucous membranes, decreased skin turgor, diminished urinary output, concentrated urine, thirst, rapid pulse, sunken eyes

- Laboratory Tests – serum electrolytes
- Diagnostic Procedures – Ultrasound reveals an elongated, sausage-shaped mass and an elongated pyloric area.

Patient-Centered Care

- Nursing Care – Prepare the child for surgery.
- Therapeutic Procedures
  - Pylorotomy – performed by laparoscope
    - Preoperative
      - IV fluids for correction of dehydration and electrolyte imbalances
      - NG for decompression
      - NPO
      - Intake and output
      - Daily weights
    - Postoperative
      - Obtain routine postoperative vital signs.
      - Administer antiemetic for vomiting.
      - Provide IV fluids.
      - Monitor daily weights and I&O.
      - Administer analgesics for pain.
      - Assess for signs of infection.
      - Start clear liquids 4 to 6 hr after surgery. Advance to breast milk or formula as tolerated.
      - Document tolerance to feedings.

HIRSCHSPRUNG DISEASE

Overview

- Hirschsprung disease (congenital aganglionic megacolon) is a structural anomaly of the gastrointestinal (GI) tract that is caused by lack of ganglionic cells in segments of the colon resulting in decreased motility and mechanical obstruction.

Assessment

- Risk Factors – family history of Hirschsprung disease
- Subjective and Objective Data
  - Newborn
    - Failure to pass meconium within 24 to 48 hr after birth
    - Episodes of vomiting bile
    - Refusal to eat
    - Abdominal distention

- ○ Infant
  - ▪ Failure to thrive
  - ▪ Abdominal distention
  - ▪ Vomiting
  - ▪ Episodes of constipation and watery diarrhea
- ○ Older child
  - ▪ Failure to thrive
  - ▪ Abdominal distention
  - ▪ Visible peristalsis
  - ▪ Palpable fecal mass
  - ▪ Constipation
  - ▪ Foul-smelling, ribbonlike stool
- Laboratory Tests
  - ○ Serum electrolytes
  - ○ CBC
- Diagnostic Procedures – rectal biopsy to confirm the absence of ganglion cells

Patient-Centered Care

- Nursing Care
  - ○ Prepare family and client for surgery.
  - ○ Assist family with improving nutritional status until surgery.
    - ▪ High-protein, high-calorie, low-fiber diet
    - ▪ Total parenteral nutrition in some cases
- Therapeutic Procedures
  - ○ Surgical removal of the aganglionic section of the bowel.
  - ○ Temporary colostomy may be required.
  - ○ Preoperative
    - ▪ Prepare the child and family for surgery using developmentally appropriate techniques.
    - ▪ Administer electrolyte and fluid replacement as prescribed.
    - ▪ Monitor for enterocolitis.
    - ▪ Bowel prep with saline enemas and oral antibiotics as prescribed.

- ○ Postoperative
  - Assess respiratory status and maintain airway.
  - Provide supplemental oxygen as prescribed.
  - Obtain vital signs.
  - Administer analgesics for pain as prescribed.
  - Assess surgical site for bleeding or any other abnormalities.
  - Provide Foley catheter care.
  - Assess bowel sounds and bowel function.
  - Provide ostomy care if appropriate.
  - Make appropriate referrals.
- ○ Client Education
  - Teach the family ostomy care if indicated.
  - Teach the family incisional care and to monitor for infection.
  - Teach the family clinical manifestations of dehydration.

Complications

- Enterocolitis – inflammation of the bowel
  - ○ Treatment is aimed at resolving enterocolitis, preventing bowel perforation, maintaining hydration, initiating antibiotic therapy, and performing surgery for colostomy or ileostomy if there is extensive bowel involvement.
  - ○ Nursing Actions
    - Monitor vital signs.
    - Assess abdominal girth.
      - □ Measure abdominal girth with a paper tape measure at the level of the umbilicus or at the widest point of the abdomen.
      - □ Mark the area with a pen to assure continuity of future measurements.
    - Monitor for signs of sepsis, peritonitis, or shock caused by enterocolitis.
    - Monitor and manage fluid, electrolyte, and blood product replacement.
    - Administer antibiotics as prescribed.
- Anal stricture and incontinence
  - ○ Bowel retaining therapy.
  - ○ May require further procedures such as dilatation.

INTUSSUSCEPTION

Overview

- One part of the intestine telescopes into another part, resulting in lymphatic and venous obstruction that results in edema in the area. With progression, ischemia and increased mucus into the intestine will occur.
- Common in infants and children between the ages of 3 months and 3 years.

Assessment

- Risk Factors – cystic fibrosis
- Subjective and Objective Data
  - Sudden episodic abdominal pain
  - Screaming with drawing knees to chest during episodes of pain
  - Abdominal mass (sausage-shaped)
  - Stools that are mixed with blood and mucus that resemble the consistency of red currant jelly
  - Vomiting
  - Fever
  - Dehydration
- Diagnostic Procedures – ultrasound

Patient-Centered Care

- Nursing Care
  - Stabilize the child prior to the procedure.
    - IV fluids to correct and prevent dehydration
    - Nasogastric (NG) tube for decompression
  - Teach the family and child about the nonsurgical procedure.
- Therapeutic Procedures
  - Air enema
    - With or without contrast
    - Performed by a radiologist

Complications

- Reoccurring intussusception
  - Surgery is required for reoccurring cases.

APPENDICITIS

Overview

- Inflammation of the vermiform appendix caused from an obstruction of the lumen of the appendix.
- Average age is 10 years

Assessment

- Subjective and Objective Data
  - Abdominal pain in the right lower quadrant
  - Rigid abdomen
  - Decreased or absent bowel sounds
  - Fever
  - Diarrhea or constipation
  - Lethargy
  - Tachycardia
  - Rapid, shallow breathing
  - Anorexia
  - Possible vomiting
- Laboratory Tests
  - CBC
  - Urinalysis
- Diagnostic Procedures – Computed tomography (CT) scan shows an enlarged diameter of appendix, as well as thickening of the appendiceal wall.

Patient-Centered Care

- Nursing Care
  - Prepare the child and family for surgery using developmentally appropriate techniques.
  - Avoid applying heat to the abdomen.
  - Avoid enemas or laxatives.
- Therapeutic Procedures
  - Laparoscopic Surgery – removal of the nonruptured appendix
    - Preoperative
      - Administer IV fluid replacement as prescribed.
      - Administer IV antibiotic.

- Postoperative
  - Assess respiratory status and maintain airway.
  - Provide supplemental oxygen as prescribed.
  - Obtain vital signs.
  - Administer analgesics for pain as prescribed.
  - Assess surgical site for bleeding or any other abnormalities.
  - Assess bowel sounds and bowel function.
- Laparoscopic or open surgery – removal of the ruptured appendix.
  - Preoperative
    - Administer electrolyte and fluid replacement as prescribed.
    - Place NG for decompression.
    - Administer IV antibiotics.
  - Postoperative
    - Assess respiratory status and maintain airway.
    - Provide supplemental oxygen as prescribed.
    - Obtain vital signs.
    - Administer analgesics for pain as prescribed.
    - Assess surgical site for bleeding or any other abnormalities.
    - Assess bowel sounds and bowel function.
    - Administer IV fluids and antibiotics as prescribed.
    - Maintain NPO status.
    - Maintain NG to low continuous suction.
    - Provide wound care for open surgical sites with antibacterial solution or saline as prescribed.
    - Provide Penrose drain care.
    - Assess for peritonitis.
      - Fever
      - Sudden increase in pain
      - Irritability
      - Rigid abdomen
      - Abdominal distention
      - Tachycardia
      - Rapid, shallow breathing
      - Pallor
      - Chills
- Client Teaching
  - Teach the family incision care
  - Teach the family clinical manifestations of infection

Complications

- Peritonitis – inflammation in the peritoneal cavity
  - Nursing Actions
    - Assess for peritonitis.
    - Provide pain management.
      - Assess for pain using a developmentally appropriate tool.
      - Administer analgesics as prescribed.
    - Manage IV fluid therapy.
    - Administer IV antibiotics for infection.
    - Manage NG tube suction.
    - Provide preoperative and postoperative nursing care.
    - Provide surgical wound care with wound irrigation and/or dressings if delayed wound closure is necessary.
    - Provide psychosocial support for the child and family.
  - Client Education
    - Educate the child and parents about preoperative care, such as the need to maintain NPO status and the need for pain medication.
    - Educate the child and parent about postoperative care, such as early ambulation, advancement of diet, wound care, and monitoring for infection.

MECKEL'S DIVERTICULUM

Overview

- Meckel's diverticulum is a complication resulting from failure of the omphalomesenteric duct to fuse during embryonic development.

Assessment

- Subjective and Objective Data
  - Can be asymptomatic
  - Abdominal pain
  - Bloody, mucus stools
- Laboratory Tests – CBC
- Diagnostic Procedures – radionucleotide scan

Patient-Centered Care

- Nursing Care
  - Prepare the child and family for surgery using developmentally appropriate techniques.
- Therapeutic Procedures
  - Surgical removal of the diverticulum
    - Preoperative
      - Provide blood transfusions to correct hypovolemia.
      - Administer fluid and electrolyte replacement as prescribed.
      - Provide oxygen as prescribed.
      - Administer IV antibiotics.
      - Maintain bedrest.
      - Closely monitor blood loss in stools.
    - Postoperative
      - Assess respiratory status and maintain airway.
      - Provide supplemental oxygen as prescribed.
      - Obtain vital signs.
      - Administer analgesics for pain as prescribed.
      - Assess surgical site for bleeding or any other abnormalities.
      - Assess bowel sounds and bowel function.
      - Administer IV fluids and antibiotics as prescribed.
      - Maintain NPO status.
      - Maintain NG to low continuous suction.
    - Client Teaching – Teach the family clinical manifestations of infection.

Complications

- GI hemorrhage and bowel obstruction (for untreated Meckel's diverticulum)

APPLICATION EXERCISES

1. A nurse is assessing an infant. Which of the following are clinical manifestations of hypertrophic pyloric stenosis? (Select all that apply.)

_____ A. Projectile vomiting

_____ B. Dry mucus membranes

_____ C. Currant jelly stools

_____ D. Sausage-shaped abdominal mass

_____ E. Constant hunger

2. A nurse is caring for a child who has Hirschsprung disease. Which of the following is an appropriate action for the nurse to take?

A. Encourage a high-fiber, low-protein, low-calorie diet.

B. Prepare the family for surgery.

C. Place an NG for decompression.

D. Initiate bedrest.

3. A nursing is caring for an infant who is postoperative following cleft lip and palate repair. Which of the following is an appropriate action for the nurse to take?

A. Remove the packing in the mouth.

B. Place the infant in an upright position.

C. Offer a pacifier with sucrose.

D. Assess mouth with a tongue blade.

4. A nurse is teaching a parent of an infant about gastrointestinal reflux disease (GERD). Which of the following should be included in the teaching? (Select all that apply.)

_____ A. Offer frequent feedings.

_____ B. Thicken formula with rice cereal.

_____ C. Use a bottle with a one-way valve.

_____ D. Position baby upright for 1 hr after feedings.

_____ E. Use a wide based nipple for feedings.

5. A nurse is caring for a child. Which of the following are clinical manifestations of Meckel's diverticulum? (Select all that apply.)

_____ A. Abdominal pain

_____ B. Fever

_____ C. Mucus, bloody stools

_____ D. Vomiting

_____ E. Rapid, shallow breathing

6. A nurse is caring for a child who is postoperative open appendectomy following a perforated appendix. Use the ATI Active Learning Template: Systems Disorder to complete this item to include the postoperative nursing interventions.

APPLICATION EXERCISES KEY

1. A. **CORRECT:** A client who has a pyloric stricture has thickening of the pyloric sphincter, resulting in projectile vomiting.

    B. **CORRECT:** A client who has pyloric stricture is unable to consume adequate food and fluid, resulting in dehydration. Dry mucous membranes is a clinical manifestation of hypertrophic pyloric stenosis.

    C. INCORRECT: A client who has intussusception have bloody mucus stools, resulting in currant jelly stools.

    D. INCORRECT: A client who has intussusception have telescoping intestine, resulting sausage shaped abdominal mass.

    E. **CORRECT:** A client who has pyloric stricture is unable to consume adequate food and fluid, resulting in constant hunger.

    ⓝ NCLEX® Connection: Physiological Adaptations, Pathophysiology

2. A. INCORRECT: A client who has Hirschsprung disease is encouraged to eat a low-fiber, high-protein, high-calorie diet.

    B. **CORRECT:** A client who has Hirschsprung disease requires surgery to remove the affected segment of the intestine. Preparing the family for surgery is an appropriate action for the nurse to take.

    C. INCORRECT: A client who has Hirschsprung disease is managed nutritionally. Placing an NG for decompression is not an appropriate action for the nurse to take.

    D. INCORRECT: A client who has Meckel's diverticulum is placed on bedrest to prevent further bleeding.

    ⓝ NCLEX® Connection: Reduction of Risk Potential, Therapeutic Procedures

3. A. INCORRECT: The packing in the mouth should stay in place for 2 to 3 days.

    B. **CORRECT:** Placing the infant in an upright position will facilitate drainage and prevent aspiration. This is an appropriate action for the nurse to take.

    C. INCORRECT: Objects in the mouth could injure the surgical site and should be avoided.

    D. INCORRECT: Objects in the mouth could injure the surgical site and should be avoided.

    ⓝ NCLEX® Connection: Physiological Adaptations, Alterations in Body Systems

4.   A. **CORRECT:** Frequent feeding will assist in decreasing the amount of vomiting episodes.

     B. **CORRECT:** Thickened formula will assist in decreasing the amount of vomiting episodes.

     C. INCORRECT: A bottle with a one-way valve is used for an infant who has cleft lip and palate.

     D. **CORRECT:** Positioning the infant in an upright position for 1 hr following feedings will assist in decreasing the amount of vomiting episodes.

     E. INCORRECT: A wide-based nipple is used for an infant who has cleft lip and palate.

     ⓝ NCLEX® Connection: Basic Care and Comfort, Nutrition and Oral Hydration

5.   A. **CORRECT:** Abdominal pain is a clinical manifestation of Meckel's diverticulum.

     B. INCORRECT: Fever is a clinical manifestation of appendicitis.

     C. **CORRECT:** Mucus, bloody stools is a clinical manifestation of Meckel's diverticulum.

     D. INCORRECT: Vomiting is a clinical manifestation of appendicitis.

     E. INCORRECT: Rapid, shallow breathing is a clinical manifestation of appendicitis.

     ⓝ NCLEX® Connection: Physiological Adaptations, Pathophysiology

6.   *Using the ATI Active Learning Template: Systems Disorder*

     • Postoperative Nursing Interventions
       ○ Assess respiratory status and maintain airway.
       ○ Provide supplemental oxygen as prescribed.
       ○ Obtain vital signs.
       ○ Administer analgesics for pain as prescribed.
       ○ Assess surgical site for bleeding or any other abnormalities.
       ○ Assess bowel sounds and bowel function.
       ○ IV fluids and antibiotics as prescribed.
       ○ Maintain NPO status.
       ○ Maintain NG to low continuous suction.
       ○ Provide wound care for open surgical sites with antibacterial solution or saline as prescribed.
       ○ Provide Penrose drain care.
       ○ Assess for peritonitis.

     ⓝ NCLEX® Connection: Physiological Adaptations, Alterations in Body Systems

UNIT 2   Nursing Care of Children with System Disorders

SECTION: GENITOURINARY AND REPRODUCTIVE DISORDERS

› Enuresis and Urinary Tract Infections
› Structural Disorders of the Genitourinary Tract and Reproductive System
› Renal Disorders

NCLEX® CONNECTIONS

When reviewing the chapters in this unit, keep in mind the relevant sections of the NCLEX® outline, in particular:

Client Needs: Basic Care and Comfort	Client Needs: Reduction of Risk Potential	Client Needs: Physiological Adaptation

› Relevant topics/tasks include:
» Elimination
  › Assess and manage the client with an alteration in elimination (e.g., bowel, urinary).
» Nutrition and Oral Hydration
  › Monitor the client's hydration status.
	› Relevant topics/tasks include:
	» Changes/Abnormalities in Vital Signs
	  › Assess and respond to changes in the client's vital signs.
	» Laboratory Values
	  › Notify the provider about laboratory test results.
	» Potential for Complications of Diagnostic Tests/Treatments/Procedures
	  › Use precautions to prevent injury and/or complications associated with a procedure or diagnosis.
		› Relevant topics/tasks include:
		» Alterations in Body Systems
		  › Monitor and maintain devices and equipment used for drainage.
		» Fluid and Electrolyte Imbalances
		  › Manage the care of the client with a fluid and electrolyte imbalance.
		» Illness Management
		  › Identify client data that need to be reported immediately.

chapter 24

Overview

- Enuresis is uncontrolled or unintentional urination that occurs after a child is beyond an age at which bladder control is achieved.

- A urinary tract infection (UTI) is an infection in any portion of the urinary tract.

ENURESIS

Overview

- Inappropriate urination must occur at least twice a week for at least 3 months. And, the child must be at least 5 years of age before there's consideration about diagnosing enuresis.

- Rule out organic causes related to genitourinary dysfunction prior to diagnosis of enuresis.

- Primary enuresis: A child has never been free of bedwetting for any extended periods of time.

- Secondary enuresis: A child who started bedwetting after development of urinary control.

Assessment

- Risk Factors
  - Enuresis has no clear etiology, but it may be related to:
    - Family history of enuresis.
    - Disorders associated with bladder dysfunction.
    - The male gender.
    - Emotional factors.
- Subjective Data
  - History of alterations in toilet training, voiding behaviors, and bowel movement patterns
  - History of chronic or acute illness (UTI, diabetes mellitus, sickle cell disease, neurologic deficits)
  - History of family disruptions or other emotional stressors
  - Family history of enuresis
  - Fluid intake, especially in the evening

Patient-Centered Care

- Nursing Care

  - Evaluate the child's self-esteem.

  - Evaluate the child's coping strategies and available support systems.

  - Evaluate the family's coping.

  - Evaluate peer and family support groups.

  - Educate the child and family regarding the management of enuresis.

    - Have the child empty his bladder prior to bedtime.

    - Encourage fluids during the day and restrict fluids in the evening.

    - Avoid fruit and fruit drinks after 1600.

    - Avoid caffeinated or carbonated drinks after 1600.

    - Allow the child to wear regular sleep wear and avoid diapers.

    - Use positive reinforcement. Avoid punishing, scolding, or teasing the child following an incident.

    - Assist the child in keeping a calendar of wet and dry days.

    - Make environmental changes to assist the child to get to the bathroom, such as avoiding the top bunk bed, use of a night light, or a clear path from the bed to the bathroom.

    - Avoid holding urine during the day.

    - Have the child change the bed linens and clothing following an incident.

    - Avoid constipation: increase fiber in diet, encourage regular bowel movements.

    - Wake the child up during the night to void.

    - Administer prescribed medications

    - Offer support to the child and the family.

- Medications

  - Antidiuretic hormone – Desmopressin acetate (DDAVP)

    - Reduces the volume of urine

    - Nursing Considerations

      - Can be prescribed either oral or nasal

      - Monitor I&O

    - Client Education

      - Encourage the family to restrict the child's fluid intake after dinner.

      - Instruct the family to administer the medication at bedtime.

      - Instruct the family to store nasal preparation in the refrigerator.

      - Inform the family of possible adverse reactions.

- ○ Tricyclic antidepressants – Imipramine hydrochloride (Tofranil)

  - ▪ Inhibits urination

  - ▪ Nursing Considerations

    - ▫ Monitor children for an increase in suicidality.

    - ▫ Monitor for therapeutic effectiveness.

    - ▫ Length of treatment is 6 to 8 weeks. Then, plan gradual withdrawal.

    - ▫ Administer with food.

  - ▪ Client Education

    - ▫ Instruct the family to administer the mediation 1 hr before bedtime.

    - ▫ Instruct the family about possible adverse reactions.

    - ▫ Instruct the family to avoid sun exposure.

    - ▫ Instruct the family to avoid using with over-the-counter medications.

- ○ Anticholinergics – Oxybutynin chloride (Ditropan)

  - ▪ Reduces bladder contractions

  - ▪ Nursing Considerations

    - ▫ Monitor for effectiveness of therapy.

  - ▪ Client Education

    - ▫ Instruct the family about possible adverse reactions.

Complications

- • Emotional problems (low self-esteem, altered body image, social isolation, fears)

  - ○ Nursing Actions

    - ▪ Support the child and family by listening to concerns and correcting misperceptions.

    - ▪ Involve the child in the teaching and management.

    - ▪ Make referrals to appropriate resources (support groups, counseling) as necessary.

  - ○ Client Education

    - ▪ Assist the child and family to understand the emotional aspects of the disorder. Early interventions can alleviate long-term emotional issues.

URINARY TRACT INFECTIONS (UTIs)

Overview

- Bacteriuria – bacteria in the urine
- Asymptomatic bacteriuria – bacteriuria with no clinical manifestations of UTI
- Symptomatic bacteriuria – bacteriuria with clinical manifestations of UTI
- Recurrent UTI – multiple occurrences of bacteriuria or symptomatic bacteriuria
- Persistent UTI – unresolved bacteriuria with antibiotic therapy
- Febrile UTI – symptomatic bacteriuria with fever
- Cystitis – inflammation of the bladder
- Urethritis – inflammation of the urethra
- Pyelonephritis – inflammation of the upper urinary tract and the kidneys
- Urosepsis – bacterial illness

Assessment

- Risk Factors
  - Urinary stasis
  - Urinary tract anomalies
  - Reflux within the urinary tract system
  - Constipation
  - Onset of toilet training
  - Uncircumcised male (inadequate hygiene)
  - Females (urethra in close proximity to rectum)
  - Synthetic, tight underwear and wet bathing suits
  - Sexual activity
- Subjective Data

  - Infants
    - Increase in irritability
    - Screaming with urination
  - Children
    - Abdominal or back pain
    - Pain with urination

- Objective Data
  - Physical Assessment Findings
    - Infants
      - Poor feeding, vomiting, or failure to gain weight
      - Increase in thirst
      - Frequent urination
      - Straining with urination
      - Foul-smelling urine
      - Fever
      - Diaper rash
      - Dehydration
      - Seizure
      - Pallor
    - Children
      - Poor appetite
      - Vomiting
      - Slowed growth
      - Increase in thirst
      - Enuresis, frequent urination
      - Swelling of the face
      - Seizures
      - Pallor
      - Fatigue
      - Blood in the urine
      - Edema
      - Hypertension
      - Tetany
  - Laboratory Tests
    - Urinalysis and urine culture and sensitivity
      - Sterile catheterization and suprapubic aspiration are the most accurate methods for obtaining urine for urinalysis and culture in children less than 2 years of age.
      - Obtain a clean-catch urine sample from children who are able to cooperate.

- ▫ Nursing Actions
  - ‣ Before performance of a suprapubic aspiration occurs, confirm that informed consent has been obtained.
  - ‣ To prevent a falsely low bacterial count, avoid having the child drink a large amount of oral fluids prior to obtaining a urine specimen.
  - ‣ Send the specimen for culture to the laboratory without delay.
  - ‣ Review findings indicative of UTI.
    - ▹ Urine culture – Positive for infecting organisms (*Escherichia coli, Proteus, Pseudomonas, Klebsiella, Haemophilus, Staphylococcus aureus*)
    - ▹ Urinalysis
      - ◆ pH: weak acid or neutral alkaline
      - ◆ Protein: positive
      - ◆ Glucose: positive
      - ◆ Ketones: positive
      - ◆ Leukocytes: positive
      - ◆ Nitrates: positive
- ▫ Client Education
  - ‣ Educate the child and family about the procedure for collecting a suprapubic aspiration, invasive urinary catheterization, or clean-voided specimen.
- ○ Diagnostic Procedures
  - ▪ Locate the primary infection site or anatomic defects
    - ▫ Percutaneous kidney tap
    - ▫ Bladder wash outs
    - ▫ Ultrasonography
    - ▫ Voiding cystourethrogram (VCUG)
    - ▫ IV pyelogram (IVP)
    - ▫ Dimercaptosuccinic acid scan (DMSA)
      - ‣ Nursing Actions
        - ▹ Educate the child and family about the procedure for the diagnostic test prescribed.
        - ▹ Assess the child for allergy to iodine or shellfish if a contrast medium is used.
        - ▹ Sedate infants and young children if required. Assist an older child to remain quiet during the examinations.
        - ▹ Maintain the child on NPO status after midnight in preparation for a cystoscopy and IVP. IVP requires bowel preparation.
        - ▹ Prepare the child if catheterization is necessary.
        - ▹ Monitor the child after the procedure, according to facility protocol.

Patient-Centered Care

- Nursing Care
  - Encourage frequent voiding and complete emptying of the bladder.
  - Encourage fluids.
  - Monitor urine output.
  - Prepare the child for diagnostic tests.
  - Administer a mild analgesic (acetaminophen [Tylenol]) for pain management.
- Medications
  - Antibiotics based on findings of urine culture and sensitivity testing (penicillins, sulfonamide, cephalosporins, and nitrofurantoin)
    - Nursing Considerations
      - Monitor for potential allergic response.
    - Client Education
      - Instruct parents to have the child complete all prescribed antibiotics, even if symptoms are no longer present.
- Client Education
  - Instruct the family to watch for signs and symptoms of recurrence of UTIs (dysuria, frequency, urgency).
  - Provide instruction to prevent recurrence.
    - Teach females to wipe the perineal area from front to back.
    - Teach parents to retract and clean the foreskin of male infants.
    - Instruct the child and parents to keep underwear dry.
    - Suggest the use of cotton underwear.
    - Tell the child to maintain adequate hydration.
    - Instruct avoidance of bubble baths.
    - Encourage frequent voiding.
    - Encourage complete emptying of bladder using double voiding.
    - Advise the child to avoid constipation and straining with bowel movements.
    - Encourage adolescents who are sexually active to void immediately after intercourse.

Complications

- Progressive kidney injury
- Urosepsis
  - Nursing Actions
    - Monitor for signs and symptoms of UTIs.
  - Client Education
    - Reinforce teaching about prevention, early identification, and treatment of UTIs.

APPLICATION EXERCISES

1. A nurse is assessing an infant who has a suspected urinary tract infection. Which of the following are anticipated findings? (Select all that apply.)

_____ A. Increase in hunger

_____ B. Irritability

_____ C. Decrease in urination

_____ D. Vomiting

_____ E. Fever

2. A nurse is assessing a child who has a urinary tract infection. Which of the following are clinical manifestations of a urinary tract infection? (Select all that apply.)

_____ A. Night sweats

_____ B. Swelling of the face

_____ C. Pallor

_____ D. Pale colored urine

_____ E. Fatigue

3. A nurse is teaching a parent of a child who has a urinary tract infection. Which of the following should the nurse include in the teaching? (Select all that apply.)

_____ A. Wear nylon underpants.

_____ B. Avoid bubble baths.

_____ C. Empty bladder completely with each void.

_____ D. Provide information about clinical manifestations of infection.

_____ E. Wipe perineal area back to front.

4. A nurse is planning care of a child who has a urinary tract infection. Which of the following should the nurse include?

A. Administer antidiuretic.

B. Restrict fluids.

C. Evaluate the child's self-esteem.

D. Encourage frequent voiding.

5. A nurse is caring for a child with enuresis. Which of the following is a complication of enuresis?

    A. Urinary tract infections

    B. Emotional problems

    C. Urosepsis

    D. Progressive kidney disease

6. A nurse educator is reviewing care of a child who has enuresis with a group of newly hired pediatric nurses. What should she include in the review? Use the ATI Active Learning Template: System Disorder to complete this item to include the following sections:

    A. Description of the Disorder

    B. Client Education: List at least 10 points to review.

APPLICATION EXERCISES KEY

1. A. INCORRECT: An increase in thirst is a clinical manifestation in an infant with a urinary tract infection.

    B. **CORRECT:** Irritability is a clinical manifestation in an infant with a urinary tract infection.

    C. INCORRECT: An increase in urination is a clinical manifestation in an infant with a urinary tract infection.

    D. **CORRECT:** Vomiting is a clinical manifestation in an infant with a urinary tract infection.

    E. **CORRECT:** Fever is a clinical manifestation in an infant with a urinary tract infection.

    Ⓝ NCLEX® Connection: Physiological Adaptations, Alterations in Body Systems

2. A. INCORRECT: Night sweats are not a clinical manifestation in children with a urinary tract infection.

    B. **CORRECT:** Swelling of the face is a clinical manifestation in children with a urinary tract infection.

    C. **CORRECT:** Pallor is a clinical manifestation in children with a urinary tract infection.

    D. INCORRECT: Bloody urine is a clinical manifestation in children with a urinary tract infection.

    E. **CORRECT:** Fatigue is a clinical manifestation in children with a urinary tract infection.

    Ⓝ NCLEX® Connection: Physiological Adaptations, Alterations in Body Systems

3. A. INCORRECT: The nurse should discuss the use of cotton underwear.

    B. **CORRECT:** The nurse should discuss avoiding bubble baths.

    C. **CORRECT:** The nurse should discuss the need to completely empty the bladder with each void.

    D. **CORRECT:** The nurse should review the clinical manifestations of infection.

    E. INCORRECT: The nurse should discuss the importance of wiping the perineal area from front to back.

    Ⓝ NCLEX® Connection: Physiological Adaptations, Medical Emergencies

4. A. INCORRECT: An antidiuretic is not indicated for a child who has a urinary tract infection.

    B. INCORRECT: The nurse should encourage fluids to a child who has a urinary tract infection.

    C. INCORRECT: The nurse should evaluate self-esteem in children with enuresis.

    D. **CORRECT:** It's important to encourage frequent voiding. This assists in flushing the bacteria through the urinary system.

    N NCLEX® Connection: Basic Care and Comfort, Elimination

5. A. INCORRECT: Urinary tract infections can occur in children; however they are not a complication of enuresis.

    B. **CORRECT:** Emotional problems are a complication of enuresis.

    C. INCORRECT: Urosepsis is a complication of urinary tract infections.

    D. INCORRECT: Progressive kidney disease is a complication of urinary tract infections.

    N NCLEX® Connection: Basic Care and Comfort, Elimination

6. *Using the ATI Active Learning Template: System Disorder*

    A. Description of the Disorder
    - Inappropriate urination must occur at least twice a week for at least 3 months, and the child must be at least 5 years of age before there's consideration about diagnosing enuresis

    B. Client Education
    - Have the child empty his bladder prior to bedtime.
    - Encourage fluids during the day, and restrict fluids in the evening.
    - Avoid fruit and fruit drinks after 1600.
    - Avoid caffeinated or carbonated drinks after 1600.
    - Allow the child to wear regular sleep wear and avoid diapers.
    - Use positive reinforcement. Avoid punishing, scolding, or teasing the child following an incident.
    - Assist the child in keeping a calendar of wet and dry days.
    - Make environmental changes to assist the child to get to the bathroom, such as avoiding the top bunk bed, providing a night light, and clearing a path from the bed to the bathroom.
    - Avoid holding urine during the day.
    - Have the child change bed linens and clothing following an incident.
    - Avoid constipation: increase fiber in the diet and encourage regular bowel movements.
    - Wake the child during the night to void.
    - Take all medications as prescribed.

    N NCLEX® Connection: Physiological Adaptations, Alterations in Body Systems

CHAPTER 25   **Structural Disorders of the Genitourinary Tract and Reproductive System**

Overview

- Various structural disorders may be evident at birth and may affect normal genitourinary and reproductive function. These disorders include
  - Obstructive uropathy: Structural or functional obstruction in the urinary system.
  - Inguinal hernia: Protrusion of abdominal organs through the inguinal canal into the scrotum.
  - Chordee: Ventral curvature of the penis.
  - Bladder exstrophy: Eversion of the posterior bladder through the anterior bladder wall and lower abdominal wall.
  - Hypospadias: Urethral opening located behind the glans of the penis or on the ventral surface of the penile shaft.
  - Epispadias: Meatal opening located on the dorsal surface of the penis.
  - Phimosis: Narrowing of the preputial opening of the foreskin.
  - Cryptorchidism: Undescended testes.
  - Hydrocele: Fluid in the scrotum.
  - Varicocele: Elongation, dilatation, and tortuosity of the veins superior to the testicle.
  - Testicular torsion: Testicle hangs free from the vascular structures.
  - Ambiguous genitalia: Erroneous or abnormal sexual differentiation.
- Children become aware of and are very interested in the genital area, normality of genital function, and gender differences between 3 and 6 years of age. Due to this, repair of structural defects ideally should be done between 6 to 15 months of age, but before 3 years of age, to minimize impact on body image and to promote healthy development.

Assessment

- Risk Factors: May have a genetic link.
- Objective and Subjective Data
  - Obstructive uropathy
    - Hydronephrosis
    - Partial obstructions may go undetected.
    - Possible other genetic disorders (prune belly syndrome, chromosomal anomalies, anorectal malformation, defects of the pinna of the ear)
    - Inability to concentrate urine
    - Urinary tract infections
    - Increased urine flow
    - Metabolic acidosis

- ○ Inguinal Hernia – Painless inguinal swelling varying in size
- ○ Chordee – Ventral curvature of the penis
- ○ Bladder exstrophy
  - ▪ Epispadias present
  - ▪ Exposed bladder, urethra, and ureteral orifices through the suprapubic area
- ○ Hypospadias
  - ▪ Meatus opening below the glans penis
  - ▪ Meatus opening along the ventral surface of the penis, scrotum, or perineum
  - ▪ Possible chordee present
- ○ Epispadias
  - ▪ Male
    - □ Widened pubic symphysis
    - □ Broad, spadelike penis
    - □ Urethra opened on dorsal surface of the penis
    - □ Possible exstrophy of the bladder
  - ▪ Female
    - □ Wide urethra
    - □ Bifid clitoris
    - □ Possible exstrophy of the bladder
- ○ Phimosis – Inability to retract foreskin of penis
- ○ Cryptorchidism – Inability to palpate testes within the scrotum
- ○ Hydrocele
  - ▪ Enlarged scrotal sac
  - ▪ Possible pain
- ○ Varicocele
  - ▪ Bulge above the testicle when bearing down
  - ▪ Mild to moderate pain
- ○ Testicular torsion
  - ▪ Enlargement of affected testicle
  - ▪ Sudden, severe onset of pain
- ○ Ambiguous genitalia
  - ▪ Possible congenital adrenal hypoplasia
  - ▪ Enlarged clitoral hood
  - ▪ Enlarged clitoris
  - ▪ Micropenis
  - ▪ Bifid scrotum

- Diagnostic/Therapeutic Procedures
  - Obstructive uropathy – Surgical procedures that divert the flow of urine to bypass the obstruction
  - Inguinal hernia
    - May resolve spontaneously.
    - Surgery is indicated for defects that have not closed by 1 year of age.
  - Chordee – Surgical release of fibrous band
  - Bladder exstrophy – Immediate surgery
  - Hypospadias/Epispadias
    - Surgery performed during the first year of life.
    - Male circumcision not performed.
  - Phimosis – Circumcision in severe cases
  - Cryptorchidism
    - Surgical orchiopexy.
    - Older children: Administration of human chorionic gonadotropin.
  - Hydrocele
    - May resolve spontaneously.
    - Surgical repair if not resolved in 1 year.
  - Varicocele – Percutaneous embolization
  - Testicular torsion – Immediate surgery
  - Ambiguous genitalia
    - Chromosomal analysis to determine genetic karyotype
    - Gonad biopsy and surgery
    - Plan for gender assignment
    - Radiographic contrast studies
    - Endoscopy
    - Ultrasonography
    - Biochemical tests
  - Nursing Actions
    - Provide support for parents during the diagnosis.
    - Administer sedation and assist with the procedure as needed.
  - Client Education
    - Advise the family and/or child about the procedure and what to expect.
    - If NPO status is necessary, explain the parameters to the family and/or child.

Patient-Centered Care

- Nursing Care
  - Nursing care should focus on education and support of the family and child.
    - Evaluate the family's perception of the child's defect, family support, and coping.
    - Assist parents to identify ways to help the child maintain a positive self-image.
    - Promote healthy growth and development.
    - Assist child with maintaining self-image.
  - Obstructive uropathy – Surgical repair with insertion of percutaneous nephrostomy or cutaneous ureterostomy tubes
  - Bladder exstrophy
    - Cover the exposed bladder with sterile, nonadherent dressing.
    - Prepare for immediate surgery.
  - Phimosis – Retract foreskin and perform cleansing, if prescribed, for mild cases.
  - Ambiguous genitalia
    - Obtain detailed family history.
    - Collaborate with genetic counseling services in preparing parents for evaluation, testing, diagnostic procedures, discussion of gender assignment, and surgery as indicated.
- Surgical Interventions
  - Structural defects will be treated with surgical intervention. The goal of most structural defect repairs is to preserve or create normal urinary and sexual function. Early intervention will minimize emotional trauma.
  - Nursing Actions
    - Preoperative
      - Provide education to the child and family related to the procedure and expectations for postoperative care.
      - Provide emotional support to the child and family.
      - Encourage parent to express concerns and fears related to the surgical procedure and outcomes.
    - Postoperative
      - Assess pain using an appropriate pain assessment tool.
      - Administer pain medication as prescribed. An antispasmodic, such as oxybutynin (Ditropan), may be prescribed to treat painful bladder spasms.
      - Monitor intake and output.
      - Monitor urinary catheters, drains, tubes, or stents.
      - Provide wound and/or dressing care.
      - Monitor for signs of infection, such as redness, warmth, drainage, or edema at surgical site. Monitor for fever, lethargy, and foul-smelling urine.
      - Do not provide tub baths for at least 1 week or as prescribed.
      - Limit activity as prescribed.

- ○ Client Education
  - ▪ Explain measures to prevent infection to include good hand hygiene, and care of wounds, drains, and urinary catheters.
  - ▪ Explain procedures at the appropriate level for child and/or parents.
  - ▪ Use age-appropriate interventions to allay fears and anxiety.
  - ▪ Help the child understand that surgery is not a punishment, and it will not mutilate the body.

Complications

- Infection
  - ○ Nursing Action
    - ▪ Observe for signs of infection including fever, skin inflammation, foul urine odor, cloudy urine, and/or urinary frequency.
  - ○ Client Education
    - ▪ Teach the family to observe for signs of infection.
    - ▪ Teach the family to report any signs of infection immediately.
- Emotional problems (poor self-esteem, altered body image, social isolation, fears)
  - ○ Nursing Actions
    - ▪ Support the child and family by listening to concerns and correcting misperceptions.
    - ▪ Use play therapy for toddlers and preschoolers.
    - ▪ Encourage peer-to-peer social networking for older children.
  - ○ Client Education
    - ▪ Educate the child and family regarding support groups.

APPLICATION EXERCISES

1. A nurse is caring for an infant who has a hydrocele. Which of the following is an appropriate action for the nurse to take?

    A. Prepare for immediate surgery.

    B. Explain to the parents that this will self-resolve.

    C. Retract foreskin and cleanse properly.

    D. Refer the family for counseling.

2. A nurse is caring for a male infant. Which of the following are clinical manifestations of an epispadias? (Select all that apply.)

_____ A. Bladder exstrophy

_____ B. Inability to retract foreskin

_____ C. Widened pubic symphysis

_____ D. Broad, spade-like penis

_____ E. Pain

3. A nurse is caring for an infant who has ambiguous genitalia. Which of the following are appropriate actions for the nurse to take? (Select all that apply.)

_____ A. Prepare for surgery.

_____ B. Obtain a detailed family history.

_____ C. Plan for a circumcision.

_____ D. Refer to genetic counseling.

_____ E. Explain the need for a chromosomal analysis.

4. A nurse is caring for an infant. Which of the following are clinical manifestations of obstructive uropathy? (Select all that apply.)

_____ A. Decreased urine flow

_____ B. Urinary tract infection

_____ C. Metabolic alkalosis

_____ D. Concentrated urine

_____ E. Hydronephrosis

5. A nurse is teaching a newly licensed nurse about structural disorders of the genitourinary tract and reproductive system. What should be included in the teaching? Use the ATI Active Learning Template: Basic Concept to complete this item to include the following:

A. Related Content/Underlying Principles:
  • Describe six structural disorders of the genitourinary tract and reproductive system.
  • Underlying Principles: Describe each structural disorder.

APPLICATION EXERCISES KEY

1. A. INCORRECT: Hydroceles are surgically repaired if they have not resolved spontaneously in 1 year.

   B. **CORRECT:** Hydrocele is fluid in the scrotum and resolves spontaneously in the majority of cases.

   C. INCORRECT: Retracting foreskin and cleansing properly is done when an infant has phimosis.

   D. INCORRECT: A referral for genetic counseling is recommended for families who have an infant with ambiguous genitalia.

   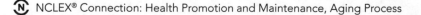 NCLEX® Connection: Reduction of Risk Potential, Therapeutic Procedures

2. A. **CORRECT:** Bladder exstrophy is a clinical manifestation of a male infant who has epispadias.

   B. INCORRECT: Inability to retract foreskin is a clinical manifestation of phimosis.

   C. **CORRECT:** Widened pubic symphysis is a clinical manifestation of a male infant who has epispadias.

   D. **CORRECT:** Broad, spade-like penis is a clinical manifestation of a male infant who has epispadias.

   E. INCORRECT: Pain is a clinical manifestation of testicular torsion, varicocele, and hydrocele.

   NCLEX® Connection: Physiological Adaptations, Pathophysiology

3. A. **CORRECT:** Infants who have ambiguous genitalia will need surgery. Preparing the family for surgery is an appropriate action for the nurse to take.

   B. **CORRECT:** A detailed family history is used for gender assignment, and is therefore an appropriate action for the nurse to take.

   C. INCORRECT: Circumcision is not recommended for an infant who has ambiguous genitalia. This is not an appropriate action for the nurse to take.

   D. **CORRECT:** Families with an infant who has ambiguous genitalia will need ongoing support. Referring to genetic counseling is an appropriate action for the nurse to take.

   E. **CORRECT:** Chromosomal analysis is used for gender assignment, and is therefore an appropriate action for the nurse to take.

   NCLEX® Connection: Health Promotion and Maintenance, Aging Process

4. A. INCORRECT: Increased urine flow is a clinical manifestation of obstructive uropathy.

    B. **CORRECT:** Urinary tract infection is a clinical manifestation of obstructive uropathy.

    C. INCORRECT: Metabolic acidosis is a clinical manifestation of obstructive uropathy.

    D. INCORRECT: Inability to concentrate urine is a clinical manifestation of obstructive uropathy.

    E. **CORRECT:** Hydronephrosis is a clinical manifestation of obstructive uropathy.

    Ⓝ NCLEX® Connection: Physiological Adaptations, Pathophysiology

5. *Using the ATI Active Learning Template: Basic Concept*

    A. Related Content/Underlying Principles
    - Describe six structural disorders of the genitourinary tract and reproductive system.
    - Underlying Principles: Describe each structural disorder.
      ○ Obstructive Uropathy: Structural or functional obstruction in the urinary system.
      ○ Inguinal hernia: Protrusion of abdominal organs through the inguinal canal into the scrotum.
      ○ Chordee: Ventral curvature of the penis.
      ○ Bladder exstrophy: Eversion of the posterior bladder through the anterior bladder wall and lower abdominal wall.
      ○ Hypospadias: Urethral opening located behind the glans of the penis or on the ventral surface of the penile shaft.
      ○ Epispadias: Meatal opening located on the dorsal surface of the penis.
      ○ Phimosis: Narrowing of the preputial opening of the foreskin.
      ○ Cryptorchidism: Undescended testes.
      ○ Hydrocele: Fluid in the scrotum.
      ○ Varicocele: Elongated, dilated, and tortuosity of the veins superior to the testicle.
      ○ Testicular torsion: Testicle hangs free from the vascular structures.
      ○ Ambiguous genitalia: Erroneous or abnormal sexual differentiation.

    Ⓝ NCLEX® Connection: Physiological Adaptations, Pathophysiology

chapter 26

Overview

- Acute glomerulonephritis (AGN)
- Nephrotic syndrome

ACUTE GLOMERULONEPHRITIS (AGN)

Overview

- Acute glomerulonephritis (AGN) – The glomeruli are inflamed, which impairs the kidney to filter the urine properly.
- Acute poststreptococcal glomerulonephritis (APSGN) is an antibody-antigen disease that occurs as a result of certain strains of the Group A ß-hemolytic streptococcal infection and is most commonly seen in children between the ages of 2 and 7 years.

Assessment

- Risk Factors
  - APSGN: streptococcal infection with a specific strain of group A ß-hemolytic streptococcus
- Subjective Data
  - Recent upper respiratory infection or streptococcal infection
- Objective Data
  - Physical Assessment Findings
    - Cloudy, tea-colored urine
    - Decreased urine output
    - Irritability
    - Ill appearance
    - Lethargy
    - Anorexia
    - Vague reports of discomfort (headache, abdominal pain, dysuria)
    - Periorbital edema
    - Facial edema that is worse in the morning but then spreads to extremities and abdomen with progression of the day
    - Mild to severe hypertension

- ○ Laboratory Tests
  - ▪ Throat culture to identify possible streptococcus infection (usually negative by the time of diagnosis)
  - ▪ Urinalysis – proteinuria, smoky or tea-colored urine, hematuria
  - ▪ Renal function – elevated BUN and creatinine
  - ▪ Antistreptolysin O (ASO) titer – positive indicator for the presence of streptococcal antibodies
  - ▪ Antihyaluronidase (AHase), antideoxyribonuclease B (ADNase-B), streptozyme antibodies – may be present
  - ▪ Serum complement (C3) – decreased initially; increases as recovery takes place; returns to normal at 8 to 10 weeks post glomerulonephritis
- ○ Diagnostic Procedures
  - ▪ Chest x-ray to identify pulmonary edema, cardiac enlargement, or pleural effusion
    - □ Nursing Actions
      - ▸ Ensure that adolescents are not pregnant.
      - ▸ Assist with proper positioning.
    - □ Client Education
      - ▸ Explain the procedure to the child and family.

Patient-Centered Care

- • Nursing Care
  - ○ Clients who have normal blood pressure and urine output can be managed at home.
  - ○ Monitor I&O.
  - ○ Monitor daily weights; weigh the child on the same scale with the same amount of clothing daily.
  - ○ Monitor vital signs.
  - ○ Monitor neurologic status and observe for behavior changes, especially in children who have edema, hypertension, and gross hematuria. Implement seizure precautions if condition indicates.
  - ○ Encourage adequate nutritional intake.
    - ▪ Possible restriction of sodium and fluid.
    - ▪ Restrict foods high in potassium during periods of oliguria.
    - ▪ Provide small, frequent meals of favorite foods due to a decrease in appetite.
    - ▪ Refer the child for dietary consultation if indicated.
    - ▪ Avoid added salt and salty foods such as chips.
  - ○ Manage fluid restrictions as prescribed. Fluids may be restricted during periods of edema and hypertension.
  - ○ Monitor skin for breakdown.
    - ▪ Encourage frequent turning and repositioning.
    - ▪ Keep skin dry.
    - ▪ Pad bony prominences and use a specialty mattress.
    - ▪ Elevate edematous body parts.

- ○ Assess tolerance for activity. Provide for frequent rest periods.

- ○ Provide for age-appropriate diversional activities.

- ○ Cluster care to facilitate rest and tolerance of activity.

- ○ Monitor and prevent infection.

  - ▪ Advise the child to turn, cough, and deep breathe to prevent pulmonary involvement.

  - ▪ Monitor vital signs, especially temperature, for changes secondary to infection.

  - ▪ Maintain good hand hygiene.

  - ▪ Administer antibiotic therapy as prescribed.

- ○ Provide emotional support.

- • Medications

  - ○ Diuretics and antihypertensives to remove accumulated fluid and manage hypertension

    - ▪ Nursing Considerations

      - ▫ Monitor blood pressure.

      - ▫ Monitor I&O.

      - ▫ Monitor for electrolyte imbalances, such as hypokalemia.

      - ▫ Observe for adverse effects of medications.

    - ▪ Client Education

      - ▫ Inform the client and family that dizziness can occur with the use of antihypertensives.

      - ▫ Instruct the client and family to take the medication as prescribed and notify the provider if adverse effects occur. Give instructions to continue the medication unless instructed otherwise.

- • Teamwork and Collaboration

  - ○ Obtain a dietary consult.

- • Ongoing Care

  - ○ Client Education

    - ▪ Encourage the child to verbalize feelings related to body image.

    - ▪ Educate the child regarding appropriate dietary management.

    - ▪ Encourage adequate rest.

    - ▪ Educate the family about the need for follow-up care.

    - ▪ Teach the family how to monitor blood pressure and daily weight.

    - ▪ Teach the family about administration and side effects of diuretics and antihypertensive medications.

    - ▪ Encourage the child and family to avoid contact with others who may be ill.

NEPHROTIC SYNDROME

Overview

- In nephrotic syndrome, alterations in the glomerular membrane allow proteins (especially albumin) to pass into the urine, resulting in decreased serum osmotic pressure.
- It can be primary, secondary, or congenital.

Assessment

- Risk Factors
  - Minimal change nephrotic syndrome (MCNS)
    - Peak incidence is between 2 and 7 years of age.
    - Cause is unknown, but it may have a multifactorial etiology (immune-mediated, biochemical).
  - Secondary nephrotic syndrome (occurs after or is associated with glomerular damage due to a known cause)
  - Congenital nephrotic syndrome (an inherited disorder)
- Subjective and Objective Data
  - Physical Assessment Findings
    - Weight gain over a period of days or weeks
    - Facial and periorbital edema – decreased throughout the day
    - Ascites
    - Edema in the ankles
    - Anorexia
    - Diarrhea
    - Irritability
    - Lethargy
    - Decreased frothy urine
    - Blood pressure within expected reference range or slightly below
  - Laboratory Tests
    - Urinalysis/24-hr urine collection
      - Proteinuria – protein greater than 2+ on dipstick
      - Hyaline casts
      - Few RBCs
      - Oval fat bodies

- Serum chemistry
  - □ Hypoalbuminemia – reduced serum protein and albumin
  - □ Hyperlipidemia – elevated serum lipid levels
  - □ Hemoconcentration – elevated Hgb, Hct, and platelets
  - □ Possible hyponatremia – reduced sodium level
  - □ Glomerular filtration rate – normal or high
- ○ Diagnostic Procedures
  - Kidney biopsy is indicated only if nephrotic syndrome is unresponsive to steroid therapy.
    - □ Biopsy will show damage to the epithelial cells lining the basement membrane of the kidney.

Patient-Centered Care

- Nursing Care
  - ○ Provide rest.
  - ○ Monitor I&O. Monitor urine for protein.
  - ○ Monitor vital signs.
  - ○ Monitor daily weights; weigh the child on the same scale with the same amount of clothing.
  - ○ Monitor edema and measure abdominal girth daily. Measure at the widest area, usually at or above the umbilicus. Assess degree of pitting, color, and texture of skin.
  - ○ Monitor and prevent infection.
    - Assist the client to turn, cough, and deep breathe to prevent pulmonary involvement.
    - Monitor vital signs, especially temperature, for changes secondary to infection.
    - Maintain good hand hygiene.
    - Administer antibiotic therapy as prescribed.
  - ○ Encourage nutritional intake within restriction guidelines. Salt and fluids may be restricted during the edematous phase.
  - ○ Cluster care to provide for rest periods.
  - ○ Assess skin for breakdown areas.
    - Avoid use of urinary collection bags in very young children.
    - Pad bony prominences or use a specialty mattress to reduce breakdown of skin.
    - Encourage frequent turning and repositioning.
    - Keep the client's skin dry.
    - Elevate edematous body parts.

- Medications
  - Corticosteroid – prednisone (Deltasone)
    - Nursing Considerations
      - 2 mg/kg/day for 6 weeks followed by 1.5 mg/kg every other day for 6 weeks.
      - Monitor for adverse effects such as hirsutism, slowed linear growth, hypertension, GI bleeding, infection, and hyperglycemia.
      - Administer with meals.
    - Client Education
      - Educate the client and family to avoid large crowds (to decrease the risk of infection).
      - Inform the client and family that using corticosteroids can increase appetite, cause weight gain (especially in the face), and cause mood swings.
      - Educate the client and the family on the medication regime.
      - Educate the client and the family on adverse effects and when to notify the provider.
  - Diuretic – furosemide (Lasix)
    - Eliminates excess fluid from the body
    - Nursing Considerations
      - Encourage the child to eat foods that are high in potassium.
      - Monitor serum electrolyte levels periodically.
  - 25% albumin
    - Increases plasma volume and decreases edema
    - Nursing Considerations
      - Administer per protocol.
      - Monitor I&O.
      - Monitor for anaphylaxis.
  - Cyclophosphamide (Cytoxan)
    - Administer for children who cannot tolerate prednisone or who have repeated relapses of MCNS.
- Teamwork and Collaboration
  - Obtain a dietary consult.
- Ongoing Care
  - Client Education
    - Encourage the client to verbalize feelings related to body image.
    - Educate the client regarding appropriate dietary management.
    - Encourage adequate rest.
    - Educate the family about the need for follow-up care.
    - Inform the family of strategies to decrease the risk of infection (good hand hygiene, up-to-date immunizations, avoidance of infected people).

- Teach the family how to monitor blood pressure, daily weight, and protein in urine. Instruct the family to notify the provider if symptoms worsen, which indicates relapse.

- Teach the family about administration and side effects of medication.

- Provide support to families and make appropriate referrals as needed. Relapses can cause physical, emotional, and financial stress for the client and family.

Complications

- Sepsis/Infection

  ○ Steroid therapy increases the risk for infection.

    - Common infections seen in children with nephrotic syndrome include pneumonia, peritonitis, and cellulitis.

  ○ Nursing Actions

    - Keep the child away from potential infection sources.

    - Monitor for signs of infection.

  ○ Client Education

    - Educate about the importance of completing the full dose of antibiotic.

    - Educate about the need for performing frequent hand hygiene.

    - Educate about signs and symptoms of infection and when to contact the provider.

    - Educate about potential infection sources (live plants, sick family members).

- Circulation insufficiency

- Thromboembolism

APPLICATION EXERCISES

1. A nurse is caring for a child. Which of the following are clinical manifestations of nephrotic syndrome? (Select all that apply.)

_____ A. Dipstick protein of 1+

_____ B. Edema in the ankles

_____ C. Hyperlipidemia

_____ D. Weight loss

_____ E. Anorexia

2. A nurse is caring for a child. Which of the following are clinical manifestations of poststreptococcal glomerulonephritis (APSGN)? (Select all that apply.)

_____ A. Frothy urine

_____ B. Periorbital edema

_____ C. Ill appearance

_____ D. Decreased creatinine

_____ E. Hypertension

3. A nurse is caring for a 10-year-old child who has acute glomerulonephritis (AGN). Which of the following findings should the nurse report to the provider?

A. Serum BUN 8 mg/dL

B. Serum creatinine 1.3 mg/dL

C. Blood pressure 100/74 mm Hg

D. Urine output 550 mL over 24 hr

4. A nurse is caring for a 10-year-old child who has nephrotic syndrome. Which of the following findings should the nurse report to the provider?

A. Serum protein 5.0 g/dL

B. Hgb 14.5 g/dL

C. Hct 40%

D. Platelet 200,000 mm³

5. A nurse is caring for a child who has a prescription for prednisone (Deltasone) 2 mg/kg/day. The child weighs 35 kg. How many mg should the nurse administer per day? (Round the answer to the nearest whole number.)

6. A nurse is teaching a parent of a child who has a new prescription for prednisone (Deltasone) for nephrotic syndrome. Use the Active Learning Template: Medication to complete this item to include the following:

A. Nursing Considerations: List three.

B. Client Education: List four teaching points.

APPLICATION EXERCISES KEY

1. A. **INCORRECT:** A client who has nephrotic syndrome will exhibit proteinuria of 2+ or greater due to the kidneys' inability to filter urine.

    B. **CORRECT:** A client who has nephrotic syndrome will exhibit edema in the ankles due to the decreasing colloidal osmotic pressure in the capillaries.

    C. **CORRECT:** A client who has nephrotic syndrome will exhibit hyperlipidemia due to the increased hepatic synthesis of proteins and lipids.

    D. **INCORRECT:** A client who has nephrotic syndrome will exhibit weight gain due to the decreasing colloidal osmotic pressure in the capillaries, which causes edema.

    E. **CORRECT:** A client who has nephrotic syndrome will exhibit anorexia due to the edema of the intestinal mucosa.

     NCLEX® Connection: Physiological Adaptations, Pathophysiology

2. A. **INCORRECT:** A client who has APSGN will exhibit cloudy, tea-colored urine due to blood and protein in the urine.

    B. **CORRECT:** A client who has APSGN will exhibit periorbital edema due to decrease in plasma filtration.

    C. **CORRECT:** A client who has APSGN will exhibit an ill appearance due to the manifestations experienced from the inadequate functioning of the kidneys.

    D. **INCORRECT:** A client who has APSGN will exhibit increased creatinine due to impaired glomerular filtration of the kidneys.

    E. **CORRECT:** A client who has APSGN will exhibit hypertension due to inadequate function of the kidneys and possibly edema.

    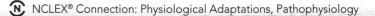 NCLEX® Connection: Physiological Adaptations, Pathophysiology

3. A. **INCORRECT:** Serum BUN 8 mg/dL is within reference range for a 10-year-old child.

    B. **CORRECT:** Serum creatinine 1.3 mg/dL is out of reference range for a 10-year-old child, therefore should be reported to the provider.

    C. **INCORRECT:** Blood pressure of 100/74 mm Hg is within reference range for a 10-year-old child.

    D. **INCORRECT:** Urine output of 550 mL over 24 hr is within reference range for a 10-year-old child.

    NCLEX® Connection: Reduction of Risk Potential, Laboratory Values

4. A. **CORRECT:** Serum protein 5.0 g/dL is out of reference range for a 10-year-old child and should be reported to the provider.

    B. INCORRECT: Hgb 14.5 g/dL is within reference range for a 10-year-old child.

    C. INCORRECT: Hct 40% is within reference range for a 10-year-old child.

    D. INCORRECT: Platelet 200,000 mm³ is within reference range for a 10-year-old child.

    (N) NCLEX® Connection: Reduction of Risk Potential, Laboratory Values

5. **70** mg

Using Ratio and Proportion, Desired Over Have, and Dimensional Analysis		
STEP 1: *What is the unit of measurement to calculate?* mg	STEP 2: *Set up an equation and solve for X.* mg x kg/day = X 2 mg x 35 kg/day = 70 mg/day STEP 3: *Round if necessary.*	STEP 4: *Reassess to determine whether the amount makes sense.* If the prescribed amount is 2 mg/kg/day and the client weighs 35 kg, it makes sense to give 70 mg/day.

(N) NCLEX® Connection: Pharmacological and Parenteral Therapies, Dosage Calculation

6. *Using the Active Learning Template: Medication*

    A. Nursing Considerations
    - Administer 2 mg/kg/day for 6 weeks followed by 1.5 mg/kg every other day for 6 weeks.
    - Monitor for adverse effects such as hirsutism, slowed linear growth, hypertension, GI bleeding, infection, and hyperglycemia.
    - Administer with meals.

    B. Client Education
    - Educate the client and family to avoid large crowds (to decrease the risk of infection).
    - Inform the client and family that using corticosteroids can increase appetite, cause weight gain (especially in the face), and cause mood swings.
    - Educate the client and the family on the medication regime.
    - Educate the client and the family on adverse effects and when to notify the provider.

    (N) NCLEX® Connection: Pharmacological and Parenteral Therapies, Medication Administration

UNIT 2 Nursing Care of Children with System Disorders

SECTION: MUSCULOSKELETAL DISORDERS

› Fractures
› Musculoskeletal Congenital Disorders
› Chronic Neuromusculoskeletal Disorders

NCLEX® CONNECTIONS

When reviewing the chapters in this unit, keep in mind the relevant sections of the NCLEX® outline, in particular:

Client Needs: Basic Care and Comfort	Client Needs: Pharmacological and Parenteral Therapies	Client Needs: Reduction of Risk Potential
› Relevant topics/tasks include: » Mobility/Immobility › Apply, maintain, or remove orthopedic devices. » Nonpharmacological Comfort Interventions › Assess client need for pain management.	› Relevant topics/tasks include: » Adverse Effects/ Contraindications/Side Effects/Interactions › Identify a contraindication to the administration of a medication to the client. » Medication Administration › Administer and document medications given by common routes. » Pharmacological Pain Management › Administer pharmacological measures for pain management.	› Relevant topics/tasks include: » Potential for Complications of Diagnostic Tests/ Treatments/Procedures › Use precautions to prevent injury and/or complications associated with a procedure or diagnosis. » System Specific Assessment › Assess the client for abnormal peripheral pulses after a procedure or treatment. » Therapeutic Procedures › Use precautions to prevent further injury when moving a client with a musculoskeletal condition.

chapter 27

Overview

- A fracture occurs when the resistance between a bone and an applied stress yields to the applied stress, resulting in a disruption to the integrity of the bone.

- Bone healing and remodeling is faster in children than in adults, due to a thicker periosteum and good blood supply.

- Epiphyseal plate injuries may result in altered bone growth.

- Radiographic evidence of previous fractures in various stages of healing or in infants may be the result of physical abuse or osteogenesis imperfecta.

Assessment

- Risk Factors

  ○ Obesity

  ○ Poor nutrition

  ○ Developmental characteristics, ordinary play activities, and recreation place children at risk for injury (falls from climbing or running; trauma to bones from skateboarding, skiing, or playing soccer or basketball)

- Subjective and Objective Data

  ○ Physical Assessment Findings

    ▪ Common types of fractures in children

      □ Plastic deformation (bend) – The bone is bent no more than 45°.

      □ Buckle (torus) – Compression of the bone resulting in a bulge or raised area at the fracture site.

      □ Greenstick – Incomplete fracture of the bone.

      □ Transverse – Break is straight across the bone.

      □ Oblique – Break is diagonal across the bone.

      □ Spiral – Break spirals around the bone.

      □ Growth plate – Injury to the end of the long bone on the growth plate.

      □ Stress – Tiny cracks in the bone.

M View Image: Fractures

      □ Complete – Bone fragments are separated.

      □ Incomplete – Bone fragments are still attached.

- □ Closed or simple – The fracture occurs without a break in the skin.

- □ Open or compound – The fracture occurs with an open wound and bone protruding.

- □ Complicated fracture – The fracture results in injury to other organs and tissues.

- Pain

- Crepitus

- Deformity

- Edema

- Ecchymosis

- Warmth or redness

○ Diagnostic Procedures

- Radiograph

  - □ Nursing Actions

    - ▸ Instruct and assist the client to remain still during the procedure.

  - □ Client Education

    - ▸ Educate the client and parents about what to expect during the procedure.

    - ▸ Provide emotional support.

Patient-Centered Care

- Nursing Care

  ○ Provide emergency care at the time of injury.

  - Maintain ABCs.

  - Monitor vital signs, pain, and neurologic status.

  - Assess the neurovascular status of the injured extremity.

  - Position the client in a supine position.

  - Stabilize the injured area, avoiding unnecessary movement.

  - Elevate the affected limb and apply ice packs.

  - Administer analgesics as prescribed.

  - Keep the client warm.

  ○ General nursing interventions

  - Assess pain frequently using an age-appropriate pain tool. Use appropriate pain management, both pharmacological and nonpharmacological.

  - Monitor neurovascular status on a regular schedule. Report any change in status.

    - □ Neurovascular Assessment

      - ▸ Sensation – Assess the client for numbness or a tingling sensation of the extremity. Loss of sensation may indicate nerve damage.

      - ▸ Skin temperature – Assess the extremity for temperature. The extremity should be warm, not cool, to touch.

- Skin color – Assess the color of the affected extremity. Check distal to the injury and look for changes in pigmentation.

- Capillary refill – Press the nail beds of the affected extremity until blanching occurs. Blood return should be within 3 seconds.

- Pulses – Pulses should be palpable and strong. Pulses should also be equal to the pulses of the unaffected extremity.

- Movement – The client should be able to move the affected extremity in passive motion.

  - Maintain proper alignment.

  - Promote range of motion of fingers, toes, and unaffected extremities.

  - Instruct the client and family regarding activity restrictions.

- Medications

  ○ Analgesics

    - Administer analgesics for pain.

    - Nursing Considerations (for use of opioid analgesia)

      □ Monitor for respiratory depression and constipation.

    - Client Education

      □ Educate the client and parents about the need for adequate pain relief.

- Teamwork and Collaboration

  ○ Orthopedic specialists are generally consulted for fracture care in children.

  ○ Notify social services in situations in which abuse is suspected.

- Therapeutic Procedures

  ○ Casting

    - Types of casts: long-leg, short-leg, bilateral long-leg, long-arm, short-arm, full spica, and single spica

    - Plaster of Paris casts are heavy, not water resistant, and can take 10 to 72 hr to dry. Synthetic fiberglass casts are light, water resistant, and dry very quickly (in 5 to 20 min).

    - Prior to casting, the skin area should be observed for integrity, cleaned, and dried. Bony prominences should be padded to prevent skin breakdown. The casting material is then applied by the provider.

    - Nursing Actions

      □ Provide atraumatic care prior to cast application by showing the procedure on a doll or toy.

      □ Assess and monitor neurovascular status.

      □ Elevate the cast above the level of the heart during the first 24 to 48 hr to prevent swelling.

      □ Apply ice for the first 24 hr to decrease swelling.

      □ Turn and position the client every 2 hr so that dry air circulates around and under the cast for faster drying. This also will prevent pressure from changing the shape of the cast.

        - Do not use heat lamps or warm hair dryers.

      □ Turn the client frequently while supporting all extremities and joints.

      □ Instruct the client to keep the affected extremity supported (with a sling) or elevated when sitting.

- Assess for increased warmth or hot spots on the cast surface, which could indicate infection.
- If a wound is present, monitor the skin through the window that has been placed in an area of the cast to allow for skin inspection.
- Monitor for drainage on the cast. Outline any drainage on the outside of the cast with a marker (and note date and time) so it can be monitored for any additional drainage.
- Assess the general skin condition and the area around the cast edges.
- Provide routine skin care and thorough perineal care to maintain skin integrity.
- Plaster casts: Use palms of hands to avoid denting, expose the case to air to promote drying.
- Use moleskin over any rough area of the cast that may rub against the client's skin.
- Cover areas of the cast with plastic to avoid soiling from urine or feces.
- Assist with proper crutch fitting and reinforce proper use.
- Client Education
  - Teach the client and parents that when the cast is applied it will feel warm, but it will not burn the client.
  - Teach the parents and client to report pain that is extremely severe or is not relieved 1 hr after the administration of pain medication.
  - Teach the parents and client how to perform neurovascular checks and when to contact the provider.
  - Give instructions for the proper use of crutches for lower-extremity casts.
  - Reinforce skin and perineal care with a spica cast.
  - Instruct the client not to place any foreign objects inside the cast to avoid trauma to the skin.
  - Reinforce use of proper restraints when transporting the client in any vehicle.
  - Teach the client and parents about cast removal and cast cutter.
  - Instruct the client to soak the extremity in warm water and then apply lotion after the cast has been removed
- Traction care – Traction, countertraction, and friction are used to align, immobilize, and reduce muscle spasms associated with certain fractures. Through the use of a forward-pulling force and a backward force, adding or removing weight controls the degree of force applied to maintain traction and alignment. The type of traction used depends on the fracture, age of the client, and associated injuries.
  - Skin traction uses a pulling force that is applied by weights (may be used intermittently). Using tape and straps applied to the skin along with boots and/or cuffs, weights are attached by a rope to the extremity (Buck, Russell, Bryant traction).
  - Skeletal traction uses a continuous pulling force that is applied directly to the skeletal structure and/or specific bone. A pin or rod is inserted through or into the bone. Force is applied through the use of weights attached by rope. Skeletal traction (90°/90° traction) allows the client to change positions without interfering with the pull of the traction and decreases complications associated with immobility and traction.
  - Balanced suspension traction suspends the leg in a flexed position. The hip and hamstring muscles are relaxed.

- Halo traction (cervical traction) uses a halo-type bar that encircles the head. Screws are inserted into the outer table of the skull. The halo is attached to either bed traction or rods that are secured to a vest worn by the client.

View Images

› Balanced Suspension Skeletal Traction   › Halo Traction

- Nursing Actions
  - Maintain body alignment.
  - Provide pharmacological and nonpharmacological interventions for the management of pain and muscle spasms.
  - Notify the provider if the client experiences severe pain from muscle spasms that is unrelieved with medications and/or repositioning.
  - Assess and monitor neurovascular status
  - Routinely monitor the client's skin integrity and document findings.
  - Assess pin sites for pain, redness, swelling, drainage, or odor. Provide pin care per facility protocol.
  - Assess for changes in elimination and maintain usual patterns of elimination.
  - Ensure that all the hardware is tight and that the bed is in the correct position.
  - Assess and maintain weights so that they hang freely and the ropes are free of knots. Do not lift or remove weights unless prescribed and supervised by the provider.
  - Assure that the wrench to release the rods is attached to the vest when using halo traction in the event that CPR is necessary.
  - Move the client in halo traction as a unit without applying pressure to the rods. This will prevent loosening of the pins and pain.
  - Consult with the provider for an overbed trapeze to assist the client to move in bed.
  - Provide range of motion and encourage activity of nonimmobilized extremities to maintain mobility and prevent contractures.
  - Encourage deep breathing and use of the incentive spirometry.
  - Promote frequent position changing within restrictions of traction.
  - Remove sheets from the head of the bed to the foot of the bed, and remake the bed in the same manner.
- Client Education
  - Educate about the need to provide adequate hydration and nutrition while in traction.
  - Educate and reinforce about the use and need for stool softeners.
  - Teach the client and parents signs of infection.
  - Teach the client to report any signs of compartment syndrome immediately.

- Surgical Interventions
  - ○ Depending on the type of fracture, surgical intervention may be required. The most common fractures requiring surgery include supracondylar fractures and fractures of the humerus and femur.
  - ○ Surgical reduction is achieved by either a closed (no incision) or open (with incision) reduction with or without pinning.
    - ▪ Nursing Actions
      - □ Monitor for signs of infection at the incision site.
      - □ Encourage mobilization as soon as prescribed.
      - □ Medicate for pain as needed.
    - ▪ Client Education
      - □ Teach and reinforce to the client and parents what to expect before and after the procedure, including NPO status.
      - □ Educate about the need for pain medication.
  - ○ Care After Discharge
    - ▪ Teach and reinforce proper cast care, as well as pin care if indicated.
    - ▪ Teach and reinforce how to perform neurovascular checks and when to call or return to the provider.
    - ▪ Instruct the client and parents about the need for and use of antipruritic medications if prescribed.
    - ▪ Instruct the parents to maintain physical restrictions as prescribed.
    - ▪ Instruct the parents in appropriate pain management.
    - ▪ Instruct the parents to report increasing pain, redness, inflammation, and/or fever to the provider.
    - ▪ Instruct the parents regarding the importance of follow-up care as instructed.

Complications

- Compartment syndrome
  - ○ Compression of nerves, blood vessels, and muscle inside a confined place.
  - ○ If untreated, tissue necrosis can result.
  - ○ Findings
    - ▪ Increased pain that is unrelieved with elevation or analgesics
    - ▪ Intense pain when passively moved
    - ▪ Paresthesia or numbness
    - ▪ Pulselessness distal to the fracture
    - ▪ Inability to move digits
    - ▪ Warm digits with skin that is tight and shiny
    - ▪ Pallor

- ○ Nursing Actions
  - Assess the extremity at frequent intervals. Notify the provider if compartment syndrome is suspected.
  - Prevention
    - □ Loosen the constrictive dressing or cut the bandage or tape.
    - □ Elevate the extremity and apply ice.
  - Prepare the client for fasciotomy.
- ○ Client Education
  - Instruct the client to report pain that is not relieved by analgesics, pain that continues to increase in intensity, numbness or tingling, or a change in color of the extremity.

- Osteomyelitis
  - ○ Infection within the bone secondary to a bacterial infection from an outside source, such as with an open fracture (endogenous) or from a bloodborne bacterial source (hematogenous)
  - ○ Clinical Manifestations
    - Appearing ill
    - Irritability
    - Fever
    - Tachycardia
    - Edema
    - Pain
    - Not wanting to use the affected extremity
    - Site of infection tender, and bone pain worsens with movement
  - ○ Nursing Actions
    - Assist in diagnostic procedures, such as obtaining skin, blood, and bone cultures.
    - Assist with joint or bone biopsy.
    - Administer IV and oral antibiotic therapy.
    - Assist with proper positioning to promote comfort.
    - Administer pain medication as prescribed.
    - Consult with the parents and provider regarding home care needs.
  - ○ Client Education
    - Educate the client and parents about the length of treatment that may be needed and long-term antibiotic therapy.
    - Remind the client and parents to avoid bearing any weight until cleared by the provider.
    - Advise the parents to provide for diversional activities consistent with the client's level of development.
    - Educate the client about the need for proper nutrition.

APPLICATION EXERCISES

1. A nurse is caring for a child who is in a plaster spica cast. Which of the following is an appropriate action for the nurse to take?

    A. Use a heat lamp to facilitate drying.

    B. Avoid turning the child until the cast is dry.

    C. Assist the client with crutch walking after the cast is dry.

    D. Apply moleskin to the edges of the cast.

2. A nurse is teaching a group of parent about fractures. Which of the following should be included in the teaching?

    A. "Children need a longer time to heal from a fracture than an adult."

    B. "Epiphyseal plate injuries may result in altered bone growth."

    C. "A greenstick fracture is a complete break in the bone."

    D. "Bones are unable to bend, so they break."

3. A nurse is caring for a child who sustained a fracture. Which of the following are appropriate actions for the nurse to take? (Select all that apply.)

    _____ A. Place a heat pack on the site of injury.

    _____ B. Elevate the affected limb.

    _____ C. Assess neurovascular status frequently.

    _____ D. Encourage ROM of the affected limb.

    _____ E. Stabilize the injury.

4. A nurse is caring for a child who has a fracture. Which of the following are clinical manifestations of a fracture? (Select all that apply.)

    _____ A. Crepitus

    _____ B. Edema

    _____ C. Pain

    _____ D. Fever

    _____ E. Ecchymosis

5. A nurse is caring for a child who is in Russell traction. Which of the following are appropriate actions for the nurse to take? (Select all that apply.)

_____ A. Remove the boots once a day for a bath.

_____ B. Assess the child's position frequently.

_____ C. Assess pin sites every 4 hr.

_____ D. Ensure the weights are hanging freely.

_____ E. Ensure the buttocks is raised off of the bed.

6. A nurse is caring for a client who has a newly placed cast. Use the ATI Active Learning Template: Systems Disorder to complete this item to include clinical manifestations of compartment syndrome.

APPLICATION EXERCISES KEY

1. A. INCORRECT: A cool fan can be used to facilitate drying of a plaster cast.

   B. INCORRECT: The child should be turned every 2 hr to expose all areas of the cast to facilitate drying.

   C. INCORRECT: A client who has a spica cast is non-weight-bearing until the cast is removed.

   D. **CORRECT:** The nurse should apply moleskin to the edges of the cast to prevent the cast from rubbing on the client's skin.

   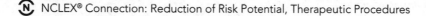 NCLEX® Connection: Reduction of Risk Potential, Therapeutic Procedures

2. A. INCORRECT: Children heal from fractures quicker than adults due to a thicker periosteum and good blood supply.

   B. **CORRECT:** Detection and early treatment is crucial for an epiphyseal plate injury to prevent altered bone growth.

   C. INCORRECT: A greenstick fracture is a partial break in the bone.

   D. INCORRECT: Children's bones are soft and pliable and can bend up to 45° before breaking.

   NCLEX® Connection: Physiological Adaptations, Pathophysiology

3. A. INCORRECT: The nurse should place a cold pack on the site of injury to decrease swelling.

   B. **CORRECT:** Elevating the affected limb can decrease swelling at the injury site. This is an appropriate action for the nurse to take.

   C. **CORRECT:** Assessing neurovascular status assists the nurse in determining if the affected limp has adequate blood supply. This is an appropriate action for the nurse to take.

   D. INCORRECT: The nurse should encourage ROM of the nonaffected limb.

   E. **CORRECT:** Stabilizing the injury will prevent further injury and damage. This is an appropriate action for the nurse to take.

   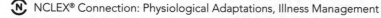 NCLEX® Connection: Physiological Adaptations, Illness Management

4. A. **CORRECT:** A fracture can leave bone fragments that will exhibit a grating sound. Crepitus is a clinical manifestation of a fracture.

    B. **CORRECT:** Swelling at the site occur related to the trauma. Edema is a clinical manifestation of a fracture.

    C. **CORRECT:** A child who has a fracture will experience pain from the trauma.

    D. INCORRECT: A child who has a fracture will not exhibit a fever related to the fracture.

    E. **CORRECT:** Bleeding under the skin can occur related to the trauma. Ecchymosis is a clinical manifestation of a fracture.

    Ⓝ NCLEX® Connection: Physiological Adaptations, Illness Management

5. A. INCORRECT: The boots should only be removed by the provider or in an emergency situation.

    B. **CORRECT:** Hip flexion must be maintained in Russell traction. The nurse should assess the child's position frequently.

    C. INCORRECT: Russell traction is a skin traction. The client will not have pin sites to assess.

    D. **CORRECT:** The nurse should ensure that the weights are hanging freely to allow for prescribed traction.

    E. INCORRECT: The buttock is raised off of the bed when Bryant traction is used.

    Ⓝ NCLEX® Connection: Basic Care and Comfort, Mobility/Immobility

6. *Using the ATI Active Learning Template: Systems Disorder*
    - Clinical Manifestations of Compartment Syndrome
      ○ Increased pain that is unrelieved with elevation or analgesics
      ○ Intense pain when passively moved
      ○ Paresthesia or numbness
      ○ Pulselessness distal to the fracture
      ○ Inability to move digits
      ○ Warm digits with skin that is tight and shiny
      ○ Pallor

    Ⓝ NCLEX® Connection: Reduction of Risk Potential, Potential for Complications from Surgical Procedures and Health Alterations

chapter 28

Overview

- Clubfoot
- Legg-Calve-Perthes
- Developmental dysplasia of the hip (DDH)
- Osteogenesis imperfecta
- Scoliosis

CLUBFOOT

Overview

- A complex deformity of the ankle and foot
- Can affect one or both feet, occur as an isolated defect, or in association with other disorders such as cerebral palsy and spinal bifida
- Categorized as positional clubfoot (occurs from intrauterine crowding), syndromic (occurs in association with other syndromes), and congenital (idiopathic)

M	View Images	
	› Club Foot	› Developmental Dysplasia of the Hip (DDH)

Assessment

- Risk Factors – presence of other syndromes
- Subjective and Objective Data
    - Talipes varus – inversion (bending inward)
    - Talipes valgus – eversion (bending outward)
    - Talipes calcaneus – dorsiflexion (toes are higher than the heels)
    - Talipes equinus – plantar flexion (toes are lower than the heels)
    - Talipes equinovarus – toes are facing inward and lower than the heel
- Diagnostic Procedures
    - Prenatal – ultrasound can identify the deformity

Patient-Centered Care

- Nursing Care
  - Encourage parents to hold and cuddle the child.
  - Encourage parents to meet the developmental needs of the child.
  - Perform neurovascular and skin integrity checks.
- Therapeutic Procedures
  - Castings
    - Series of castings starting shortly after birth and continuing until maximum correction is accomplished.
    - Nursing Care
      - Assess neurovascular status.
      - Perform cast care.
    - Client Education
      - Teach cast care.
      - Teach the family on follow-up care for cast changes.
- Surgical Interventions (congenital clubfoot and syndromic clubfoot)
  - Osteotomy – removing part of the bone
  - Fusion – fusing two or more bones together
  - Tendon lengthening or shortening
- Complications
  - Growth and development delays
    - Nursing Care – Monitor growth and development.
    - Client Education – Teach the family strategies to enhance normal growth and development.
  - Effects of casting
    - Skin breakdown
    - Neurovascular alterations

LEGG-CALVE-PERTHES DISEASE

Overview

- Aseptic necrosis of the femoral head can be unilateral or bilateral

Assessment

- Risk Factors
  - Trauma, inflammation to the femoral head
  - Coagulation defects

- Subjective and Objective Data
  - Intermittent painless limp
  - Hip stiffness
  - Limited ROM
  - Thigh pain
  - Shortening of the affected leg
  - Muscle wasting
- Diagnostic Procedures – radiographs of the hip and pelvis

Patient-Centered Care

- Nursing Care
  - Treatment varies with the child's age and the appearance of the femoral head.
  - Administer NSAIDs as prescribed.
  - Maintain rest and nonweightbearing.
    - Abduction brace
    - Casts
    - Leather harness sling
    - Traction
  - Advance to active motion as prescribed.
- Surgical Interventions
  - Total hip resurfacing
    - Replace the hip joint.
- Client Education
  - Teach about the nonweightbearing treatment prescribed.
  - Offer developmental appropriate strategies for learning and activities during the nonweightbearing periods.

DEVELOPMENTAL DYSPLASIA OF THE HIP (DDH)

Overview

- A variety of disorders resulting in abnormal development of the hip structures that can affect infants or children
- Acetabular dysplasia – delay in acetabular development
- Subluxation – incomplete dislocation of the hip
- Dislocation – femoral head does not have contact with the acetabulum

Assessment

- Risk Factors
  - Birth order
  - Family history
  - Intrauterine position
  - Delivery type
  - Joint stability
- Subjective and Objective Data
  - Infant
    - Asymmetry of gluteal and thigh folds
    - Limited hip abduction
    - Shortening of the femur
    - Positive Ortolani test (hip is reduced by abduction)
    - Positive Barlow test (hip is dislocated by adduction)
  - Child
    - One leg shorter than the other
    - Positive Trendelenburg sign (while bearing weight on the affected side, the pelvis tilts downward)
    - Walking on toes on one foot
    - Walk with a limp
- Diagnostic Procedures
  - Ultrasound – should be performed at 2 weeks of age to determine the cartilaginous head of the femur
  - X-ray – can diagnose DDH in infants older than 4 months of age

Patient-Centered Care

- Nursing Care
  - Treatment starts as soon as it is diagnosed and depends on the child's age and the extent of the dysplasia.
  - Encourage parents to hold and cuddle the infant/child.
  - Encourage parents to meet the developmental needs of the infant/child.
  - Newborn to 6 months
    - Pavlik harness
      - Maintain harness placement for to 12 weeks.
      - Check straps every 1 to 2 weeks for adjustment.
      - Perform neurovascular and skin integrity checks.

- □ Removing the harness is dependent on the client.
- □ Client Teaching

  - ‣ Teach the family not to adjust the straps.
  - ‣ Teach the family how to place the harness if removal is prescribed.
  - ‣ Teach the family skin care (use an undershirt, knee socks, assess skin, gently massage skin under straps, avoid lotions and powders, place diaper under the straps).
- ■ Bryant traction or hip spica cast (when adduction contracture is present)
  - □ Bryant traction
    - ‣ Skin traction
    - ‣ Hips are flexed at a 90° angle with the buttock raised off of the bed
    - ‣ Nursing Actions
      - ▷ Neurovascular checks
      - ▷ Maintain traction (ropes, boots, pulleys, and weights)
      - ▷ Ensure the client maintains alignment
      - ▷ Skin care
  - □ Hip spica cast
    - ‣ Needs to be changed to accommodate growth
    - ‣ Nursing Actions
      - ▷ Assess and maintain the hip spica cast.
      - ▷ Perform frequent neurovascular checks.
      - ▷ Perform range of motion with the unaffected extremities.
      - ▷ Perform frequent assessment of skin integrity, especially in the diaper area.
      - ▷ Assess for pain control using an age-appropriate pain tool. Intervene as indicated.
      - ▷ Evaluate hydration status frequently.
      - ▷ Assess elimination status daily.
    - ‣ Client Education
      - ▷ Reinforce teaching regarding positioning, turning, neurovascular assessments, and care of the cast.
      - ▷ Position casts on pillows.
      - ▷ Keep the casts elevated until dry.
      - ▷ Encourage frequent position changes to allow for drying.
      - ▷ Handle the casts with the palm of the hand until dry.
      - ▷ Note color and temperature of toes on casted extremity.
      - ▷ Give sponge baths to avoid wetting the cast.
      - ▷ Use a waterproof barrier around the genital opening of spica cast to prevent soiling with urine or feces.
      - ▷ Educate regarding care after discharge with emphasis on using appropriate equipment (stroller, wagon, car seat) for maintaining mobility.

- 6 months to 2 years
  - Surgical closed reduction with placement of hip spica cast
    - Nursing Actions
      - Prepare family and client for surgery
      - Perform neurovascular checks
      - Manage postoperative pain
      - Skin care
      - Cast care
    - Client Education
      - Teach about spica cast and home cares
- Older children
  - Surgical reduction with presurgical traction
  - Femoral osteotomy, reconstruction, and tenotomy are often needed

Complications

- Postoperative complications (atelectasis, ileus, infection)
- Effects of immobilization (decreased muscle strength, bone demineralization, altered bowel motility)
- Effects of casting (skin breakdown, neurovascular alterations)
- Infection
  - Infection may be caused by bacteria, such as Staphylococcus aureus.
  - Nursing Actions
    - Monitor vital signs. Observe changes in temperature that could be associated with complications of infection.
    - Keep the cast dry and intact.
    - Monitor for changes in neurovascular status (numbness; tingling; decreased mobility, sensation, or capillary refill).
    - Reposition the child frequently.
    - Maintain a high-fiber diet and promote adequate hydration.
    - Monitor bowel and bladder elimination. Report any changes, especially the decrease or absence of bowel sounds or distention.
    - Report any foul odor from cast or urine.
    - Observe changes in behavior, especially increasing irritability in infants.
  - Client Education
    - Reinforce expected complications of specific treatment or procedure with the child and/or family.
    - Reinforce the need to notify the provider with any concerns or signs of complications.
    - Educate the child and/or family about follow up.

OSTEOGENESIS IMPERFECTA (OI)

Overview

- Heterogeneous, autosomal dominant disorder of the bones resulting in fractures and deformity.
- Several classifications of OI

Assessment

- Risk Factors
  - Parent with OI
- Subjective and Objective Data
  - Classic manifestations
    - Multiple bone fractures
    - Blue sclera
    - Early hearing loss
  - More severe manifestations
    - Bowed legs and arms
    - Kyphosis
    - Scoliosis
- Diagnostic Procedures
  - Bone biopsy
    - Nursing Actions
      - Prepare the client for the procedure.
      - Assist with positioning the client.

Patient-Centered Care

- Nursing Care
  - Treatment is supportive.
  - Medication
    - Pamidronate (Aredia)
      - Increase bone density
      - Nursing Actions
        - Administer IV.
        - Monitor for adverse effects (hypokalemia, hypomagnesemia, hypocalcemia, hypophosphatemia, general malaise).
      - Client Education
        - Teach adverse effects and when to call the provider.

- ○ Teach the family and client low-impact exercises.
- ○ Teach the family about medication regime as prescribed.
- ○ Consult with physical therapy.
- ○ Assist with braces and splints as prescribed.
- ○ Assist client with meeting developmental milestones.
- ○ Education the parents on the client's limitations.
- ○ Encourage support groups.
- Surgical Interventions (for severe cases)
  - ○ Correct bone deformities, placement of rods.

Complications

- Disuse osteoporosis
  - ○ Limit time in casts.
  - ○ Encourage activity.
- Hearing loss
- Permanent deformities

SCOLIOSIS

Overview

- Scoliosis is a complex deformity of the spine that also affects the ribs.
- Characterized by a lateral curvature of the spine and spinal rotation that causes rib asymmetry.
- A curve needs to be at least 10° for diagnosis and mild curves (less than 25°) are monitored.
- Idiopathic or structural scoliosis is the most common form of scoliosis and can be seen in isolation or associated with other conditions.
  - ○ Scoliosis – bracing and exercise

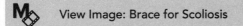
M◇   View Image: Brace for Scoliosis

Assessment

- Risk Factors
  - ○ Genetic tendency
- Subjective and Objective Data
  - ○ Asymmetry in scapula, ribs, flanks, shoulders, and hips
  - ○ Improperly fitting clothing (one leg shorter than the other)

- Diagnostic Procedures
  - Screen during preadolescence for boys and girls.
    - Observe the child, who should be wearing only underwear, from the back.
    - Have the child bend over at the waist with arms hanging down and observe for asymmetry of ribs and flank.
    - Measure truncal rotation with a scoliometer.
  - Radiographs
    - Use the Cobb technique to determine the degree of curvature.
    - Use the Risser scale to determine the skeletal maturity.

Patient-Centered Care

- Nursing Care
  - Treatment depends on the degree, location, and type of curvature.
- Therapeutic Procedures
  - Bracing
    - Customized braces that slow the progression of the curve
    - Nursing Actions
      - Assist with fitting the client with a brace.
      - Assess skin.
      - Assist the client with self-image.
    - Client Education
      - Teach the client how to apply the brace.
- Surgical Interventions
  - Spinal fusion with rod placement
  - Used for curvatures greater than 45°
  - Nursing Actions
    - Preoperative
      - Inform the adolescent to obtain autologous (self-donated) blood donations and assist them.
      - Obtain routine laboratory studies, including a type and cross match for blood as prescribed.
      - Orient the adolescent and family to the ICU.
      - Inform the adolescent and/or family about what can be expected during the postoperative period, such as monitoring equipment, NG tube, chest tubes, indwelling urinary catheters, and self-administering analgesic pumps.
    - Postoperative
      - Monitor the adolescent initially in the intensive care unit.
      - Perform standard postoperative care to prevent complications.
      - Monitor pain using an age-appropriate pain tool.

◻ Administer analgesia using a patient-controlled analgesic pump as prescribed.

◻ Perform frequent neurovascular checks.

◻ Turn the adolescent frequently by log rolling to prevent damage to the spinal fusion.

◻ Assess skin for pressure areas, especially if a brace has been prescribed.

◻ Provide skin care by keeping skin clean and dry.

◻ Monitor surgical and drain sites for signs of infection. Provide wound care as prescribed.

◻ Assess bowel sounds and monitor, observing for paralytic ileus.

◻ Monitor for decreases in Hgb and Hct. Observe for indications of bleeding.

◻ Administer blood transfusion as prescribed. The adolescent may have self-donated blood available for transfusion.

◻ Encourage mobility as soon as tolerated.

◻ Assess for infection.

◻ Perform range of motion on unaffected extremities.

◻ Provide age-appropriate activities and opportunities to visit with friends and family during the hospital stay.

○ Client Education

■ Preoperative

◻ Reinforce teaching (use of incentive spirometer, turning, coughing, deep breathing) to prevent complications.

◻ Perform extensive preoperative teaching to educate the adolescent and/or family and to promote cooperation and participation in recovery.

◻ Demonstrate the use of a patient-controlled analgesic pump if age-appropriate.

◻ Demonstrate log rolling that will be used after surgery.

◻ Demonstrate the respiratory therapy techniques that will be used postoperatively to reduce complications of anesthesia.

◻ Discuss medical terms that are unfamiliar to the adolescent and/or family.

■ Postoperative

◻ Emphasize the importance of physical therapy and proper positioning of the spine.

◻ Encourage independence following surgery for the adolescent who has a brace.

◻ Encourage the adolescent to contact friends when able.

◻ Emphasize the necessity of follow-up care.

○ Care After Discharge

■ Client Education

◻ Reinforce the expected course of treatment and recovery.

◻ Suggest that the family arrange the environment to facilitate the adolescent's ability to be as independent as possible (keep favorite items within reach).

◻ Emphasize the necessity of follow-up care.

Complications

- Breathing difficulties (with severe curvatures)
- Lower self-esteem
  - Assist the client with age-appropriate actions with self-esteem.
- Infection following surgery
  - Infection may be caused by bacteria, such as Staphylococcus aureus.
  - Nursing Actions
    - Monitor vital signs. Observe changes in temperature that could be associated with complications of infection.
    - Monitor for changes in neurovascular status (numbness; tingling; decreased mobility, sensation, or capillary refill).
    - Reposition the child frequently.
    - Maintain a high-fiber diet and promote adequate hydration.
  - Client Education
    - Reinforce expected complications of specific treatment or procedure with the child and/or family.
    - Reinforce the need to notify the provider with any concerns or signs of complications.
    - Educate the child and/or family about follow up.
- Spine or nerve damage (uncorrected scoliosis)

APPLICATION EXERCISES

1. A nurse is caring for a toddler who is diagnosed with hip dysplasia and has been placed in a hip spica cast. The child's mother asks the nurse why a Pavlik harness is not being used. Which of the following responses by the nurse appropriately addresses the mother's question?

    A. "The Pavlik harness is used for children with scoliosis, not hip dysplasia."

    B. "The Pavlik harness is used for school-age children."

    C. "The Pavlik harness cannot be used for your child because her condition is too severe."

    D. "The Pavlik harness is used for infants less than 6 months of age."

2. A nurse is completing preoperative teaching with an adolescent client who is going to receive spinal instrumentation for scoliosis. Which of the following information should the nurse include in the teaching?

    A. "You will go home the same day of surgery."

    B. "You will have minimal pain."

    C. "You will need to receive blood."

    D. "You will not be able to eat until the day after surgery."

3. A nurse is assessing a child. Which of the following are clinical manifestations of Legg-Calve-Perthes disease? (Select all that apply.)

    _____ A. Longer affected leg

    _____ B. Hip stiffness

    _____ C. Intense pain

    _____ D. Limited ROM

    _____ E. Limp with walking

4. A nurse is caring for a preschool-age child. Which of the following assessments should the nurse use to assess for developmental dysplasia of the hip?

    A. Barlow test

    B. Trendelenburg sign

    C. Manipulation of foot and ankle

    D. Ortolani test

5. A nurse is caring for a child. Which of the following diagnostic procedure should the nurse prepare the child for to determine if the child has Legg-Calve-Perthes disease?

    A. Bone biopsy

    B. Genetic testing

    C. MRI

    D. Radiographs

6. A nurse is caring for a child in a hip spica cast. What should the nurse include in the care of this client? Use the ATI Active Learning Template: Therapeutic Procedure to complete this item to include the following:

    A. Nursing Actions: List seven.

    B. Client Education: List eight.

APPLICATION EXERCISES KEY

1. A. INCORRECT: The Pavlik harness is for infants with hip dysplasia. This is not an appropriate response for the nurse to make.

    B. INCORRECT: The Pavlik harness is for infants with hip dysplasia. This is not an appropriate response for the nurse to make.

    C. INCORRECT: The Pavlik harness is for infants with hip dysplasia. This is not an appropriate response for the nurse to make.

    D. **CORRECT:** The Pavlik harness is a soft brace designed for infants less than 6 months of age. A toddler is too large to fit into the brace.

     NCLEX® Connection: Physiological Adaptations, Illness Management

2. A. INCORRECT: Clients who have spinal instrumentation for scoliosis are hospitalized for approximately 1 week.

    B. INCORRECT: Clients who have spinal instrumentation for scoliosis experience intense pain that require a PCA pump.

    C. **CORRECT:** Clients who have spinal instrumentation for scoliosis have a lengthy surgery with blood loss and require blood replacements.

    D. INCORRECT: Clients who have spinal instrumentation for scoliosis are allowed to advance diet as tolerated.

     NCLEX® Connection: Reduction of Risk Potential, Therapeutic Procedures

3. A. INCORRECT: A child who has Legg-Calve-Perthes exhibit shortening of the affected leg.

    B. **CORRECT:** A child who has Legg-Calve-Perthes exhibits hip stiffness due to the necrosis of the femoral head.

    C. INCORRECT: A child who has Legg-Calve-Perthes exhibits a painless intermitted limp.

    D. **CORRECT:** A child who has Legg-Calve-Perthes exhibits limited ROM due to the necrosis of the femoral head.

    E. **CORRECT:** E. A child who has Legg-Calve-Perthes exhibits a limp with walking due to the necrosis of the femoral head.

     NCLEX® Connection: Physiological Adaptations, Pathophysiology

4. A. INCORRECT: Use a Barlow test to assess developmental dysplasia of the hip for infants.

    B. **CORRECT:** The Trendelenburg sign assesses for developmental dysplasia of the hip. The preschooler bears weight on the affected leg while holding on to something for balance. The examiner observes from behind for abnormal downward tilting of the pelvis on the unaffected side.

    C. INCORRECT: Manipulation of the foot and ankle is a test that assesses for clubfoot.

    D. INCORRECT: The Ortolani test assesses developmental dysplasia of the hip for infants.

    Ⓝ NCLEX® Connection: Reduction of Risk Potential, Diagnostic Tests

5. A. INCORRECT: A bone biopsy is used to diagnosis cancer, infection, and other bone disorders. It is not indicated to diagnosis Legg-Calve-Perthes.

    B. INCORRECT: Legg-Calve-Perthes is necrosis of the femoral head and is not genetic. Therefore, genetic testing is not indicated to diagnosis Legg-Calve-Perthes.

    C. INCORRECT: An MRI is used to visualize structures inside the body. Legg-Calve-Perthes is necrosis of the femoral head. An MRI is not indicated to diagnosis Legg-Calve-Perthes.

    D. **CORRECT:** A child who has Legg-Calve-Perthes exhibits necrosis of the femoral head and can be diagnosed by radiographs of the hip and pelvis.

    Ⓝ NCLEX® Connection: Reduction of Risk Potential, Diagnostic Tests

6. *Using the ATI Active Learning Template: Therapeutic Procedure*

    A. Nursing Actions

    - Assess and maintain the hip spica cast.
    - Perform frequent neurovascular checks.
    - Perform range of motion with the unaffected extremities.
    - Perform frequent assessment of skin integrity, especially in the diaper area.
    - Assess for pain control using an age-appropriate pain tool. Intervene as indicated.
    - Evaluate hydration status frequently.
    - Assess elimination status daily.

    B. Client Education

    - Reinforce teaching regarding positioning, turning, neurovascular assessments, and care of the cast.
    - Position casts on pillows.
    - Keep the casts elevated until dry.
    - Encourage frequent position changes to allow for drying.
    - Handle the casts with the palm of the hand until dry.
    - Note color and temperature of toes on casted extremity.
    - Give sponge baths to avoid wetting the cast.
    - Use a waterproof barrier around the genital opening of spica cast to prevent soiling with urine or feces.
    - Educate regarding care after discharge with emphasis on using appropriate equipment (stroller, wagon, car seat) for maintaining mobility.

    Ⓝ NCLEX® Connection: Reduction of Risk Potential, Therapeutic Procedures

chapter 29

Overview

- Chronic neuromusculoskeletal disorders affect the brain, muscles, joints, and skeletal structures of the body.
  - Cerebral palsy (CP)
  - Spina bifida
  - Down syndrome
  - Juvenile idiopathic arthritis (JIA)
  - Muscular dystrophy (MD)

CEREBRAL PALSY (CP)

Overview

- Cerebral palsy (CP) is a nonprogressive impairment of motor function, especially that of muscle control, coordination, and posture.
- CP may cause abnormal perception and sensation; visual, hearing, and speech impairments; seizures; and cognitive disabilities.
- CP manifests differently in each child. Developmental outcomes vary and are dependent on the severity of the injury.

Assessment

- Risk Factors
  - The exact cause of CP is not known. Prenatal, perinatal, and postnatal risk factors known to be associated with CP include:
    - Existing brain anomalies, cerebral infections, head trauma (shaken baby syndrome), and/or anoxia to the brain.
    - Maternal chorioamnionitis.
    - Premature birth.
    - Multiple births.
    - Extremely low or very low birth weights in newborns.
    - Inability of the placenta to provide the developing fetus with oxygen and nutrients.
    - Interruption of oxygen delivery to the fetus during birth.
    - Kernicterus as a result of high levels of bilirubin in the neonatal period.

- Subjective Data
  - Parents may describe concerns with development.
- Objective Data
  - Physical Assessment Findings
    - Failure to meet developmental milestones
    - Persistent primitive reflexes (Moro or tonic neck)
    - Gagging or choking with feeding, poor suck reflex
    - Tongue thrust
    - Poor head control
    - Rigid posture and extremities, abnormal posturing
    - Asymmetric crawl
    - Hyperreflexia
    - Vision or hearing impairments
    - Seizures
    - Impaired social relationships
    - Assessment findings associated with specific types of CP
      - Spastic (Pyramidal)
        - Hypertonicity (muscle tightness or spasticity); increased deep tendon reflexes; clonus; and poor control of motion, balance, and posture.
        - Impairments of fine and gross motor skills.
        - May present in all extremities (quadriplegia), similar parts of the body (diplegia), three limbs (triplegia), one limb (monoplegia), or one side of the body (hemiplegia); often causes affected limbs to be shorter and thinner.
        - Gait may appear crouched with a scissoring motion of the legs with intoeing and use of primarily the balls of the feet in a tip-toe fashion.
      - Dyskinetic (Nonspastic, Extrapyramidal)
        - Athetoid: Findings include involuntary jerking movements that appear slow, writhing, and wormlike. These movements involve the trunk, neck, face, and tongue.
        - Dystonic: Slow, twisting movements affect the trunk and extremities with abnormal posturing from muscle contractions.
      - Ataxic (Nonspastic, Extrapyramidal)
        - Evidence of wide-based gait and difficulty with coordination
        - Poor ability to do repetitive movements
        - Difficulty with quick or precise movements (writing or buttoning a shirt)
        - Shakiness
        - Low muscle tone

- ○ Diagnostic Procedures
  - ▪ Complete neurological assessment
  - ▪ MRI
    - □ Used to evaluate structures or abnormal areas located near bone, and sedation may be necessary.
    - □ Nursing Actions
      - ▸ Assist the child to remain during the procedure.
      - ▸ Sedate the child if prescribed.
    - □ Client Education
      - ▸ Provide emotional support.
  - ▪ Metabolic and genetic testing

Patient-Centered Care

- Nursing Care
  - ○ Individualize care to meet a client's needs.
  - ○ Monitor developmental milestones.
  - ○ Evaluate the need for hearing and speech evaluations.
  - ○ Promote independence with self-care activities as much as possible. Assist the client to maintain a positive self-image and a high level of self-esteem.
  - ○ Determine the extent of family coping and support.
  - ○ Assess the family's awareness of available resources.
  - ○ Assess the client's developmental level.
  - ○ Structure interventions and communications around the client's developmental level, rather than chronological age.
  - ○ Communicate with the child directly, but include parents as needed.
  - ○ Help the child to use augmented communication, such as electronic devices for speech and other types of communication tools.
  - ○ Include the family in physical care during hospitalization.
    - ▪ Ask the family about routine care, and encourage them to provide it if appropriate.
    - ▪ Encourage the family to help verify the client's needs if communication is impaired.
  - ○ Maintain an open airway by elevating the head of the child's bed. (This is especially important if the child has increased oral secretions.)
  - ○ Ensure suction equipment is available if required. Suction oral secretions as needed.
  - ○ Monitor for pain (especially with muscle spasms) using a developmentally appropriate pain tool.
  - ○ Administer medication for pain and/or spasms as prescribed.

- ○ Ensure adequate nutrition.
  - Assess for the possibility of aspiration for children who are severely disabled.
  - Determine the child's ability to take oral nutrition.
  - Ascertain the correct positioning for feeding the child. Use head positioning and manual jaw control methods as needed.
  - Provide foods that are similar to foods eaten at home when possible. Administer supplements as prescribed.
  - Administer feedings by gastric tube as prescribed.
  - Maintain weight/height chart.
  - Provide skin care.
    - □ Assess skin under splints and braces if applicable.
    - □ Maintain skin integrity by turning the child to keep pressure off bony prominences.
    - □ Keep skin clean and dry.
  - Provide rest periods as needed.
- Medications
  - ○ Baclofen (Lioresal)
    - Used as a centrally acting skeletal muscle relaxant that decreases muscle spasm and severe spasticity
    - Nursing Considerations
      - □ Administer orally or intrathecally via a specialized, surgically implanted pump.
      - □ Monitor effectiveness of the medication.
      - □ Monitor for muscle weakness, increased fatigue, or less-common adverse effects (diaphoresis, constipation).
    - Client Education
      - □ Educate the family about expected responses of medications.
      - □ Reinforce with the family the adverse effects of medications and when to call the provider.
  - ○ Diazepam (Valium)
    - Skeletal muscle relaxant used to decrease muscle spasms and severe spasticity
    - Nursing Considerations
      - □ Use in older children and adolescents.
      - □ Monitor for drowsiness and fatigue.
    - Client Education
      - □ Educate the family about expected responses to medications.
      - □ Reinforce with the family the adverse effects of the medication and when to call the provider.

- ○ Botulinum toxin A (Botox)
  - ■ Reduces spasticity in specific muscle groups
  - ■ Used primarily for client's with spasticity only in the lower extremities
  - ■ Nursing Considerations – Monitor for temporary weakness.
  - ■ Client Education – Teach the family that onset of the medication is 24 to 72 hr, with a peak of 2 weeks, lasting 3 to 6 months.
- ○ Antiepileptics
  - ■ Control seizure activity
- Teamwork and Collaboration
  - ○ Coordinate care with other professionals such as speech, physical and recreational therapists, and education and/or medical specialists.
  - ○ Initiate referral for technical aids that can assist with coordination, speaking, mobility, and an increased level of independence. This may be achieved with the use of a voice activated wheelchair.
  - ○ Surgical intervention may be needed for tendon release to correct contractures or other spastic deformities.
  - ○ Care after Discharge
    - ■ Client Education
      - □ Reinforce the therapeutic plan of care.
      - □ Reinforce the need for rest periods.
      - □ Reinforce feeding schedule and feeding techniques if changes were made during hospitalization.
      - □ Reinforce adherence to medication regimen.
      - □ Encourage regular dental care.
      - □ Encourage parents to provide developmental stimulation.
      - □ Teach wound care if needed.
      - □ Teach the family and client about ankle-foot orthoses if prescribed.
      - □ Teach self-urinary catheterization if needed.
      - □ Teach pulmonary hygiene techniques.
      - □ Coordinate interdisciplinary team with cares.
      - □ Help the family identify resources needed (respite care).
      - □ Suggest participation in a support group for CP.

Complications

- Aspiration
  - ○ Nursing Actions
    - ■ Keep the child's head elevated.
    - ■ Keep suction available if copious oral secretions are present or the child has difficulty with swallowing foods and/or fluids.
  - ○ Client Education
    - ■ Educate the family about feeding techniques to decrease the risk of aspiration.
    - ■ Encourage the family to take CPR classes.

- Potential for injury
  - Nursing Actions
    - Make sure the child's bed rails are raised to prevent falls from the bed.
    - Pad side rails and wheelchair arms to prevent injury.
    - Secure the child in mobility devices, such as wheelchairs.
    - Encourage the child to receive adequate rest to prevent injury at times of fatigue.
    - Encourage the use of helmets, seat belts, and other safety equipment.
  - Client Education
    - Educate the child and family about safety precautions.

SPINA BIFIDA

Overview

- Spinal bifida is failure of the osseous spine to close.
- Neural tube defects (NTDs) are present at birth and affect the CNS and osseous spine.
  - Spina bifida occulta – Mostly affects the lumbosacral area and is not visible
  - Spina bifida cystica – Has an visual sac protrusion
    - Meningocele – The sac contains spinal fluid and meninges.
    - Myelomeningocele – The sac includes meninges, spinal fluid, and nerves.

 View Image: Spina Bifida

Assessment

- Risk Factors
  - Medications/drugs taken during pregnancy
  - Maternal malnutrition
  - Insufficient folic acid intake during pregnancy
  - Exposure to radiation or chemicals during pregnancy
  - Prepregnancy obesity, diabetes mellitus, hyperthermia, low vitamin B_{12}
- Subjective Data
  - Assess prenatal history.
  - Assess family history for neural tube defects.

- Objective Data
  - Physical Assessment Findings
    - Protruding sac midline of the osseous spine
    - Dimpling in the lumbosacral area
  - Laboratory Tests
    - Maternal blood tests – Serum alpha-fetoprotein between 16 and 18 weeks of gestation indicate possible NTD.
    - Infant blood tests – Blood cultures to determine causative pathogen if appropriate.
  - Diagnostic Procedures
    - Prenatal
      - Ultrasound may show visual defect.
      - Amniocentesis is done following elevated alpha-fetoprotein levels to detect anencephaly or myelomeningocele.
    - Infant following birth
      - MRI, ultrasonography, and CT to evaluate spinal cord and brain

Patient-Centered Care

- Nursing Care
  - Assess for infant-parent attachment.
  - Assess the sac.
  - Perform a routine newborn assessment.
  - Assess the level of neurologic involvement.
  - Obtain accurate output measurements.
  - Assess head circumference and fontanels.
- Teamwork and Collaboration
  - Neurosurgery, neurology, urology, orthopedics, physical therapy, occupational therapy and social services
- Surgical Interventions
  - Closure of a myelomeningocele sac is done as soon as possible to prevent complications of injury and infection.
  - Nursing Actions
    - Preoperative
      - Prepare the family for surgery (within the first 24 to 48 hr after birth).
      - Protect the sac from injury.
      - Place infant in a warmer, without clothing.
      - Apply a sterile, moist, nonadhering dressing with 0.9% sodium chloride on the sac, changing it every 2 hr.

- □ Inspect the sac closely for leaks, irritation.
- □ Assess for signs of infection (fever, irritability, and lethargy).
- □ Place infant in the prone position with hips flexed, legs abducted.
- □ Administer IV antibiotic as prescribed.
- □ Avoid rectal temperatures.
- □ Avoid cuddling or putting pressure on the sac.
- Postoperative
  - □ Monitor vital signs
  - □ Monitor I&O.
  - □ Assess for signs of infection.
  - □ Provide pain management as prescribed.
  - □ Provide incision care as prescribed.
  - □ Assess for CSF leakage.
  - □ Maintain prone position until other positions are prescribed.
  - □ Resume oral feedings.
  - □ Provide range of motion (ROM) to extremities.
- Care After Discharge
  - ○ Provide teaching on postoperative care at home.
  - ○ Depending on disability teach ROM techniques.
  - ○ Ongoing care
    - Assess head circumference.
    - Assess skin integrity.
    - Assess for allergies such as latex allergy.
    - Assess cognitive development.
    - Assess bladder and bowl functioning.
    - Assess motor development.
    - Monitor for infections.
    - Address body image concerns.
    - Offer support to the family.
    - Assist the client with independence through lifespan.
    - Assist the family with obtaining medical equipment/services needed at home.

Complications

- Skin ulceration
  - Caused by prolonged pressure in one area
  - Nursing Actions
    - Monitor skin for breakdown.
    - Reposition frequently to prevent pressure on bony prominences.
    - Monitor skin under splints and braces.
  - Client Education
    - Teach the child and parents to monitor skin integrity.
- Latex allergy
  - The child may have a high risk of allergy to latex. Allergy responses range from urticaria to wheezing, which may progress to anaphylaxis. There also may be an allergy to certain foods (bananas, avocados, kiwi, and chestnuts).
  - Nursing Actions
    - Assist with testing for allergy.
    - Reduce exposure.
  - Client Education
    - Educate the parents to avoid exposing the child to latex.
    - Provide the family with a list of household items that may contain latex (disposable diapers, cleaning or kitchen gloves, elastic found in clothing).
    - Educate the family about how to identify signs and symptoms of allergic reaction and report them to the provider.
    - Provide instruction about the use of epinephrine (EpiPen).
- Increased intracranial pressure
  - Caused by shunt malfunction or hydrocephalus.
  - Prepare for surgery for shunt or shunt revision.
  - Clinical manifestations
    - Infants – high-pitched cry, lethargy, vomiting, bulging fontanels, and/or widening cranial suture lines, increase head circumference
    - Children – headache, lethargy, nausea, vomiting, double vision, decreased school performance of learned tasks, decreased level of consciousness, seizures
    - Nursing Actions
      - Use gentle movements when performing ROM exercises.
      - Minimize environmental stressors (noise, frequent visitors).
      - Assess and manage pain.
    - Client Education
      - Teach the clinical manifestation of shunt malfunction and hydrocephalus and when to notify the provider.

- Bladder issues
  - May be performed to manage bladder dysfunction (either spasms or flaccidity)
  - Nursing Actions
    - Monitor for signs of bladder dysfunction.
    - Monitor for signs of bladder infection.
    - Monitor for bleeding.
    - Prepare the family and client for surgery if needed.
    - Teach the child and family care of stoma (vesicostomy) if applicable.
- Orthopedic issues
  - Corrections of associated potential problems, such as clubfoot, scoliosis, and other malformations of the feet and legs
  - Nursing Actions
    - Monitor for signs of infection.
    - Administer pain medications.
    - Prepare the family and client for surgery if needed.
    - Provide cast care if cast is present.
    - Monitor for neurosensory deficits.
  - Client Education
    - Educate the family about signs and symptoms of infection.
    - Educate the family about cast and splint care if indicated.

DOWN SYNDROME

Overview

- Down syndrome is a chromosomal abnormality.
- Many medical conditions accompany Down syndrome (congenital heart malformation, hypotonicity, dysfunction of the immune system, thyroid dysfunction, leukemia).

Assessment

- Risk Factors
  - Maternal age greater than 35
- Objective Data
  - Physical Assessment Findings
    - Separated sagittal suture
    - Enlarged anterior fontanel
    - Small round head

- Flattened forehead
- Upward, outward slant to eyes
- Small nose with depressed nasal bridge
- Small ears with short pinna
- High-arched narrow palate
- Protruding tongue
- Short, broad neck
- Shortened rib cage
- Possible congenital heart defect
- Protruding abdomen
- Broad, short feet and hands with stubby toes and fingers
- Transverse palmar crease
- Large space between big and second toes with plantar crease
- Short stature
- Hyperflexibility and hypotonia

○ Diagnostic Procedures
  - Prenatal – testing for alpha-fetoprotein in maternal serum
  - Infant – chromosome analysis and echocardiography

Patient-Centered Care

- Nursing Care
  ○ Support family at the time of diagnosis.
  ○ Make appropriate referrals.
  ○ Assist the parents in holding and bonding with the infant.
  ○ Manage secretions and prevention of upper respiratory infections.
- Surgical Interventions – depend on the associated congenital anomalies. These may include cardiac defects or strabismus.
- Teamwork and Collaboration
  ○ Social work, home health, school early intervention, genetic counseling, speech therapy, physical therapy, occupational therapy
  ○ Nursing Actions
    - Listen to concerns of the parents and discuss ethical dilemmas regarding treatment for physical defects.
    - Provide standard postoperative care with emphasis on wound care, respiratory care, and pain management.
  ○ Client Education
    - Teach postoperative and home-care management.
    - Reinforce the therapeutic plan of care.

- Ongoing Care
  - Teach the family how to aspirate nasal secretions.
  - Teach the family to rinse the mouth after feedings.
  - Teach the family to use cool mist in the room to assist in moistening secretions.
  - Encourage the family to change the infant's position frequently.
  - Teach the family pulmonary hygiene by performing postural drainage with percussion.
  - Teach the family feeding strategies to accommodate for the protruding tongue.
  - Teach the family skin care and the need for moisturizing creams daily.
  - Encourage a diet high in fiber and fluid to prevent constipation, and monitor calorie intake to prevent obesity.
  - Encourage regular health care visits.
  - Monitor developmental milestones.
  - Monitor height and weight by plotting growth on a Down syndrome growth chart.
  - Prepare for surgery for cardiac problems or strabismus if indicated.
  - Evaluate eyesight and hearing frequently.
  - Perform frequent thyroid functioning tests.
  - Assess for atlantoaxial instability (neck pain, weakness, and torticollis).
  - Teach the family how to prevent complications.

Complications

- Respiratory infections
  - Respiratory infections are common due to decreased muscle tone and poor drainage of mucus because of hypotonicity and associated underdeveloped nasal bone.
  - Nursing Actions
    - Rinse the child's mouth with water after feeding and at other times of the day when it is dry. Mucous membranes are dry due to constant mouth breathing, which also increases the risk for respiratory infection.
    - Provide cool mist humidification and clearing of the nasal passages with a bulb syringe as needed.
    - Encourage exercise in older children.
  - Client Education
    - Teach the parents and child good hand hygiene. Encourage frequent repositioning of the child to promote respiratory function.
    - Teach parents to perform postural drainage and percussion if needed.
    - Reinforce the need for routine immunizations.
    - Teach parents to seek health care at the earliest sign of infection.
    - Reinforce the need to follow the antibiotic schedule if prescribed.

JUVENILE IDIOPATHIC ARTHRITIS (JIA)

Overview

- Juvenile idiopathic arthritis (JIA) is a chronic autoimmune inflammatory disease affecting joints and other tissues.
- The chronic inflammation of the synovium of the joints leads to wearing down and damage to the articular cartilage.
- JIA is rarely life-threatening, and it may subside over time, but it can result in residual joint deformities and altered joint function.
- There are multiple classifications of JIA with or without a rheumatoid factor.

Assessment

- Risk Factors
  - Immunogenic susceptibility
  - Environmental triggers
- Subjective and Objective Data
  - Physical Assessment Findings
    - Joint swelling, stiffness, redness, and warmth that tend to be worse in the morning or after naps
    - Mobility limitations
    - Fever
    - Rash
    - Limp in the morning
    - Enlarged lymph nodes
    - Delayed growth
  - Laboratory Tests
    - Anticyclic citrullinated peptide (anti-CCP) antibodies can be detected before symptoms of disease occur.
    - Erythrocyte sedimentation rate (ESR) may or may not be elevated.
    - CBC with differential may demonstrate elevated WBCs, especially during exacerbations.
    - Antinuclear antibodies (ANA) indicate an increased risk for uveitis.
    - Rheumatoid factor is rarely detected in children.
  - Diagnostic Procedures
    - Radiographic studies may be used for baseline comparison. X-rays may demonstrate increased synovial fluid in the joint, which causes soft tissue swelling or widening of the joint. Later findings may include osteoporosis and narrowed joint spaces.
    - Slit lamp eye examination is used to diagnosis uveitis.

Patient-Centered Care

- Nursing Care

  - Care is primarily in an outpatient setting.

  - Assist the client with an exercise program.

  - Teach the client relaxation techniques and nonpharmacological pain management.

  - Evaluate the child's pain and response to prescribed analgesics.

  - Encourage a support group.

  - Encourage the child to participate in a physical therapy program to increase mobility and prevent deformities.

  - Encourage activity as tolerated.

  - Teach parents to apply splints for nighttime sleep. Splints should be applied to knees, wrists, and hands to decrease pain and prevent flexion deformities.

  - Encourage proper positioning with sleep. Encourage the use of electric blankets or sleeping bags for extra warmth.

  - Provide firm mattress and discourage use of pillows under knees. Use no pillow or flat pillow for head.

  - Encourage full ROM exercises.

  - Apply heat or warm moist packs to the child's affected joints prior to exercise.

  - Encourage warm baths.

  - Identify alternate ways for the child to meet developmental needs, especially during periods of exacerbation.

  - Encourage self-care by allowing adequate time for completion.

  - Encourage a well-balanced diet with adequate fluid intake.

  - Encourage participation in school and contact with peers.

  - Collaborate with the school nurse and teachers to arrange for care during the school day (medication administration, rest periods, extra time to get to classes, extra sets of books, split days).

  - Teach the family that exacerbation worsens with illnesses.

  - Teach the family about routine follow up with provider and regular eye exams.

- Medications

  - Nonsteroidal anti-inflammatory medications (NSAIDs)

    - Ibuprofen (Motrin), naproxen (Naprelan), and tolmetin (Tolectin)

    - Control pain and inflammation

    - Nursing Considerations

      - Instruct the child and family to administer NSAIDs as prescribed.

      - Instruct the child and family that NSAIDs should be taken with food to minimize gastric irritation.

- Client Education
  - Teach the child and family to report changes in stool and GI discomfort or increase in bruising immediately.
- Methotrexate (Rheumatrex)
  - A cytotoxic disease-modifying antirheumatic drug (DMARD) that slows joint degeneration and progression of rheumatoid arthritis when NSAIDs do not work alone
  - Nursing Considerations
    - ▸ Monitor liver function tests and CBC regularly.
  - Client Education
    - ▸ Teach adolescents to avoid alcohol.
    - ▸ Discuss the use of effective birth control to avoid birth defects while taking this medication.
- Corticosteroids: prednisone (Deltasone)
  - Provide symptomatic relief of inflammation and pain. They are reserved for life-threatening complications, severe arthritis, and uveitis.
  - Nursing Considerations
    - ▸ Administer as eye solution, orally, or IV. An injection into the intra-articular space may provide effective pain relief.
    - ▸ Administer at the lowest effective dose for short-term therapy and then discontinue by tapering the dose.
  - Client Education
    - ▸ Advise the child and family that weight gain, especially in the face, is a common adverse effect.
    - ▸ Monitor height and weight.
    - ▸ Advise the family that an alteration in growth is a possible long-term complication of corticosteroids.
    - ▸ Advise the child to avoid exposure to potentially infectious agents.
    - ▸ Advise the child and family to practice healthy eating habits.
  - Etanercept (Enbrel)
    - Etanercept is a tumor necrosis factor alpha-receptor blocker, another DMARD, that is used when methotrexate is not effective for immunosuppressive action.
    - Nursing Considerations
      - Administer etanercept once or twice each week by subcutaneous injection.
    - Client Education
      - Educate about the potential for allergic reactions.
      - Teach the child and family to avoid exposure to infectious agents.
- Teamwork and Collaboration
  - Physical therapist, occupational therapist, ophthalmologist, dentist, dietitian, social worker, school nurse

Complications

- Joint deformity and functional disability
  - Nursing Actions
    - Reinforce the individualized therapeutic plan of care.
    - Advocate for the child when treatments are not producing expected results.
  - Client Education
    - Encourage the child and family to adhere to the treatment regimen.
    - Encourage self-care and active participation in an exercise program.

MUSCULAR DYSTROPHY (MD)

Overview

- Muscular dystrophy (MD) is a group of inherited disorders with progressive degeneration of symmetric skeletal muscle groups.
- Onset of disease, pace of progression, and muscle group affected depend on the type of MD.
  - Duchenne (pseudohypertrophic) muscular dystrophy (DMD) is the most common form of MD. Inherited as an X-linked recessive trait, DMD has an onset between 3 and 7 years of age. Progressive disease with life expectancy with current technology for DMD reaches into early adulthood.
  - Facioscapulohumeral muscular dystrophy is an autosomal dominant inherited disorder. Progression is slow with normal life span.
  - Limb-girdle muscular dystrophy (LGMD) is an autosomal dominant and recessive, heterogeneous disorder. It appears later in childhood with a slow progression.

DUCHENNE MUSCULAR DYSTROPHY (DMD)

Assessment

- Risk Factors
  - Family genetic history
- Subjective and Objective Data
  - Physical Assessment Findings
    - Fatigue
    - Muscle weakness beginning in the lower extremities
    - Unsteady gait, with a waddle
    - Lordosis
    - Delayed motor skill development

- Frequent falling
- Difficulty getting out of bed, rising from a seated position, or climbing stairs
- Learning difficulties
- Mild cognitive delays that do not worsen with disease
- Progressive difficulty walking with possible loss of ability to walk by the age of 12 years
- Progressive muscle atrophy
- Respiratory and cardiac difficulties usually start by age 20

○ Laboratory Tests
- Serum polymerase chain reaction (PCR) to detect the dystrophin gene mutation
- Serum creatine kinase (CK) – elevated and can be elevated prior to clinical manifestations

○ Diagnostic Procedures
- Muscle biopsy
- EMG

Patient-Centered Care

- Nursing Care
  - ○ Encourage and provide for genetic counseling.
  - ○ Assess and monitor:
    - The child's ability to perform ADLs.
    - The child's respiratory function, including depth, rhythm, and rate of respirations during sleep and daytime hours.
    - The child's cardiac function.
    - The child and parent's understanding of long-term effects.
    - The child and parent's coping and support.
  - ○ Maintain optimal physical function for as long possible.
    - Encourage the child to be independent for as long as possible and to perform ADLs.
    - Perform ROM exercises and provide appropriate physical activity. Include stretching exercises, strength and muscle training, and breathing exercises.
    - Maintain proper body alignment and encourage the child to reposition self frequently to avoid skin breakdown.
    - Assist with splints and braces as prescribed.
  - ○ Maintain respiratory functioning.
    - Encourage the use of incentive spirometry.
    - Position the child to enhance expansion of lungs.
    - Teach the client how to use a mechanical cough device.
    - Provide oxygen as prescribed.
    - Provide noninvasive ventilation as prescribed.

- ○ Encourage adequate fluid intake.
- ○ Monitor and encourage adequate nutritional intake.
- ○ Encourage routine physical exams and immunizations.
- ○ Facilitate discussion of end-of-life decisions when appropriate.
- • Medications
  - ○ Corticosteroids – prednisone (Deltasone)
    - ▪ Increases muscle strength
    - ▪ Nursing Considerations
      - □ Monitor for infection.
      - □ Monitor for adverse effects.
    - ▪ Client Education
      - □ Instruct the child and parents to avoid potentially infectious agents.
      - □ Teach the child and family to practice healthy eating habits.
      - □ Teach the family about adverse effects and when to notify the provider.
  - ○ Other medications can include bronchodilators, amino acids, vitamins, and mineral supplements.
- • Teamwork and Collaboration
  - ○ Neurologist; genetic counselor; physical, occupational, and respiratory therapists; dietitian; social worker; school teacher.
  - ○ Encourage parents to consider assistance with care as disease progresses (respite care, long-term care, and home-health care).
  - ○ Refer the child and parents to support groups for MD.
- • Surgical Interventions
  - ○ Surgery may be indicated for release or repair of contractures or for insertion of a gastrostomy tube or tracheostomy.

Complications

- • Respiratory compromise
  - ○ Respiratory muscles unable the child to maintain adequate respirations
  - ○ Nursing Actions
    - ▪ Help the child turn hourly or more frequently.
    - ▪ Have the child use deep breathing and coughing.
    - ▪ Suction as needed.
    - ▪ Administer oxygen as prescribed.
    - ▪ Use intermittent positive pressure ventilation and mechanically-assisted cough devices if indicated.
    - ▪ Administer antibiotics as prescribed.
  - ○ Client Education
    - ▪ Discuss mechanical ventilation options with the child and parents.

APPLICATION EXERCISES

1. A nurse is caring for a child who has cerebral palsy. Which of the following medications should the nurse expect to administer to treat painful muscle spasms? (Select all that apply.)

_____ A. Baclofen (Lioresal)

_____ B. Diazepam (Valium)

_____ C. Oxybutynin chloride (Ditropan)

_____ D. Methotrexate (Rheumatrex)

_____ E. Prednisone (Deltasone)

2. A nurse is caring for a school-age child who has juvenile idiopathic arthritis. Which of the following are appropriate home care instructions? (Select all that apply.)

_____ A. Sleep on a firm mattress.

_____ B. Use cold compresses for joint pain.

_____ C. Take ibuprofen (Motrin) on an empty stomach.

_____ D. Take frequent rest periods throughout the day.

_____ E. Perform range-of-motion exercises.

3. A nurse is teaching a group of parents about possible manifestations of Down syndrome. Which of the following should she include in the teaching? (Select all that apply.)

_____ A. A large head with bulging fontanelles

_____ B. Larger ears that are set back

_____ C. Protruding abdomen

_____ D. Broad, short feet and hands

_____ E. Hypotonia

4. A nurse is caring for a child who has muscular dystrophy. For which of the following findings should the nurse assess? (Select all that apply.)

_____ A. Purposeless, involuntary, abnormal movements

_____ B. Spinal defect and saclike protrusion

_____ C. Muscular weakness in lower extremities

_____ D. Unsteady, wide-based or waddling gait

_____ E. Upward slant to the eyes

5. A nurse is caring for an infant who has a myelomeningocele. Which of the following should she include in the plan of care?

   A. Assist the mother with breastfeeding.

   B. Assess the infant's temperature rectally.

   C. Place the infant in a supine position.

   D. Apply a moist dressing on the sac.

6. A nurse is caring for a child who has a new prescription for baclofen (Lioresal). Use the ATI Active Learning Template: Medication to complete this item to include the following sections:

   A. Therapeutic Uses

   B. Nursing Administration

   C. Adverse Effects

   D. Client Education

APPLICATION EXERCISES KEY

1. A. **CORRECT:** Baclofen is a centrally acting skeletal muscle relaxant that decreases muscle spasm and severe spasticity.

    B. **CORRECT:** Diazepam is a skeletal muscle relaxant that decreases muscle spasms and severe spasticity.

    C. INCORRECT: Oxybutynin chloride is an antispasmodic, anticholinergic medication that decreases bladder spasms.

    D. INCORRECT: Methotrexate is a cytotoxic disease-modifying antirheumatic drug (DMARD) that slows joint degeneration and progression of rheumatoid arthritis. It is used for children with juvenile idiopathic arthritis (JIA).

    E. INCORRECT: Prednisone is a corticosteroid that increases muscle strength for children with muscular dystrophy. It decreases inflammation in children with JIA.

    Ⓝ NCLEX® Connection: Pharmacological and Parenteral Therapies, Expected Actions/Outcomes

2. A. **CORRECT:** A firm mattress can help prevent joint deformities and maintain body alignment.

    B. INCORRECT: Using a warm compresses or moist packs can provide comfort and relieve stiffness.

    C. INCORRECT: Ibuprofen should be taken with food to prevent GI distress.

    D. **CORRECT:** Frequent rest periods are necessary to conserve energy.

    E. **CORRECT:** Range of motion will assist in maintaining function of the joints.

    Ⓝ NCLEX® Connection: Physiological Adaptations, Alterations in Body Systems

3. A. INCORRECT: A child with hydrocephalus will exhibit a large head with bulging fontanelles because of the increased CSF in the head.

    B. INCORRECT: A child with Down syndrome will exhibit small features such as small ears with a short pinna.

    C. **CORRECT:** A child with Down syndrome will exhibit small features such as short stature. The child will exhibit a protruding abdomen.

    D. **CORRECT:** A child with Down syndrome will exhibit small features such as broad, short feet and hands.

    E. **CORRECT:** A child with Down syndrome will exhibit hyperflexibility and hypotonia.

    Ⓝ NCLEX® Connection: Physiological Adaptations, Pathophysiology

4. A. INCORRECT: A child who has cerebral palsy exhibit purposeless, involuntary, abnormal movements.

    B. INCORRECT: An infant who has the spinal defect myelomeningocele will exhibit a saclike protrusion.

    C. **CORRECT:** A child with MD will exhibit muscular weakness in the lower extremities as one of the first clinical signs.

    D. **CORRECT:** A child with MD will exhibit an unsteady, wide-based, or waddling gait because of the progressive muscle weakness.

    E. INCORRECT: A child with Down syndrome may exhibit an upward slant to the eyes.

    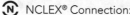 NCLEX® Connection: Physiological Adaptations, Alterations in Body Systems

5. A. INCORRECT: Breastfeeding could cause pressure on the sac, which could cause rupture. This should not be in the plan of care.

    B. INCORRECT: Rectal temperatures could cause irritation or rectal prolapse. This should not be in the plan of care.

    C. INCORRECT: Placing the infant in supine position could cause pressure on the sac, which could cause rupture. This should not be in the plan of care.

    D. **CORRECT:** A sterile, moist, nonadhering dressing is placed on the sac to keep it moist until surgery. This should be in the plan of care.

    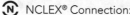 NCLEX® Connection: Physiological Adaptations, Illness Management

6. *Using the ATI Active Learning Template: Medication*

    A. Therapeutic Uses
        *   Used as a centrally acting skeletal muscle relaxant that decreases muscle spasm and severe spasticity.

    B. Nursing Administration
        *   Administer orally or intrathecally via a specialized, surgically implanted pump.
        *   Monitor effectiveness of the medication.

    C. Adverse Effects
        *   Muscle weakness
        *   Increased fatigue
        *   Less-common adverse effects (diaphoresis, constipation)

    D. Client Education
        *   Educate the family about expected responses of medications.
        *   Reinforce with the family the adverse effects of medications and when to call the provider.

    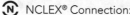 NCLEX® Connection: Pharmacological and Parenteral Therapies, Medication Administration

UNIT 2 ## Nursing Care of Children with System Disorders

SECTION: INTEGUMENTARY DISORDERS

› Skin Infections and Infestations
› Dermatitis and Acne
› Burns

NCLEX® CONNECTIONS

When reviewing the chapters in this unit, keep in mind the relevant sections of the NCLEX® outline, in particular:

Client Needs: Pharmacological and Parenteral Therapies

› Relevant topics/tasks include:
  » Dosage Calculation
    › Perform calculations needed for medication administration.
  » Parenteral/Intravenous Therapy
    › Apply knowledge and concepts of mathematics/ nursing procedures/ psychomotor skills when caring for a client receiving intravenous and parenteral therapy.
  » Pharmacological Pain Management
    › Assess the client's need for administration of a PRN pain medication.

Client Needs: Reduction of Risk Potential

› Relevant topics/tasks include:
  » Changes/Abnormalities in Vital Signs
    › Apply knowledge of client pathophysiology when measuring vital signs.
  » Laboratory Values
    › Recognize deviations from normal for values of albumin, ALT, AST, ammonia, bilirubin, bleeding time, calcium, cholesterol, digoxin, ESR, lithium, magnesium, phosphorous/phosphate, protein, urine.
  » Potential for Complications of Diagnostic Tests/ Treatments/Procedures
    › Evaluate responses to procedures and treatments.

Client Needs: Physiological Adaptation

› Relevant topics/tasks include:
  » Alterations in Body Systems
    › Provide care for the client with an infectious disease.
  » Fluid and Electrolyte Imbalances
    › Apply knowledge of pathophysiology when caring for the client with fluid and electrolyte imbalances.
  » Medical Emergencies
    › Apply knowledge of nursing procedures and psychomotor skills when caring for a client experiencing a medical emergency.

chapter 30

Overview

- Skin infections can be bacterial, viral, or fungal.
- Arthropod bites and stings can be due to flies, mosquitoes, chiggers, bees, fire ants, mites, ticks, spiders, and scorpions.
- Skin infestations include scabies and lice.

SKIN INFECTION

Overview

- Bacterial infections include impetigo contagiosa, pyoderma, folliculitis, furuncle, carbuncle, cellulitis, and staphylococcal scalded skin syndrome.
- Viral infections include verruca, verruca plantaris, herpes simplex virus, varicella-zoster virus, and molluscum contagiosum.
- Fungal infections include tinea capitis, tinea corporis, tinea cruris, tinea pedis, and candidiasis.

Assessment

- Risk Factors
  - Bacterial
    - Congenital or acquired immunodeficiency disorders
    - Immunosuppression
    - Generalized malignancy
  - Viral
    - Contact with infected person
  - Fungal
    - Geographic area
- Subjective Data
  - History of causative agent/exposure

- Objective Data
  - History of causative agent/exposure

BACTERIAL INFECTION/CAUSATIVE AGENTS CLINICAL MANIFESTATIONS

Impetigo contagiosa – *Staphylococcus*

› Reddish macule becomes vesicular	› Spreads peripherally and by direct contact
› Erupts easily leaving moist erosion on the skin, dries leaving crusty secretions	› Pruritus common

Pyoderma – *Staphylococcus, Streptococcus*

› Deeper infection into the dermis	› Possible systemic effects (fever, lymphangitis)

Folliculitis (pimple) – *Staphylococcus aureus*

› Infection of a hair follicle

Furuncle (boil) – *Staphylococcus aureus*

› Larger swollen, red lesion of a single hair follicle

Carbuncle (multiple boils) – *Staphylococcus aureus*

› More extensive swollen, red lesions involving multiple hair follicles

Cellulitis – Streptococcus, *Staphylococcus, Haemophilus influenzae*

› Firm, swollen, red area of the skin and subcutaneous tissue	› Possible systemic effects (fever, malaise)

Staphylococcal scalded skin syndrome – *Staphylococcus aureus*

› Rough-textured skin with macular erythema	› Epidermis becomes wrinkled within 2 days with large bullae appearing

VIRAL INFECTION/CAUSATIVE AGENTS CLINICAL MANIFESTATIONS

Verruca (warts) – Human papillomavirus

› Elevated, rough, gray-brown firm papules	› Can be single or in groups
› Can occur anywhere on the skin	

Verruca plantaris (plantar warts)

› Flat warts on the plantar surface of the feet	› Possibly surrounded by hyperkeratosis

Herpes simplex virus – Type I: cold sore, fever blister; Type II: genital

› Near a mucocutaneous area (lips, nose, buttock, genitalia)	› After drying, form a crusty area followed by exfoliation
› Group of vesicles that itch and burn	› Healing occurs in 8 to 10 days
	› Possible lymphadenopathy

Varicella-zoster virus (herpes zoster, shingles)

› Neurologic pain, hyperesthesias, or itching	› Same virus as chicken pox

Molluscum contagiosum (pox virus)

› Asymptomatic flesh-colored papules on stalks

FUNGAL INFECTION/CAUSATIVE AGENTS CLINICAL MANIFESTATIONS	
Tinea capitis – *Trichophyton tonsurans, Microsporum audouinii, Microsporum canis*	
› Scaly, circumscribed lesion with alopecia on the scalp	
Tinea corporis – *Trichophyton rubrum, Trichophyton mentagrophytes, Microsporum canis*	
› Round erythematous scaling patch	› Spreads peripherally and clears centrally
Tinea cruris (jock itch) – *Epidermophyton floccosum, Trichophyton rubrum, Trichophyton mentagrophytes*	
› Medial and proximal aspect of the thigh and crural folds › May include the scrotum	› Pruritic › Round erythematous scaling patch › Spreads peripherally and clears centrally
Tinea pedis (athlete's foot) – *Trichophyton rubrum, Trichophyton interdigitale, Epidermophyton floccosum*	
› Between toes or on the plantar surface of the feet	› Maceration and fissuring lesions between the toes and patches with tiny vesicles on the plantar surface of the foot
Candidiasis (moniliasis) – *Candida albicans*	
› Found in moist areas of the skin surface › White exudate, peeling inflamed areas that bleed easily	› Pruritic

- ○ Laboratory Tests
  - Cultures (bacterial, viral, fungal)

Patient-Centered Care

- Nursing Care
  - ○ Assess the general condition of the affected area.
  - ○ Assess for evidence of associated infection.
  - ○ Assist in preventing the child to itch or touch the affected areas.

BACTERIAL INFECTION/CAUSATIVE AGENTS MANAGEMENT

Impetigo contagiosa – *Staphylococcus*

› Use compresses of 1:20 aluminum acetate in water (Burow's solution) to remove crusted exudate.	› Use topical antibacterial ointment › Oral or parenteral antibiotics for severe cases

Pyoderma – *Staphylococcus, Streptococcus*

› Cleanse with soap and water › Apply wet compresses › Bathe using antibacterial soap	› Launder washcloths and towels to prevent bacterial spread › Apply mupirocin (Bactroban) to lesions as prescribed › Systemic antibiotics, as prescribed in severe cases

Folliculitis (pimple) – *Staphylococcus aureus*
Furuncle (boil) – *Staphylococcus aureus*
Carbuncle (multiple boils) – *Staphylococcus aureus*

› Apply warm moist compresses › Clean skin often › Topical antibiotic medications	› Systemic antibiotics for severe cases › Incision, draining, and irrigation of severe lesions

Cellulitis – *Streptococcus, Staphylococcus, Haemophilus influenzae*

› Oral or parenteral antibiotics, as prescribed › Rest and immobilize affected area	› Apply warm, moist compresses

Staphylococcal scalded skin syndrome – *Staphylococcus aureus*

› Use systemic antibiotics	› Gentle cleansing with saline, Burow's solution, or 0.25% silver nitrate compresses

VIRAL INFECTION/CAUSATIVE AGENTS MANAGEMENT

Verruca (warts) – Human papillomavirus

› Individualized destructive therapy such as surgical removal, electrocautery, cryotherapy, laser

Verruca plantaris (plantar warts)

› Caustic solution applied to wart › Wear insoles with holes to decrease pressure for 2 to 3 days	› Soak affected area for 20 min › Repeat treatment until wart falls off

Herpes simplex virus – Type I: cold sore, fever blister; Type II: genital

› Apply Burow's solution during weeping stage › Apply penciclovir (Denavir) cream to oral lesion	› Oral antiviral (acyclovir) to reduce duration › Oral antiviral (valacyclovir) for genital herpes

Varicella-zoster virus (herpes zoster, shingles)

› Use oral or topical analgesics › Apply moist compresses	› Oral antiviral (acyclovir)

Molluscum contagiosum (pox virus)

› Resolves spontaneously in 18 months	› Complicated cases: remove pox

FUNGAL INFECTION/CAUSATIVE AGENTS MANAGEMENT	
Tinea capitis – *Trichophyton tonsurans, Microsporum audouinii, Microsporum canis*	
› Use of selenium sulfide shampoos	› Complicated cases: oral ketoconazole
› Topical antifungal medications (clotrimazole)	› Treat infected pets, if necessary
› Oral griseofulvin	
Candidiasis (moniliasis) – *Candida albicans*	
› Topical antifungal ointment (Amphotericin B, nystatin)	
Tinea corporis – *Trichophyton rubrum, Trichophyton mentagrophytes, Microsporum canis* **Tinea cruris (jock itch)** – *Epidermophyton floccosum, Trichophyton rubrum, Trichophyton mentagrophytes* **Tinea pedis (athlete's foot)** – *Trichophyton rubrum, Trichophyton interdigitale, Epidermophyton floccosum*	
› Oral griseofulvin	› Wear light-colored socks, well-ventilated shoes
› Topical antifungal (tolnaftate, clotrimazole)	› Treat infected pets (Tinea corporis)
› Apply wet compresses or take sitz bath	

- Client Teaching
  - Teach client and family how to avoid the spread of infections.
    - Use appropriate hand hygiene.
    - Avoid sharing clothing, hats, combs, brushes, and/or towels.
    - Keep the child from touching the affected area by using distraction.
    - Do not squeeze vesicles.
    - Apply topical medications as prescribed.
    - Administer oral medications as prescribed.

ARTHROPOD BITES AND STINGS

Overview

- Scorpions, black widow, and brown recluse spiders inject venom that requires immediate attention.

Assessment

- Risk Factors
  - Geographic area
- Assessment Data
  - Subjective Data
    - History of causative agent/exposure

○ Objective Data

CAUSATIVE AGENT	CLINICAL MANIFESTATIONS
Mosquitoes, fleas, flies	› Variable, from no reaction to hypersensitivity reaction › Papular urticaria › Firm papules
Bees, wasps, hornets, fire ants, yellow jackets	› Local reaction: small red itchy wheal that is warm to the touch › Systemic reaction: mild to severe – generalized edema, pain, nausea and vomiting, confusion, respiratory problems, and shock
Chiggers	› Bites on warm parts of the body › Variable, from no reaction to hypersensitivity reaction › Papular urticaria › Firm papules
Ticks	› Attaches to the skin with head embedded › Firm, discrete, pruritic nodule at site › Possible urticaria or persistent localized edema
Brown recluse spiders	› Mild sting leads to transient erythema and to blister › Pain 2 to 8 hr following bite › Star-shaped purple area in 3 to 4 days › Necrotic ulceration in 7 to 14 days
Black widow spiders	› Mild sting leads to swollen, painful, and erythematous site › Dizziness, weakness, and abdominal pain › Possible delirium, paralysis, seizures, and death
Scorpions	› Intense pain › Erythema, burning, numbness › Restlessness and vomiting › Ascending paralysis: seizures, weakness, increase in pulse, thirst, salivation, dysuria, pulmonary edema leading to coma and death › Death for children less than age 4 in the first 24 hr

Lyme disease (tick infected with *Borrelia burgdorferi*)	› May appear in any of these stages:
	» Stage 1:
	  › 3 to 31 days following bite – erythema migrans at site
	  › Chills, fever, itching, headache, fainting, stiff neck, muscle weakness; bull's eye rash at the site of the bite
	» Stage 2: systematic involvement begins (neurologic, cardiac and musculoskeletal); occurs several weeks following bite
	  › Paralysis or weakness in the face, muscle pain, swelling in large joints (knees), heart problems
	» Stage 3: systemic involvement is advanced (musculoskeletal pain that includes the muscles, tendons, bursae and synovia); possible arthritis, deafness and encephalopathy.
	  › Abnormal muscle movement and weakness, numbness and tingling, speech problems

- Patient-Centered Care
  - Nursing Care

CAUSATIVE AGENT	MANAGEMENT
Mosquitoes, fleas, flies	› Use antipruritic agent › Administer oral and topical antihistamines › Baths
Bees, wasps, hornets, fire ants, yellow jackets	› Remove the stinger › Cleanse with soap and water › Apply cool compresses › Apply home products (baking soda, lemon juice) › Administer topical and oral antihistamines › Epinephrine and corticosteroids for severe cases
Chiggers	› Systemic steroids for severe cases
Ticks	› Remove by pulling straight up with steady, even pressure with tweezers to remove the tick › Remove any remaining parts using a sterile needle › Cleanse site with soap and disinfectant
Brown recluse spiders	› Apply cool compresses › Administer antibiotic, corticosteroids › Analgesic for pain › Possible skin graft
Black widow spiders	› Cleanse bite with antiseptic › Apply cool compresses › Administer antivenom › Administer muscle relaxant
Scorpions	› Position site in dependant position › Keep child calm › Administer antivenom › Analgesic for pain › Admit to intensive care unit
Lyme disease (tick infected with *Borrelia burgdorferi*)	› Observe clients bitten by a tick for 30 days › Antibiotic (single dose) for clients who meet criteria › Antibiotic (2- to 3-week course) for clients who have confirmed disease › Doxycycline for children older than 8 years and amoxicillin for children under 8 years; cefuroxime or erythromycin for children who have an allergy to penicillin

- Client Teaching
  - Prevent secondary infections.
  - Wear medical alert bracelet for severe reactions.
  - Inspect skin after possible exposure.
  - Prevent bites.
    - Avoid areas of tall grass.
    - Use insect repellent.
    - Avoid contact with insects.
    - Avoid wood piles.
    - Inspect and treat pets, carpets, and furniture.
    - Avoid flowery prints and bright clothing.
    - Avoid perfumes and colognes.

SKIN INFESTATIONS

Overview

- Scabies mite, *Sarcoptes scabiei*, is spread by direct contact with an infected person. The mite burrows into the skin and lay eggs. The eggs mature in 21 days.
- Pediculosis capitis (head lice), *Pediculus humanus capitis*, is spread by direct contact with an infected person, bedding, and clothing. The life span of the adult louse life is 1 month and they can live up to 48 hr without a human host. The female lays eggs at night, close to the skin surface and at the junction of the hair shaft. The nits hatch in 7 to 10 days.
- Pediculosis corporis (body lice), *Pediculus humanus corporis*, is spread by direct contact with an infected person, bedding, and clothing. The adult louse feeds on human blood and can live in folds of clothing for 1 month. They die at room temperature in 5 to 7 days.

Assessment

- Risk Factors
  - Scabies: nursing homes, nursing facilities, and day care settings
  - Head lice: day care and schools; overcrowded conditions; sharing of combs, brushes, or hats
  - Body lice: overcrowded conditions and poor hygiene
  - Pubic lice: multiple sex partners

- Assessment Data
  - ○ Subjective Data
    - ▪ Itching
  - ○ Objective Data

CAUSATIVE AGENT	CLINICAL MANIFESTATIONS
Scabies mite – Sarcoptes scabiei	› Itchy, especially at night
	› Rash, especially between fingers
	› Thin, pencil marks lines on the skin
	› Infants:
	» Widespread on the body
	» Pimples on the trunk
	» Blisters on the palms of the hands and soles of the feet
	› Young children: Most common on head, neck, shoulders, palms, and soles
	› Older Children: Most common on hands, wrists, genitals, and abdomen
Pediculosis capitis (head lice) – *Pediculus humanus capitis*	› Intense itching
	› Small, red bumps on the scalp
	› Nits (white specks) on the hair shaft
Pediculosis corporis (body lice) – *Pediculus humanus corporis*	› Intense itching, worse around the waist, under the arms and anywhere clothing is tight
	› Red bumps on the skin
	› Changes in skin if lice have been present for extended period
Pediculosis pubis (pubic lice) – *Pediculus humanus pubis*	› Intense itching
	› Bluish-gray skin
	› Sores

  - ○ Diagnostic tests
    - ▪ Scabies: examination under a microscope or skin biopsy
- Patient-Centered Care
  - ○ Nursing Care
    - ▪ Assess for infestation.
      - □ Scabies: Pencil-like mark on skin
      - □ Head Lice: Adult lice are hard to see. They're small, greyish-tan, and have no wings. Nits look like dandruff on the hair shaft and are firmly attached.
      - □ Body Lice: Adult lice are larger than other lice. They are the size of a sesame seed, tan to greyish-white with six legs. Nits are small grey-white ovals seen on clothing, around the waist or armpits.
      - □ Pubic Lice: Adult lice have a crab-like appearance. Nits are small grey-white ovals attached to the hair shaft

■ Assess for secondary skin infection.

CAUSATIVE AGENT	NURSING INTERVENTIONS
Scabies mite – Sarcoptes scabiei	› Apply 5% permethrin cream (Elimite) over the entire body as a one-time treatment; may need to repeat in 1 week › Treat entire family and persons that have been in contact with infected person during and 60 days after infection › Wash underwear, towels, clothing, and sleepwear in hot water › Vacuum carpets and furniture › Apply calamine lotion or cool compresses until itching subsides following treatment › Difficult cases: May use oral ivermectin
Pediculosis capitis (head lice) – *Pediculus humanus capitis*	› Shampoos containing 1% permethrin as prescribed › Remove nits with a nit comb, repeat in 7 days after shampoo treatment › Wash clothing, bedding in hot water with detergent › Difficult cases: use malathion 0.5% in isopropanol
Pediculosis corporis (body lice) – *Pediculus humanus corporis*	› Lotions containing 1% permethrin as prescribed › Wash clothing, bedding, and towels in hot water (130° or more) then machine dry in hot cycle › Proper hygiene practices
Pediculosis pubis (pubic lice) – *Pediculus humanus pubis*	› Shampoos containing 1% permethrin as prescribed › Remove nits with a nit comb, repeat in 7 days after shampoo treatment › Wash clothing, bedding in hot water with detergent › Assess for other STIs › Difficult cases: Repeat shampoo in 4 to 7 days

Q
PCC

- Client Teaching
  - Teach the child and parents about medications.
  - Teach the child and parents to avoid home remedies, as it may worsen infection.
  - Teach the parent about correct laundering of potentially infected clothing, bedding.
  - Teach the parent to bag items that cannot be laundered into tightly sealed bag for 14 days.
  - Teach the parents to boil combs, brushes and hair accessories in lice-killing products for 1 hr.
  - Discourage sharing of personal items.
- Complications
  - Secondary infections
    - Examples include *staphylococcus, streptococcus, Haemophilus influenzae*
    - Nursing Actions
      □ Ensure the family understands prescribed plan of care to prevent secondary infections.
      □ Monitor for secondary infections.
      □ Administer medications as prescribed for secondary infection.
      □ Teach about clinical manifestations of secondary infections.

APPLICATION EXERCISES

1. A nurse is assessing an infant who has scabies. Which of the following are expected findings? (Select all that apply.)

_____ A. Presence of nits on the hair shaft

_____ B. Pencil-like marks on hands

_____ C. Blisters on the soles of the feet

_____ D. Bluish-gray skin color

_____ E. Pimples on the trunk

2. A nurse is teaching a group of parents about preventing insect bites. Which of the following should the nurse include in the teaching? (Select all that apply.)

_____ A. Wear perfumes when outside.

_____ B. Avoid areas of tall grass.

_____ C. Wear bright-colored clothing.

_____ D. Wear insect repellent.

_____ E. Check house pets frequently.

3. A nurse is teaching a parent of a child who has pediculosis capitis. Which of the following should the nurse include in the teaching?

A. Apply mayonnaise to the affected area at night.

B. Treat all household pets.

C. Use an over-the-counter medication containing 1% permethrin.

D. Discard the child's stuffed animals.

4. A nurse is caring for a child who has cellulitis on the hand. Which of the following is an appropriate action for the nurse to take?

A. Apply hot compresses.

B. Cleanse area using Burow's solution.

C. Prepare for cryotherapy.

D. Administer antifungal medication.

5. A nurse is planning care for a child who has tinea capitis. Which of the following should the nurse include in the plan of care? (Select all that apply.)

_____ A. Treat infected house pets.

_____ B. Use selenium sulfide shampoo.

_____ C. Cleanse area with Burow's solution.

_____ D. Administer antiviral medication.

_____ E. Use moist, warm compresses.

6. A nurse is teaching a group of parents about preventing skin infections. Use the ATI Active Learning Template: Systems Disorder to complete this item to include Client Education: Describe five teaching points.

APPLICATION EXERCISES KEY

1. A. INCORRECT: Presence of nits on the hair shaft is a clinical manifestation of pediculosis capitis.

    B. **CORRECT:** Pencil-like marks on hands is a clinical manifestation of scabies.

    C. **CORRECT:** Blisters on the soles of the feet is a clinical manifestation of scabies.

    D. INCORRECT: Bluish-gray skin color is a clinical manifestation of pediculosis pubis.

    E. **CORRECT:** Pimples on the trunk is a clinical manifestation of scabies.

    Ⓝ NCLEX® Connection: Physiological Adaptations, Pathophysiology

2. A. INCORRECT: Perfumes attract insects and should be avoided.

    B. **CORRECT:** Insects live in tall grasses; therefore, these areas should be avoided.

    C. INCORRECT: Bright colored clothing attracts insects and should be avoided.

    D. **CORRECT:** Insect repellent should be applied to prevent insect bites.

    E. **CORRECT:** House pets should be inspected and treated for insects to prevent exposing family members.

    Ⓝ NCLEX® Connection: Health Promotion and Maintenance, Health Promotion/Disease Prevention

3. A. INCORRECT: Home remedies such as mayonnaise increase the risk of infection and should be avoided.

    B. INCORRECT: Pediculosis capitis is transmitted person-to-person and does not host on household pets.

    C. **CORRECT:** Pediculosis capitis is treated with 1% permethrin, which can be purchased over the counter.

    D. INCORRECT: Items that cannot be placed in the laundry can be placed in a sealed bag for 14 days to kill the lice.

    Ⓝ NCLEX® Connection: Physiological Adaptations, Alterations in Body Systems

4. A. **CORRECT:** Hot compresses increase circulation and promote healing, and are an appropriate action for the nurse to take.

    B. INCORRECT: Cleansing with Burow's solution is recommended for impetigo contagiosa or herpes simplex virus.

    C. INCORRECT: Cryotherapy is recommended for human papillomavirus.

    D. INCORRECT: Cellulitis is a bacterial infection and requires antibiotic therapy.

    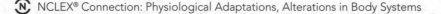 NCLEX® Connection: Physiological Adaptations, Alterations in Body Systems

5. A. **CORRECT:** Tinea capitis can be transmitted from household pets to persons. Therefore, pets should be treated, if infected.

    B. **CORRECT:** Selenium sulfide shampoo is recommended for use for children who have tinea capitis.

    C. INCORRECT: A topical antifungal medication is recommended for children who have tinea capitis.

    D. INCORRECT: Tinea capitis is a fungal infection. Therefore, antifungal medications are administered.

    E. INCORRECT: Moist, warm compresses are applied for bacterial skin infections and not recommended for children who have tinea capitis.

    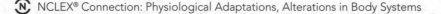 NCLEX® Connection: Physiological Adaptations, Alterations in Body Systems

6. *Using the ATI Active Learning Template: Systems Disorder*
    - Client Education
      - Use good hand hygiene.
      - Avoid sharing clothing, hats, combs, brushes, and towels.
      - Keep the child from touching the affected area by using distraction.
      - Do not squeeze vesicles.
      - Apply topical medications as prescribed.
      - Administer oral medications as prescribed.

    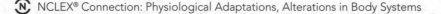 NCLEX® Connection: Health Promotion and Maintenance, Health Promotion/Disease Prevention

chapter 31

Overview

- Common skin conditions of the pediatric population include the following:
  - Contact dermatitis
  - Atopic dermatitis
  - Acne

CONTACT DERMATITIS

Overview

- Contact dermatitis is an inflammatory reaction of the skin. It is caused when the skin comes into contact with chemicals or other irritants (feces, urine, soaps, poison ivy, animals, metals, dyes, medications).
  - Diaper dermatitis may be caused by detergents, soaps, and/or chemicals that come in contact with the genital area. It may also be a result of *Candida albicans*.
  - Seborrheic dermatitis (cradle cap, blepharitis, otitis externa) has an unknown etiology but is most common in infancy and then again at puberty.

Assessment

- Risk Factors
  - Use of diapers
  - Exposure to an irritant
- Subjective Data
  - Pruritus
- Objective Data
  - Physical Assessment Findings (depends on the cause of the irritant and the client)
    - Contact dermatitis
      - Red bumps that may form moist, weeping blisters
      - Skin warm and tender to the touch
      - Presence of oozing, drainage, or crusts
      - Skin becomes scaly, raw, or thickened

- Diaper dermatitis
  - Bright red rash that extends gradually
  - Fiery red and scaly areas on the scrotum and penis
  - Red or scaly areas on the labia
  - Pimples, blisters, ulcers, large bumps, or pus-filled sores
  - Smaller red patches that blend together

Patient-Centered Care

- Nursing Care
  - Diaper dermatitis
    - Promptly remove the wet diaper.
    - Clean urine off the perineal area with a nonirritating cleanser. Cleanse the perineal area of feces with warm water and mild soap.
    - Wash skin folds and the genital area frequently with water.
    - Expose the affected area to air.
    - Use superabsorbent disposable diapers to reduce skin exposure.
    - Apply a skin barrier, such as zinc oxide. Do not wash it off with each diaper change.
    - Use cornstarch to reduce friction between the diaper and the skin.
  - Contact dermatitis
    - Remove irritant, and limit further exposure.
    - Poisonous Plant Exposure
      - Cleanse exposed area as soon as possible with isopropyl alcohol followed by water, then soap and water shower.
      - Clothes, shoes should be cleansed in alcohol.
      - Apply calamine lotion, Burrow's solution compresses, or Aveeno baths.
      - Use topical corticosteroid gel.
      - Oral corticosteroids for severe reactions.
  - Seborrheic dermatitis
    - Treat by gently scrubbing the scalp with mild pressure, and shampoo daily with mild soap or antiseborrheic shampoo.
    - Use a fine-tooth comb to remove the loosened crusts from the hair.
- Medications
  - Antihistamines – Hydroxyzine (Atarax) or diphenhydramine (Benadryl)
    - Administer in cases of allergic/medication reactions.
    - Nursing Considerations
      - Administer the medication as prescribed.

- Client Education
    - Educate the family on the importance of the medication and administering on schedule.

    - Reinforce the sedating effect of some antihistamines and the need for parents to monitor the child and provide for safety during use.
  - Antibiotics
    - Use to treat secondary infections.
    - Nursing Considerations
      - Administer medications as prescribed.
    - Client Education
      - Educate the family about the importance of continuing the medication as prescribed.
  - Antifungal Ointments – clotrimazole (Lotrimin)
    - Used to treat *Candida albicans*.
    - Nursing Considerations
      - Administer the medication as prescribed.
    - Client Education
      - Educate the family on the importance of the medication and administering schedule.
- Care After Discharge
  - Client Education
    - Encourage frequent diaper changes.
    - Advise parents that their child should avoid bubble baths and harsh soaps.
    - Encourage children to wear long sleeves and pants when there is risk of possible exposure to irritants.
    - Educate parents to remove an offending agent as soon as exposure takes place.

Complications

- Bacterial Infections
  - Caused by breaks in the skin from scratching
  - Nursing Actions
    - Monitor the area for signs of infection.
    - Keep fingernails trimmed short.
    - Cleanse the area with mild soap and water.
    - Administer antipruritics and antibiotics as prescribed.

  - Client Education
    - Educate the family and child about avoiding offending agents.

ATOPIC DERMATITIS (AD)

Overview

- Atopic dermatitis (AD) is a type of eczema (eczema describes a category of integumentary disorders, not a specific disorder with a determined etiology) that is characterized by pruritus and associated with a history of allergies that are of an inherited tendency (atopy).

- Lesions disappear if the scratching is stopped.

- Classifications of atopic dermatitis are based on the child's age, how the lesions are distributed, and the appearance of the lesions.

- AD cannot be cured but can be well controlled.

Assessment

- Risk Factors

  ○ Presence of allergic condition and family history of atopy

  ○ Previous skin disorder and exacerbation of present skin disorder

  ○ Exposure to irritating and/or causative agents

- Subjective Data

  ○ Recent exposure to any irritant (medication, food, soap, contact with animals)

  ○ Intense pruritus

- Objective Data

  ○ Physical Assessment Findings

CLASSIFICATION	DISTRIBUTION	LESIONS
› Infants – Onset at 2 to 6 months of age with spontaneous remission by 3 years of age	› Generalized distribution of lesions on cheeks, scalp, trunk, hands and feet, as well as extensor surfaces of extremities	› Erythema › Vesicles, papules › Weeping, oozing, crusting, scaling
› Children – Onset at 2 to 3 years of age with 90% of children having manifestations by 5 years of age; may follow infantile eczema	› Lesions in the flexural areas (antecubital and popliteal fossae, neck), wrists, ankles, and feet with symmetric involvement	› Clusters › Erythematous or flesh-colored papules › Dry › Lichenification › Keratosis pilaris
› Adolescents – Onset at age 12 and may continue into adulthood	› Similar distribution to children	› Same as for children › Dry, thick › Confluent papules

  - Unaffected skin may appear dry and rough.

  - Hypopigmentation of skin may occur in small, diffuse areas.

  - Pallor surrounds the nose, mouth, and ears.

- A bluish discoloration is present underneath the eyes.
- Numerous infections of the nails are present.
- Lymphadenopathy occurs, especially around affected areas.
- Signs of a wound infection are present (swelling, purulent drainage, pain, increased temperature, redness extending beyond the wound margin).

Patient-Centered Care

- Nursing Care
  - Keep skin hydrated with tepid baths (with/without mild soap or emulsifying oil), then apply an emollient within 3 min of bathing. Two or three baths may be given daily with one prior to bedtime.
  - Dress the child in cotton clothing. Avoid wool and synthetic fabrics.
  - Avoid excessive heat and perspiration, which increases itching.
  - Avoid irritants (bubble baths, soaps, perfumes, fabric softeners).
  - Provide support to the child and family.
  - Wash skin folds and genital area frequently with water.
    - Assist in identifying causative agent.
- Medications
  - Antihistamines – Hydroxyzine (Atarax) or diphenhydramine (Benadryl)
    - Client Education
      - Reinforce the sedating effect of some antihistamines and the need for parents to monitor the child during use.
      - Reinforce safety of the child when using sedating antihistamines.
  - Antihistamines – Loratadine (Claritin) or fexofenadine (Allegra)
    - Oral antihistamine for antipruritic effect
    - Nursing Considerations
      - Administer the medication as prescribed.
    - Client Education
      - Inform the parents that it is preferred for use during the daytime.
  - Antibiotics
    - Antibiotics should be used to treat secondary infections.
  - Topical corticosteroids
    - Topical corticosteroids may be used intermittently to reduce or control flare-ups. They may be low, moderate, or high potency and are prescribed based on the degree of skin involvement (extremity versus eyelids), age of the child, and consequences from side effects.

- Nonsteroidal agents
  - Used to decrease inflammation during flare-ups
  - Nursing Considerations
    - Use for children older than 2 years of age.
    - Use at the start of an exacerbation of AD when skin turns red and starts to itch.
- Client Education
  - Signs of infection
  - Instruct the family to:
    - Change diapers when wet or soiled.
    - Keep nails short and trimmed.
    - Place gloves or cotton socks over hands for sleeping.
    - Dress young children in soft, cotton, one-piece, long-sleeve, long-pant outfits.
    - Remove items that may promote itching (woolen blankets, scratchy fabrics). Use cotton items whenever possible.
    - Use mild detergents to wash clothing and linens. The wash cycle may be repeated without soap.
    - Avoid latex products, second-hand smoke, furry pets, dust, and molds.
    - Encourage tepid baths without the use of soap. Avoid oils and powders.
    - Follow specific directions regarding topical medications, soaks, and baths. Emphasize the importance of understanding the sequence of treatments to maximize the benefit of therapy and prevent complications.
    - Avoid overheating the bedroom during winter months. Use a room humidifier.
    - Maintain treatment to prevent flare-up.
    - Follow up with the health care provider as directed.
    - Participate in support groups.

Complications

- Infection
  - Caused by breaks in the skin from scratching
  - Nursing Actions
    - Keep nails trimmed.
    - Administer antipruritics as prescribed.
    - Monitor the area for signs of infection.
    - Cleanse the area with mild soap and water.

  - Client Education
    - Educate the family and child to avoid offending agents.

ACNE

Overview

- Acne is the most common skin condition during adolescence.

- Acne is self-limiting and non life-threatening. However, it poses a threat to self-image for adolescents.

- Acne involves the pilosebaceous follicles (hair follicle and sebaceous gland complex) of the face, neck, chest, and upper back.

- *Propionibacterium acnes* (*P. acnes*) is the bacteria associated with inflammation in acne.

Assessment

- Risk Factors

  - Acne may be genetic.

  - Acne is more common in males than in females.

  - Hormonal fluctuations may result in acne flares in females.

  - The use of cosmetic products containing ingredients such as petrolatum and lanolin may increase acne outbreaks.

  - Although there is no dietary intake link with acne, adolescents working at fast food restaurants may have an increased incidence of acne due to exposure to cooking grease.

- Subjective and Objective Data

  - Report of exacerbations and remissions

  - Physical Assessment Findings

    - Lesions (comedones) are either open (blackheads) or closed (whiteheads). Both are most often found on the face, neck, back, and chest.

    - *P. acnes* may lead to inflammation manifesting as papules, pustules, nodules, or cysts.

Patient-Centered Care

- Nursing Care

  - Discuss the process of acne with the child and family.

  - Discuss the importance of adherence with the prescribed plan of care.

  - Provide written instructions to accompany verbal instructions.

  - Teach the child to gently wash the face and other affected areas, avoiding scrubbing and abrasive cleaners.

  - Teach the child and family about medications prescribed, especially side effects.

  - Monitor for signs of mood changes or suicidal ideation in adolescents who are taking isotretinoin 13-cis-retinoic acid (Amnesteem)

  - Provide support and encouragement to the child and family.

MEDICATION	ACTION	NURSING CONSIDERATIONS
Tretinoin (Retin-A)	› Interrupts abnormal keratinization that causes microcomedones	› Inform the client that tretinoin may irritate the skin. Instruct the client to apply within 20 to 30 min after washing the face. › Tell the client to: » Use a pea-size amount of medication and apply at night. » Avoid sun exposure. » Use sunscreen (SPF 15 or greater) to avoid sunburn.
Benzoyl peroxide	› Antibacterial agent › Inhibits growth of *P. acnes*	› Benzoyl peroxide may bleach bed linens, towels, and clothing, but not skin.
Topical antibacterial agents	› Inhibits growth of *P. acnes*	› Various topical or oral antibacterial agents may be used. However, be alert to allergic reactions. › Avoid overexposure to the sun. › Use sunscreen with an SPF of 15 or greater when exposure to sun is unavoidable.
Isotretinoin 13-cis-retinoic acid (Amnesteem)	› Affects factors involved in the development of acne	› Isotretinoin 13-cis-retinoic acid is only prescribed by dermatologists. › Side effects include dry skin and mucous membranes, dry eyes, decreased night vision, headaches, photosensitivity, elevated cholesterol and triglycerides, depression, suicidal ideation, and/or violent behaviors. › Monitor for behavioral changes. › Isotretinoin 13-cis-retinoic acid is teratogenic. Therefore, it is contraindicated in women of childbearing age who are not taking oral contraceptives.

- Care After Discharge
  - Client Education
    - Reinforce that adherence to the therapeutic plan is essential to preventing acne flares.
    - Encourage the child to eat a balanced, healthy diet.
    - Encourage sleep, rest, and daily exercise.
    - Teach the child to wash the affected area gently with a mild cleanser once or twice daily, and not to pick or squeeze comedones.
    - Encourage frequent shampooing.
    - Encourage family support of the child and family members to assist the child in coping with body-image changes.
    - Instruct the child to wear protective clothing and sunscreen when outside.
    - Teach the child to avoid the use of tanning beds.
    - Reinforce the need for follow-up and monitoring of cholesterol and triglycerides, especially in adolescents who are taking isotretinoin 13-cis-retinoic acid.
    - Reinforce the importance of using oral contraceptives while taking isotretinoin 13-cis-retinoic acid

Complications

- Infection and cellulitis
  - Caused by lesions of dermatitis and/or acne or breaks in the skin from scratching
  - Nursing Actions
    - Monitor the area for signs of infection.
    - Cleanse the area with mild soap and water.
    - Assess for signs of redness, swelling, and pain, which may indicate cellulitis.
    - Assess for fever.

  - Client Education
    - Educate the family and child on avoidance of offending agents.
    - Instruct the child and family to keep fingernails trimmed and short.
    - Use antipruritics as prescribed.
    - Teach the family signs and symptoms of cellulitis and to notify the health care provider if they occur.

APPLICATION EXERCISES

1. A nurse is teaching the parent of an infant who has seborrheic dermatitis. Which of the following should be included in the teaching?

 A. "The patches are from not washing the infant's head regularly."

 B. "The cause is unknown and not contagious."

 C. "The patches are due to an infection the infant has."

 D. "The cause is due to the infant acquiring it from another child at day care."

2. A nurse is caring for a child who has contact dermatitis due to poison ivy. Which of the following should be included in the plan of care? (Select all that apply.)

 _____ A. Remove the clothing over the rash.

 _____ B. Initiate contact isolation precautions.

 _____ C. Expose the rash to a heat lamp for 15 min.

 _____ D. Cleanse the affected skin with hydrogen peroxide solution.

 _____ E. Apply calamine lotion to the skin.

3. A nurse is caring for an adolescent who has acne and is prescribed isotretinoin 13-cis-retinoic acid (Amnesteem). Which of the following laboratory findings should be monitored?

 A. Cholesterol and triglycerides

 B. BUN and creatinine

 C. Serum potassium

 D. Serum sodium

4. A nurse is caring for an infant who has diaper dermatitis. Which of the following should be included in the plan of care? (Select all that apply.)

 _____ A. Apply talcum powder with every diaper change.

 _____ B. Allow the buttocks to air dry.

 _____ C. Use commercial baby wipes to cleanse the area.

 _____ D. Use cloth diapers until the rash is gone.

 _____ E. Apply zinc oxide ointment to the affected area.

5. A nurse is assessing an infant who has eczema. Which of the following are clinical manifestations of eczema in an infant? (Select all that apply.)

_____ A. Generalized distribution

_____ B. Papules

_____ C. Clusters

_____ D. Crusting lesions

_____ E. Lichenification

6. A nurse is teaching a parent of a child who has eczema. Use the ATI Active Learning Template: Systems Disorder to complete this item to include the following sections:

A. Description of the Disorder/Disease Process

B. Client Education

APPLICATION EXERCISES KEY

1. A. INCORRECT: The cause of seborrheic dermatitis is unknown. Not washing the infant's head regularly should not be included in the teaching.

    B. **CORRECT:** The cause of seborrheic dermatitis is unknown. The condition is not contagious; therefore, this should be included in the teaching.

    C. INCORRECT: The cause of seborrheic dermatitis is unknown. It is not due to infection; therefore, this should not be included in the teaching.

    D. INCORRECT: Seborrheic dermatitis is not contagious and not acquired from another child; therefore, this should not be included in the teaching.

     NCLEX® Connection: Physiological Adaptations, Alterations in Body Systems

2. A. **CORRECT:** Removing the irritant from the skin will decrease the exposure. Therefore, removing the clothing over the rash should be included in the plan of care.

    B. INCORRECT: The irritant chemical in poison ivy is not spread by contact or scratching. Therefore, contact isolation precautions are not necessary.

    C. INCORRECT: Using a heat lamp can cause skin burns and should be avoided.

    D. INCORRECT: The affected area should be cleansed with isopropyl alcohol followed by water.

    E. **CORRECT:** Calamine lotion will assist in relieving discomfort and should be included in the plan of care.

     NCLEX® Connection: Physiological Adaptations, Alterations in Body Systems

3. A. **CORRECT:** Adverse effects of 13-cis-retinoic acid include elevated cholesterol and triglycerides; therefore, these laboratory findings should be monitored.

    B. INCORRECT: Medications such as cephalosporins and furosemide can alter serum BUN and creatinine levels. However, they do not to be monitored in clients taking 13-cis-retinoic acid.

    C. INCORRECT: Medications such as diuretics and corticosteriods can alter serum potassium levels. However, it does not need to be monitored in clients taking 13-cis-retinoic acid.

    D. INCORRECT: Medications such as IV fluids and corticosteriods can alter the serum sodium level. However, it does not need to be monitored in clients taking 13-cis-retinoic acid.

     NCLEX® Connection: Pharmacological and Parenteral Therapies, Expected Actions/Outcomes

4. A. INCORRECT: Talcum powder can cake and cause inhalation injury. Therefore, it should not be used for infants who have diaper dermatitis.

   B. **CORRECT:** Allowing the buttocks to air dry facilitates thorough drying of the skin and should be included in the plan of care.

   C. INCORRECT: Commercial baby wipes contain chemicals that can irritate the skin. Therefore, they should not be used for infants who have diaper dermatitis.

   D. INCORRECT: Superabsorbant diapers should be used for infants who have diaper dermatitis to assist in keeping the skin dry.

   E. **CORRECT:** Zinc oxide ointment protects the skin from moisture and irritation and should be included in the plan of care.

   Ⓝ NCLEX® Connection: Basic Care and Comfort, Elimination

5. A. **CORRECT:** Generalized distribution is a clinical manifestation found in infants who have eczema.

   B. **CORRECT:** Papules are a clinical manifestation found in infants who have eczema.

   C. INCORRECT: Clusters are a clinical manifestation found in children who have eczema.

   D. **CORRECT:** Crusting lesions are a clinical manifestation found in infants who have eczema.

   E. INCORRECT: Lichenification is a clinical manifestation found in children who have eczema.

   Ⓝ NCLEX® Connection: Physiological Adaptations, Pathophysiology

6. *Using ATI Active Learning Template: Systems Disorder*

A. Description of the Disorder/Disease Process
   - Eczema describes a category of integumentary disorders, not a specific disorder with a determined etiology, that is characterized by pruritus and associated with a history of allergies that are of an inherited tendency (atopy).

B. Client Education
   - Clinical signs of infection
   - Change diapers when wet or soiled.
   - Keep nails short and trimmed.
   - Place gloves or cotton socks over hands for sleeping.
   - Dress young children in soft, cotton, one-piece, long-sleeve, long-pant outfits.
   - Remove items that may promote itching (woolen blankets, scratchy fabrics). Use cotton items whenever possible.
   - Use mild detergent to wash clothing and linens. The wash cycle may be repeated without soap.
   - Avoid latex products, secondhand smoke, furry pets, dust, and molds.
   - Encourage tepid baths without the use of soap. Avoid oils and powders.
   - Follow specific directions regarding topical medications, soaks, and baths.
   - Emphasize the importance of understanding the sequence of treatments to maximize the benefit of therapy and prevent complications.
   - Avoid overheating the bedroom during winter months. Use a room humidifier.
   - Maintain treatment to prevent flare-up.
   - Follow up with the health care provider as directed.
   - Participate in support groups.

(N) NCLEX® Connection: Physiological Adaptations, Illness Management

chapter 32

Overview

- Thermal, chemical, electrical, and radioactive agents can cause burns, which result in cellular destruction of the skin layers and underlying tissue. The type and severity of the burn impact the treatment plan.

  - Thermal burns occur when there is exposure to flames, steam, or hot liquids.

  - Chemical burns occur when there is exposure to a caustic agent. Cleaning agents used in the home (drain cleaner, bleach) and agents used in the industrial setting (caustic soda, sulfuric acid) cause chemical burns.

  - Electrical burns occur when an electrical current passes through the body. This type of burn may result in severe damage, including loss of organ function, tissue destruction with the subsequent need for amputation of a limb, and cardiac and/or respiratory arrest.

 View Image: Percentage of Burns

Assessment

- Risk Factors

  - Lack of supervision, abuse, or neglect

  - Developmental growth of the child

- Subjective Data

  - Type of burning agent (dry heat, moist heat, chemical, electrical, ionizing radiation)

  - Duration of contact

  - Area of the body in which the burn occurred

- Objective Data

  - Physical Assessment Findings

DEPTH	APPEARANCE	SENSATION/HEALING
› Superficial (first-degree) » Damage to epidermis	› Pink to red in color with no blisters, mild edema, and no eschar › Blanches with pressure	› Painful. › Heals within 5 to 10 days. › No scarring.
› Superficial partial thickness (second-degree) » Damage to the entire epidermis » Dermal elements are intact	› Pink to red in color with blisters, mild to moderate edema, and no eschar › Blanches with pressure	› Pain is present. › Heals within 14 to 21 days. › Variable amounts of scarring. › Sensitive to temperature changes and light touch.

DEPTH	APPEARANCE	SENSATION/HEALING
› Deep partial thickness (second-degree) » Damage to the entire epidermis and some parts of the dermis » Sweat glands and hair follicles remain intact	› Red to white in color with blisters and moderate edema › Blanches with pressure	› Pain is present. › Sensitive to temperature changes and light touch. › Healing time may extend beyond 21 days. › Scarring is likely.
› Full thickness (third-degree) » Damage to the entire epidermis and dermis and possible damage to the subcutaneous tissue » Nerve endings, hair follicles, and sweat glands are destroyed	› Red to tan, black, brown, or white in color › Dry, leathery appearance › No blanching	› As burn heals, painful sensations return and severity of pain increases. › Heals within weeks to months. › Scarring is present. › Grafting is required.
› Deep full thickness (fourth-degree) » Damage to all layers of the skin that extends to muscle, tendons, and bones	› Color variable › Dull and dry › Charring › Possible visible ligaments, bone or tendons	› No pain is present. › Heals within weeks to months. › Scarring is present. › Grafting is required. › Amputation possible.

 View Image: Stages of Burns

- Extent of Injury
  - Total Body Surface Area (TBSA)
    - Age-related charts determine the extent of injury to body surface, which is expressed in percentages.
    - Infant's skin is thin. Therefore, injury is likely to be deeper
  - Burns are classified as minor, moderate, or major.
    - Minor: treated in a clinic setting
    - Moderate: treated in a hospital with expertise in burn care
    - Major: require medical services of a burn center
- Laboratory Tests (for injury greater than 30% TBSA)
  - CBC, serum electrolytes, BUN, ABGs, fasting blood glucose, random blood glucose, liver enzymes, urinalysis, and clotting studies.

Patient-Centered Care

- Nursing Care
  - Minor burns
    - Stop the burning process.
      - Remove clothing or jewelry that may conduct heat.
      - Apply cool water soaks or run cool water over the injury. Do not use ice.
      - Flush chemical burns with large amounts of water.
    - Cover the burn with a clean cloth to prevent contamination.
    - Cleanse with mild soap and tepid water (avoid excess friction).
    - Removing blisters is controversial.
    - Use antimicrobial ointment.
    - Apply dressing (nonadherent, hydrocolloid).
    - Provide warmth.
    - If necessary, child is seen in a health care facility for medical care.
    - Provide analgesia.
    - Check immunization status and determine the need for immunization. Administer tetanus vaccine if it has been more than 5 years since last immunization.
    - Educate the family to avoid using greasy lotions or butter on burns.
    - Educate the family to monitor for signs of infection.
  - Moderate and major burns
    - Maintain airway and ventilation.
    - Provide humidified 100% supplemental oxygen as prescribed.
    - Monitor vital signs.
    - Maintain cardiac output.
      - Initiate IV access with large-bore catheter. Multiple access points may be necessary.
      - Fluid replacement is important during the first 24 hr.
        - Isotonic crystalloid solutions, such as 0.9% sodium chloride or lactated Ringer's solution, are used during the early stage of burn recovery.
        - Colloid solutions, such as albumin or synthetic plasma expanders (Hespan), may be used after the first 24 hr of burn recovery.
        - Maintain urine output of 1 to 2 mL/kg/hr if the child weighs less than 30 kg (66 lb).
        - Maintain urine output of 30 mL/hr if the child weighs more than 30 kg (66 lb).
        - Be prepared to administer blood products as prescribed.
      - Monitor for manifestations of septic shock.
        - Alterations in sensorium (confusion)
        - Increased capillary refill
        - Spiking fever
        - Decreased bowel sounds
        - Decreased urine output
      - Notify the provider of findings.

- Manage pain.
  - Establish ongoing monitoring of pain and effectiveness of pain management.
  - Avoid IM or subcutaneous injections.
  - Use intravenous opioid analgesics, such as morphine sulfate, hydromorphone (Dilaudid), and fentanyl (Sublimaze).
  - Monitor for respiratory depression when using opioid analgesics.
  - Administer pain medications prior to dressing changes or procedures.
  - Use nonpharmacologic methods for pain control (guided imagery, music therapy, therapeutic touch) to enhance the effects of analgesics and promote improved pain management.
- Prevent infection.
  - Follow standard precautions when performing wound care.
  - Restrict plants and flowers due to the risk of contact with pseudomonas.
  - Change position frequently to prevent contractures and prolonged pressure.
  - Limit visitors.
  - Use reverse isolation if prescribed.
  - Monitor for manifestations of infection and report to the provider.
  - Use client-designated equipment, such as blood pressure cuffs and thermometers.
  - Administer tetanus toxoid if indicated.
  - Administer antibiotics if infection is present.
- Provide nutritional support.
  - Increase caloric intake to meet increased metabolic demands and prevent hypoglycemia.
  - Increase protein intake to prevent tissue breakdown and promote healing.
  - Provide enteral therapy or total parenteral nutrition (TPN) if necessary due to decreased gastrointestinal motility and increased caloric needs.
  - Administer vitamins A and C to facilitate cell growth, and zinc for wound healing.
- Restore mobility.
  - Maintain correct body alignment, splint extremities, and facilitate position changes to prevent contractures.
  - Maintain active and passive range of motion.
  - Assist with ambulation as soon as the child is stable.
  - Apply pressure dressings to prevent contractures and scarring.
  - Closely monitor areas at high risk for pressure sores (heels, sacrum, back of head).
- Provide psychological support.
  - Provide developmentally appropriate support for the child.
  - Assist with coping.
  - Use family-centered approach.
  - Make referrals as needed.

- Medications
  - Topical agents
    - Silver sulfadiazine (Silvadene)
      - Use with second- and third-degree burns.
      - Apply to cleansed, debrided area.
      - Wear sterile gloves for application.
      - Apply thickness of 1/16th inch.
    - Mafenide acetate (Sulfamylon)
      - Use with second- and third-degree burns.
      - Apply to cleansed, debrided area.
      - Wear sterile gloves for application.
      - Apply thickness of 16 mm.
    - Bacitracin
      - Use for prevention of secondary infection.
      - Apply thin film two to four times per day.
  - Morphine sulfate
    - Analgesia
    - Nursing Considerations
      - Administer via continuous IV infusion with boluses prior to procedures.
      - Monitor for respiratory depression.
      - Monitor pain relief.
    - Client Education
      - Educate the child and family on the safety precautions needed with opioid administration.
  - Midazolam (Versed), fentanyl (Sublimaze), propofol (Diprivan), and nitrous oxide
    - Sedation and analgesia
    - Nursing Considerations
      - Administer IV just prior to the start of a procedure.
      - Monitor the need for sedation.
      - Monitor pain relief.
    - Client Education
      - Educate the child and the family about the safety precautions needed with opioid administration.
- Teamwork and Collaboration – Referral to services such as nutrition, child life, social support, respiratory therapy, occupational/physical therapy, and individual and family counseling as prescribed.

- Therapeutic Procedures
  - Wound care
    - Nursing Actions
      - Premedicate as prescribed prior to wound care.
        - ▸ Administer analgesics.
        - ▸ Administer hydroxyzine (Vistaril) or diphenhydramine (Benadryl) for pruritus.
      - Remove previous dressings.
      - Assess for odors, drainage, and discharge.
      - Cleanse the wound as prescribed.
      - Assist with debridement.
        - ▸ Provide hydrotherapy (place client or affected extremity in a warm tub of water or use warm running water, as if to shower) to cleanse the wound. Use once or twice a day for up to 20 min.
          - ▹ Use mild soap or detergent to gently wash burns and then rinse with room-temperature water.
          - ▹ Encourage active range of motion during hydrotherapy.
          - ▹ Monitor for cold stress and hypothermia.
  - Skin coverings
    - Biologic skin coverings may be used to promote healing of large burns. Requires repeated surgical application.
      - Allograft (homograft) – Skin from human cadavers that is used for partial and full thickness burn wounds
      - Xenograft – Obtained from animals, such as pigs, for partial thickness burn wounds
      - Synthetic skin coverings – Used for partial thickness burn wounds
    - Permanent skin coverings may be the treatment of choice for burns covering large areas of the body.
      - Autografts (client's skin)
        - ▸ Sheet graft – Sheet of skin used to cover the wound
        - ▸ Mesh graft – Sheet of skin placed in a mesher so skin graft has small slits in it; allows graft to cover larger areas of burn wound
        - ▸ Cultured epithelium – Epithelial cells cultured for use when grafting sites are limited
      - Artificial skin – Synthetic product that is used for partial and full thickness burn wounds (healing is faster)
    - Nursing Actions
      - Maintain immobilization of the graft site.
      - Elevate the extremity.
      - Provide wound care to the donor site.
      - Administer analgesics.

☐ Monitor for infection before and after skin coverings or grafts are applied.

▸ Discoloration of unburned skin surrounding burn wound

▸ Green color to subcutaneous fat

▸ Degeneration of granulation tissue

▸ Development of subeschar hemorrhage

▸ Hyperventilation indicating systemic involvement of infection

▸ Unstable body temperature

- Client Education

☐ Instruct the child to keep the extremity elevated.

☐ Instruct the family to report evidence of infection.

● Care After Discharge

○ Initiate a referral for home health services.

○ Initiate a referral to occupational therapy for evaluation of the home environment and assistance to relearn how to perform ADLs.

○ Initiate a referral to social services for community support services.

○ Client Education

- Instruct the child to continue to perform range-of-motion exercises and to work with a physical therapist to prevent contractures.

- Provide instructions about how to assess the wound for infection and how to perform wound care.

- Teach age-appropriate safety measures for the home (covering electrical outlets, supervising children when in the bath, keeping irons out of reach of children, teaching the dangers of playing with matches).

- Teach the family to avoid sun exposure between 1000 and 1600, wear protective clothing, and apply sunscreen to prevent sunburn.

Complications

● Inhalation injury

○ Direct thermal injury

- Occurs with burns to the face and lips.

- Can be delayed 24 to 48 hr.

- Findings include wheezing, increased secretions, hoarseness, wet crackles in the lungs, singed nasal hairs, laryngeal edema, and carbonaceous secretions.

○ Carbon monoxide injury

- Occurs when incident took place in an enclosed area.

- Findings include mucosal erythema and edema followed by sloughing of the mucosa.

○ Nursing Actions

- Maintain airway and ventilation, and provide 100% oxygen as prescribed.

- Shock/Systemic Sepsis
  - Nursing Actions
    - Administer IV crystalloid solutions for the first 24 hr followed by colloid solutions.
    - Meticulous monitoring of intake and output.
    - Monitor laboratory findings, noting indications of anemia and infection.
    - Monitor vital signs.
    - Assess sensorium.
    - Assess capillary refill in extremities.
- Pulmonary problems include edema, infections, aspiration, embolus, and posttraumatic pulmonary insufficiency.
  - Nursing Actions
    - Maintain airway via intubation, sometimes tracheostomy.
    - Administer oxygen as prescribed.
- Wound infections
  - Nursing Actions
    - Assess for discoloration, edema, odor, and drainage.
    - Assess for fluctuations in temperature and heart rate.
    - Obtain a wound culture.
    - Administer antibiotics as prescribed.
    - Monitor laboratory findings, noting indications of anemia and infection.
    - Maintain surgical aseptic technique with dressing changes.

APPLICATION EXERCISES

1. A nurse is caring for a client who has a superficial partial thickness burn. Which of the following is an appropriate action for the nurse to take?

    A. Administer an IV infusion of 0.9% sodium chloride.

    B. Apply cool, wet compresses to affected area.

    C. Clean the affected area using a soft-bristle brush.

    D. Administer morphine sulfate.

2. A nurse is caring for a client who has major burns and suspected septic shock. Which of the following findings are consistent with septic shock? (Select all that apply.)

_____ A. Increased body temperature

_____ B. Altered sensorium

_____ C. Decreased capillary refill

_____ D. Decreased urine output

_____ E. Increased bowel sounds

3. A nurse is caring for a client who has a major burn and is experiencing severe pain. Which of the following is an appropriate nursing intervention to manage this client's pain?

    A. Administer morphine sulfate IV via continuous infusion.

    B. Administer meperidine (Demerol) IM as needed.

    C. Administer acetaminophen (Tylenol) PO every 4 hr.

    D. Administer hydrocodone (Vicodin) PO every 6 hr.

4. A nurse is caring for a client who has a skin graft. Which of the following clinical manifestations indicate infection? (Select all that apply.)

_____ A. Green color to subcutaneous fat

_____ B. Unstable body temperature

_____ C. Generation of granulation tissue

_____ D. Subeschar hemorrhage

_____ E. Change in skin color around the affected area

5. A nurse is caring for a client who has a moderate burn. Which of the following is an appropriate action for the nurse to take?

    A. Maintain immobilization of the affected area.

    B. Expose affected area to the air.

    C. Initiate a high-protein, high-calorie diet.

    D. Implement contact isolation.

6. A nurse is teaching a newly licensed nurse about clinical manifestations of burns. Use the ATI Active Learning Template: Basic Concept to complete this item to include Underlying Principles. List the depth, appearance, sensation, and healing of first-, second-, third-, and fourth-degree burns.

APPLICATION EXERCISES KEY

1. A. INCORRECT: Fluid replacement is indicated for clients who have sustained moderate to major burns.

   B. **CORRECT:** Applying cool, wet compresses stops the burn process. Therefore, this is an appropriate action for the nurse to take.

   C. INCORRECT: Gentle cleansing with tepid water, not a soft-bristle brush, is recommended for a superficial partial thickness burn.

   D. INCORRECT: Morphine sulfate for pain relief is indicated for clients who have sustained moderate to major burns.

   Ⓝ NCLEX® Connection: Physiological Adaptations, Illness Management

2. A. **CORRECT:** Increased body temperature is a clinical manifestation of septic shock.

   B. **CORRECT:** Altered sensorium is a clinical manifestation of septic shock.

   C. INCORRECT: Increased capillary refill is a clinical manifestation of septic shock.

   D. **CORRECT:** Decreased urine output is a clinical manifestation of septic shock.

   E. INCORRECT: Decreased bowel sounds is a clinical manifestation of septic shock.

   Ⓝ NCLEX® Connection: Physiological Adaptations, Hemodynamics

3. A. **CORRECT:** Opioids administered IV via continuous infusion are recommended for clients who have major burns.

   B. INCORRECT: IM medications are contraindicated for clients who have major burns.

   C. INCORRECT: Oral acetaminophen is recommended for clients who have minor burns.

   D. INCORRECT: IV opioid medications are recommended for clients who have major burns.

   Ⓝ NCLEX® Connection: Pharmacological and Parenteral Therapies, Pharmacological Pain Management

4. A. **CORRECT:** Green color to subcutaneous fat is a clinical manifestation of infection.

   B. **CORRECT:** Unstable body temperature is a clinical manifestation of infection.

   C. INCORRECT: Degeneration of granulation tissues is a clinical manifestation of infection.

   D. **CORRECT:** Subeschar hemorrhage is a clinical manifestation of infection.

   E. **CORRECT:** A discoloration of the skin around the burn is a clinical manifestation of infection.

   Ⓝ NCLEX® Connection: Physiological Adaptations, Unexpected Response to Therapies

5. A. INCORRECT: Active and passive range of motion of the affected area is recommended to prevent contractures.

    B. INCORRECT: Dressings should be applied to the burned area to prevent infection.

    C. **CORRECT:** A high-protein, high-calorie diet is initiated to meet increased metabolic demands and promote healing.

    D. INCORRECT: Reverse isolation precautions are recommended to prevent wound infections.

    (N) NCLEX® Connection: Physiological Adaptations, Pathophysiology

6. *Using the ATI Active Learning Template: Basic Concept*
    - Underlying Principles
        - Superficial (first-degree)
            - Damage to the epidermis.
            - Pink to red in color with no blisters.
            - Blanches with pressure.
            - Mild edema.
            - No eschar.
            - Painful.
            - Heals within 5 to 10 days with no scarring.
        - Superficial partial thickness (second-degree)
            - Damage to the entire epidermis with intact dermal elements.
            - Pink to red in color with blisters.
            - Blanches with pressure.
            - Mild to moderate edema.
            - No eschar.
            - Painful, sensitive to temperature changes and light touch.
            - Heals within 14 to 21 days with variable scarring.
        - Deep partial thickness (second-degree)
            - Damage to the entire epidermis and some parts of the dermis. Sweat glands and hair follicles remain intact.
            - Red to white in color with blisters.
            - Blanches with pressure.
            - Moderate edema.
            - Painful, sensitive to temperature changes and light touch.
            - Healing can go beyond 21 days with scarring.
        - Full thickness (third degree)
            - Damage to the entire epidermis and dermis with possible damage to the subcutaneous tissue. Nerve endings, hair follicles, and sweat glands are destroyed.
            - Red to tan, black, brown, or white in color.
            - Dry, leathery appearance.
            - No blanching.
            - As burn heals, painful sensations return and severity of pain increases.
            - It heals within weeks to months. Scarring is present. Grafting is required.
        - Deep full thickness (fourth-degree)
            - Damage to all layers of the skin that extends to the muscle, tendons, and bones.
            - Color variable, dull, and dry with charring. Possible visible ligaments, bone, or tendons.
            - No pain is present.
            - Heals within weeks to months. Scarring is present and grafting is required. Amputation possible.

    (N) NCLEX® Connection: Physiological Adaptations, Pathophysiology

UNIT 2 Nursing Care of Children with System Disorders

SECTION: ENDOCRINE DISORDERS

› Diabetes Mellitus
› Growth Hormone Deficiency

NCLEX® CONNECTIONS

When reviewing the chapters in this unit, keep in mind the relevant sections of the NCLEX® outline, in particular:

Client Needs: Pharmacological and Parenteral Therapies	Client Needs: Reduction of Risk Potential	Client Needs: Physiological Adaptation
› Relevant topics/tasks include: » Adverse Effects/ Contraindications/Side Effects/Interactions › Notify the provider of side effects, adverse effects, and contraindications of medications and parenteral therapy. » Expected Actions/Outcomes › Evaluate client response to medication. » Medication Administration › Titrate dosage of medication based on assessment and ordered parameters.	› Relevant topics/tasks include: » Diagnostic Tests › Monitor the results of diagnostic testing and intervene as needed. » System Specific Assessment › Assess the client for signs of hypoglycemia or hyperglycemia. » Therapeutic Procedures › Educate the client about treatments and procedures.	› Relevant topics/tasks include: » Alterations in Body Systems › Educate the client about managing health problems. » Fluid and Electrolyte Imbalances › Evaluate the client's response to interventions to correct fluid or electrolyte imbalance. » Illness Management › Apply knowledge of client pathophysiology to illness management.

chapter 33

Overview

- Diabetes mellitus is characterized by a partial or complete metabolic deficiency of insulin.
- Diabetes mellitus is a contributing factor for the development of cardiovascular disease, hypertension, renal failure, blindness, and stroke as individuals age.

Assessment

- Risk Factors
  - Genetics can predispose a person to the occurrence of type 1 and type 2 diabetes mellitus.
  - Toxins and viruses can predispose an individual to diabetes by destroying the beta cells, leading to type 1 diabetes mellitus.
  - Obesity, physical inactivity, high triglycerides (greater than 250 mg/dL), and hypertension may lead to the development of insulin resistance and type 2 diabetes mellitus.
- Subjective and Objective Data
  - Blood glucose alterations
    - Hypoglycemia – blood glucose level less than 60 mg/dL

AUTONOMIC NERVOUS SYSTEM RESPONSES RAPID ONSET	IMPAIRED CEREBRAL FUNCTION GRADUAL ONSET
› Hunger, lightheadedness, and shakiness	› Strange or unusual feelings
› Headache	› Decreasing level of consciousness
› Anxiety and irritability	› Difficulty in thinking and inability to concentrate
› Pale, cool skin	› Change in emotional behavior
› Diaphoresis	› Slurred speech
› Irritability	› Headache and blurred vision
› Normal or shallow respirations	› Seizures leading to coma
› Tachycardia and palpitations	

- Hyperglycemia – blood glucose levels usually greater than 250 mg/dL
    - Thirst
    - Polyuria (early), oliguria (late)
    - Nausea, vomiting, abdominal pain
    - Skin that is warm, dry, and flushed with poor turgor
    - Dry mucous membranes
    - Confusion
    - Weakness
    - Lethargy
    - Weak pulse
    - Diminished reflexes
    - Rapid, deep respirations with acetone/fruity odor due to ketones (Kussmaul respirations)
- Laboratory Tests
    - Diagnostic criteria for diabetes
        - An 8-hr fasting blood glucose level of 126 mg/dL or more
        - A random blood glucose of 200 mg/dL or more with classic signs of diabetes
        - An oral glucose tolerance test of 200 mg/dL or more in the 2-hr sample
    - Fasting blood glucose
        - Client Education
            - Ensure that the child has fasted (no food or drink other than water) for 8 hr prior to the blood draw. Antidiabetic medications should be postponed until after the level is drawn.
    - Oral glucose tolerance test
        - Client Education
            - Instruct the client to consume a balanced diet for the 3 days prior to the test. Then instruct the client to fast for 8 hr prior to the test. A fasting blood glucose level is drawn at the start of the test. The client is then instructed to consume a specified amount of glucose. Blood glucose levels are drawn every 30 min for 2 hr. The child must be assessed for hypoglycemia throughout the procedure.
    - Glycosylated hemoglobin (HbA1c)
        - The expected reference range is 4% to 6%, but an acceptable target for children who have diabetes may be 6.5% to 8% with a total target goal of less than 7%.

- Diagnostic Procedures
    - Self-monitored blood glucose (SMBG)
        - Blood glucose monitoring is essential to management of diabetes. Measurements should be assessed at a minimum before meals and at bedtime.
        - Follow or ensure that the child follows the proper procedure for blood sample collection and use of a glucose meter.
        - Client Education
            - Instruct the child to check the accuracy of the strips with the control solution provided.
            - Advise the child to keep a record of the SMBG that includes time, date, serum glucose level, insulin dose, food intake, and other events that may alter glucose metabolism, such as activity level or illness.

Patient-Centered Care

QTC

- Nursing Care
  - Monitor the following:
    - Vital signs
    - Blood glucose levels and factors affecting levels (other medications, diet, and/or activity)
    - Intake and output and weight
    - Skin integrity and healing status of any wounds, paying close attention to the feet and folds of the skin
    - Sensory alterations (tingling, numbness)
    - Visual alterations
    - Presence of recurrent infections
    - Dietary practices
    - Exercise patterns
    - The child's proficiency at self-monitoring blood glucose
    - The child's proficiency at self-administering medication
  - Follow agency policy for nail care. Some protocols allow for trimming toenails straight across with clippers and filing edges with a nail file. If clippers or scissors are contraindicated, the child should file the nails straight across.
  - Teach proper foot care.
    - Inspect feet daily. Wash feet daily with mild soap and warm water.
    - Pat feet dry gently, especially between the toes.
    - Use mild foot powder (powder with cornstarch) on sweaty feet.
    - Do not use commercial remedies for the removal of calluses or corns.
    - Perform nail care after a bath/shower if possible.
    - Separate overlapping toes with cotton or lambs' wool.
    - Avoid open-toe, open-heel shoes. Leather shoes are preferred to plastic ones. Wear slippers with soles. Do not go barefoot. Shake out shoes before putting them on.
    - Wear clean, absorbent socks or stockings that are made of cotton or wool and have not been mended.
    - Do not use hot water bottles or heating pads to warm feet. Wear socks for warmth.
    - Avoid prolonged sitting, standing, and crossing of legs.
  - Teach the child to cleanse cuts with warm water and mild soap, gently dry, and apply a dry dressing. Instruct the child and parents to monitor healing and to seek intervention promptly.
  - Have the child's eyes examined yearly.
  - Emphasize the importance of regular dental and health care visits.

- ○ Provide nutritional guidelines.
  - Read labels for nutritional value.
  - Meal planning is based on the requirements of growth and development of the child.
  - Plan meals to achieve appropriate timing of food intake, activity, onset, and peak of insulin. Calories and food composition should be similar each day.
  - Eat at regular intervals and do not skip meals.
  - Count grams of carbohydrates consumed.
  - Recognize that 15 g of carbohydrates are equal to 1 carbohydrate exchange.
  - Avoid high-fat and high-sugar/high-carbohydrate food items.
  - Use artificial sweeteners in moderation.
- ○ Teach appropriate techniques for SMBG, including obtaining blood samples, recording and responding to results, and correctly handling supplies and equipment.
- ○ Assist with an exercise plan
  - Children active with team sports will require a snack 30 min prior to activity.
  - Adjustment in diet and insulin may be required with changes in activities.
- ○ Teach the child guidelines to follow when sick.
  - Monitor blood glucose levels every 3 hr.
  - Continue to take insulin or oral antidiabetic agents.
  - Encourage sugar-free, non-caffeinated liquids to prevent dehydration.
  - Meet carbohydrate needs by eating soft foods if possible. If not, consume liquids that are equal to the usual carbohydrate content.
  - Test urine for ketones every 3 hr.
  - Rest.
  - Call the health care provider if:
    - □ Blood glucose is higher than 240 mg/dL.
    - □ Fever higher than 38.9° C (102° F), fever does not respond to acetaminophen (Tylenol), or fever lasts more than 12 hr.
    - □ Positive ketones in the urine.
    - □ Disorientation or confusion occurs.
    - □ Rapid breathing is experienced.
    - □ Vomiting occurs more than once.
    - □ Diarrhea occurs more than five times or for longer than 24 hr.
    - □ Liquids cannot be tolerated.
    - □ Illness lasts longer than 2 days.

- Teach signs and symptoms of hypoglycemia (e.g., shakiness, diaphoresis, anxiety, nervousness, chills, headache, confusion, labile, difficulty focusing, hunger, dizziness, pallor, palpations).
  - Check blood glucose levels.
  - Follow guidelines outlined by the health care provider/diabetes educator. Guidelines may include:
    - Treat with 10 to 15 g simple carbohydrate (1 tbsp sugar).
      - Examples of 15 g of carbohydrate are 4 oz orange juice, 8 oz milk, 3 to 4 glucose tablets, 4 oz regular soft drink.
    - For mild reactions, use milk or fruit juice.
    - Monitor blood glucose frequently
    - Follow with complex carbohydrate
    - If the child is unconscious or unable to swallow, administer glucagon SC or IM and notify the health care provider. Administer simple carbohydrate as soon as tolerated. Watch for vomiting and take precaution against aspiration.
  - Teach signs and symptoms of hyperglycemia (lethargy, confusion, thirst, nausea, vomiting, abdominal pain, signs of dehydration, rapid respirations, fruity breath).
    - Encourage oral fluid intake.
    - Administer insulin as prescribed.
    - Test urine for ketones and report if findings are abnormal.
    - Consult the health care provider if symptoms progress.
  - Encourage the child to wear a medical identification wristband.
- Medications
  - Insulin is used to manage type 1 diabetes.
    - Insulin pumps
      - Regular insulin
      - Delivers a programmed amount of insulin on a consistent basis.
    - Insulin injections
      - Self-administered injections 2 or more times per day
      - Mixing insulin: usually rapid-acting and intermediate-acting
  - The rate of onset, peak, and duration of action varies for each different type of insulin.

TYPE	TRADE NAME	ONSET	PEAK	DURATION
Rapid acting	› Insulin lispro (Humalog)	Less than 15 min	0.5 to 1 hr	3 to 4 hr
Short acting	› Regular insulin (Humulin R)	0.5 to 1 hr	2 to 4 hr	5 to 7 hr
Intermediate acting	› NPH insulin (Humulin N)	1 to 2 hr	4 to 12 hr	18 to 24 hr
Long acting	› Insulin glargine (Lantus)	3-4 hr	none	10.4 to 24 hr

- Nursing Considerations
  - Observe the child and/or parent drawing up and administering the insulin injection, and offer additional instruction as indicated.
  - Do not mix insulin glargine (Lantus) with other insulins due to incompatibility.
  - Observe the child and/or parent using the insulin pump and offer additional instruction as indicated.

- Client Education
  - Provide information regarding self-administration of insulin.
    - Rotate injection sites (prevent lipohypertrophy) within one anatomic site (prevent day-to-day changes in absorption rates).
    - Inject at a 90° angle (45° angle if thin). Aspiration for blood is not necessary.
    - When mixing a rapid- or short-acting insulin with a longer-acting insulin, draw up the shorter-acting insulin into the syringe first and then the longer-acting insulin (this reduces the risk of introducing the longer-acting insulin into the vial of the shorter-acting insulin).
- Teamwork and Collaboration
  - Refer the child and family to a diabetes educator for comprehensive education in diabetes management.

Complications

- Diabetic ketoacidosis (DKA)
  - DKA is an acute, life-threatening condition characterized by hyperglycemia (greater than 300 mg/dL), resulting in the breakdown of body fat for energy and an accumulation of ketones in the blood and urine. The onset is rapid, and the mortality rate is high.
  - Causes of DKA include insufficient insulin (usually failure to take the appropriate dose), acute stress (as from trauma or surgery), and poor management of acute illness.
  - Nursing Actions
    - Admit to an intensive care unit.
      - Place on a cardiac monitor.
    - Assess subjective and objective data for DKA.
      - Ketones in the blood and urine
      - Fruity scent to the breath
      - Mental confusion
      - Dyspnea
      - Nausea and vomiting
      - Dehydration
      - Weight loss
      - Electrolyte imbalances
      - Untreated: Coma
    - Provide rapid isotonic fluid (0.9% sodium chloride) replacement to maintain perfusion to vital organs. Often large quantities are required to replace losses. Monitor the child for evidence of fluid volume excess.
    - Follow with a hypotonic fluid (0.45% sodium chloride) to continue replacing losses to total body fluid.

- When serum glucose levels approach 250 mg/dL, add glucose to IV fluids to minimize the risk of cerebral edema associated with drastic changes in serum osmolality.

    □ Administer Regular insulin 0.1 unit/kg as an IV bolus dose and then follow with a continuous intravenous infusion of regular insulin at 0.1 unit/kg/hr.

- Monitor glucose levels hourly.

- Monitor serum potassium levels. Potassium levels will initially be elevated. With insulin therapy, potassium will shift into cells and the child will need to be monitored for hypokalemia. Provide potassium replacement therapy in all replacement IV fluids as indicated by lab values. Make sure urinary output is adequate before administering potassium.

- Administer sodium bicarbonate by slow IV infusion for severe acidosis (pH of less than 7.0). Monitor potassium levels because a correction of acidosis that occurs too quickly may lead to hypokalemia.

- Administer oxygen to client whose arterial oxygen level is less than 90%.

- ○ Client Education

    - Reinforce instructions to manage diabetes.

- Long-Term Complications
  - ○ Nephropathy
  - ○ Retinopathy
  - ○ Neuropathy
  - ○ Cardiovascular disease
  - ○ Altered thyroid function
  - ○ Limited mobility of the small joints

APPLICATION EXERCISES

1. A nurse is reviewing sick day management with a parent of a child who has type 1 diabetes mellitus. Which of the following should the nurse include in the teaching? (Select all that apply.)

_____ A. Monitor blood glucose levels every 3 hr.

_____ B. Discontinue taking insulin until feeling better.

_____ C. Drink 8 oz of fruit juice every hour.

_____ D. Test urine for ketones.

_____ E. Call the health care provider if blood glucose is greater than 240 mg/dL.

2. A nurse is teaching a child who has type 1 diabetes mellitus about self care. Which of the following statements by the child indicates understanding of the teaching?

A. "I should skip breakfast when I am not hungry."

B. "I should increase my insulin with exercise."

C. "I should drink a glass of milk when I am feeling irritable."

D. "I should draw up the NPH insulin into the syringe before the regular insulin."

3. A nurse is caring for a child who has type 1 diabetes. Which of the following is a clinical manifestation of diabetic ketoacidosis? (Select all that apply.)

_____ A. Blood glucose 58 mg/dL

_____ B. Weight gain

_____ C. Dehydration

_____ D. Mental confusion

_____ E. Fruity breath

4. A nurse is teaching an adolescent who has diabetes about foot care. Which of the following should the nurse include in the teaching?

A. "You should inspect your feet once a week."

B. "You should cut your toe nails in a rounded fashion."

C. "You can use cornstarch on your feet."

D. "You can use over-the-counter callus removers."

5. A nurse is teaching an adolescent who has diabetes about clinical manifestations of hypoglycemia. Which of the following should be included in the teaching? (Select all that apply.)

_____ A. Increased urination

_____ B. Hunger

_____ C. Signs of dehydration

_____ D. Irritability

_____ E. Sweating and pallor

_____ F. Kussmaul respirations

6. A nurse is teaching parent of a child who has type 1 diabetes mellitus. Use the ATI Active Learning Template: Systems Disorder to complete this item to include the following:

A. Description of the Disorder/Disease Process

B. Collaborative Care: Medications: List the types of insulin used for children who have type 1 diabetes mellitus.

C. Nursing Care: Describe eight interventions.

D. Client Outcomes: Describe three.

APPLICATION EXERCISES KEY

1. A. **CORRECT:** A client who is experiencing illness can have waning blood glucose levels. Therefore, frequent monitoring of blood glucose levels is done to identify hyper- or hypoglycemic episodes.

   B. INCORRECT: A client who is experiencing illness should continue taking insulin during to prevent hyperglycemic episodes.

   C. INCORRECT: A client who is experiencing illness should drink fluids without sugars.

   D. **CORRECT:** A client who is experiencing an illness should test her urine for ketones to assist in early detection of ketoacidosis.

   E. **CORRECT:** A client who is experiencing illness should notify the provider of blood glucose levels greater than 240 mg/dL to obtain further instructions in caring for the hyperglycemia.

    NCLEX® Connection: Physiological Adaptations, Alterations in Body Systems

2. A. INCORRECT: A client who has diabetes should eat three meals a day with snacks and should avoid skipping meals to prevent hypoglycemic episodes.

   B. INCORRECT: The insulin requirements of a client who has type 1 diabetes will decrease with exercise, therefore increasing the amount of insulin with exercise could precipitate a hypoglycemic episode.

   C. **CORRECT:** An early clinical manifestation of hypoglycemia is irritability. Therefore, drinking a glass of milk, which is approximately 15 g of carbohydrates, indicates understanding of the teaching.

   D. INCORRECT: Regular insulin should be drawn up into the syringe prior to drawing up NPH to avoid altering the regular insulin.

    NCLEX® Connection: Physiological Adaptations, Alterations in Body Systems

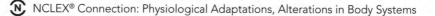

3. A. INCORRECT: Diabetic ketoacidosis is classified as a blood glucose level greater than 300 mg/dL.

    B. INCORRECT: Clients who have diabetic ketoacidosis display weight loss.

    C. **CORRECT:** Clients who have diabetic ketoacidosis experience osmotic diuresis because of the electrolyte shift.

    D. **CORRECT:** Clients who have diabetic ketoacidosis experience mental confusion because of the electrolyte shift.

    E. **CORRECT:** Clients who have diabetic ketoacidosis experience fruity breath because of the body's attempt to eliminate ketones.

    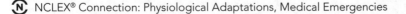 NCLEX® Connection: Physiological Adaptations, Medical Emergencies

4. A. INCORRECT: Clients who have diabetes should inspect their feet daily.

    B. INCORRECT: Clients who have diabetes should cut their toenails straight across.

    C. **CORRECT:** Clients who have diabetes can use cornstarch to aid in moisture absorption.

    D. INCORRECT: Clients who have diabetes should avoid commercial remedies for callus removal.

    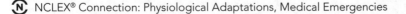 NCLEX® Connection: Health Promotion and Maintenance, Health Promotion/Disease Prevention

5. A. INCORRECT: An increase in urination is a clinical manifestation of hyperglycemia.

    B. **CORRECT:** Hunger is a clinical manifestation of hypoglycemia because of the increased adrenergic nervous system activity.

    C. INCORRECT: Signs of dehydration is a clinical manifestation of hyperglycemia.

    D. **CORRECT:** Irritability is a clinical manifestation of hypoglycemia because of the depleted glucose in the CNS.

    E. **CORRECT:** Sweating and pallor is a clinical manifestation of hypoglycemia because of the increased adrenergic nervous system activity.

    F. INCORRECT: Kussmaul respirations is a clinical manifestation of hyperglycemia.

    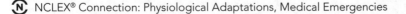 NCLEX® Connection: Physiological Adaptations, Medical Emergencies

6. *Using the ATI Active Learning Template: Systems Disorder*

    A. Description of the Disorder/Disease Process
        * Diabetes mellitus is characterized by a partial or complete metabolic deficiency of insulin.

    B. Collaborative Care: Medications
        * Insulin lispro (Humalog): Rapid-acting
        * Regular Insulin (Humulin R): Short-acting
        * NPH insulin (Humulin N): Intermediate-acting
        * Insulin glargine (Lantus): Long-acting

    C. Nursing Care
        * Monitor clinical manifestations of hyper and hypoglycemia.
        * Provide nail care according to policy.
        * Teach proper foot care.
        * Teach wound care.
        * Provide nutritional guidelines.
        * Encourage yearly eye exams.
        * Encourage dental and medical follow up.
        * Teach self monitoring of blood glucose.
        * Teach guidelines to follow when sick.
        * Teach hypo and hyperglycemia.
        * Teach about medications.

    D. Client Outcomes
        * The child will have blood glucose levels within an acceptable range levels less than 126 mg/dl.
        * The child will have a glycosylated hemoglobin of 7% or less.
        * The child and/or family will be able to self-administer insulin.
        * The child and/or family will be able to monitor for complications and intervene as necessary.
        * The child and/or family will maintain adequate dietary intake to support growth and development.

    ⓝ NCLEX® Connection: Physiological Adaptations, Alterations in Body Systems

chapter 34

Overview

- Human growth hormone (GH), somatotropin, is a naturally occurring substance that is secreted by the pituitary gland.
- GH is important for normal growth, development, and cellular metabolism.
- A deficiency in GH prevents somatic growth throughout the body.
- Other hormones that work with GH to control metabolic processes include adrenocorticotropic hormone (ACTH), thyroid stimulating hormone (TSH), and the gonadotropins (follicle-stimulating hormone [FSH] and luteinizing hormone [LH]).
- Hypopituitarism is the diminished or deficient secretion of pituitary hormones (primarily GH). Consequences of the condition depend on the degree of the deficiency.

Assessment

- Risk Factors
  - Structural factors (tumors, trauma, structural defects, surgery)
  - Heredity disorders
  - Other pituitary hormone deficiencies (deficiencies of TSH or ACTH)
  - Most often, GH deficiencies are idiopathic.
- Objective Data
  - Physical Assessment Findings
    - Short stature but proportional height and weight
    - Delayed epiphyseal closure
    - Increased insulin sensitivity
    - Delayed dentition
    - Underdeveloped jaw
    - Delayed sexual development
  - Laboratory Tests
    - Plasma insulin-like growth factor-1 (IGF-1) and IGF binding protein-3 (IGFBP-3) levels
      - Further evaluation is indicated if the values are one standard deviation below the mean for age.
    - Nursing Actions
      - Collect the appropriate amount of blood for the test.
      - Explain the laboratory procedure to the family and child.
    - Client Education
      - The child should fast the night before the test.

- ○ Diagnostic Procedures
  - ▪ GH stimulation
    - □ GH stimulation testing is generally done for children who have a low level of IGF-1 and IGFBP-3, and short stature.
    - □ Nursing Actions
      - ▸ Draw baseline blood sample between 0600 and 0800.
      - ▸ Administer medication that triggers the release of GH (arginine or GH-releasing hormone).
      - ▸ Obtain blood sample every 30 min for a 3-hr period following medication administration.
    - □ Client Education
      - ▸ Nothing to eat or drink 10 to 12 hr before the test.
      - ▸ Limit activity 10 to 12 hr before the test.
  - ▪ Radiologic assessments
    - □ Assess the child's skeletal maturity by comparing epiphyseal centers on an x-ray to age-appropriate published standards.
    - □ Perform a general skeletal survey in children under 3 years of age, or survey the hands and wrists in older children. This will provide information about growth as well as epiphyseal function.
    - □ Nursing Actions
      - ▸ Assist in positioning the child.
  - ▪ Computed tomographic (CT) scanning, magnetic resonance imaging (MRI), and skull x-rays
    - □ Used to identify tumors or other structural defects
    - □ Nursing Actions
      - ▸ Monitor the child during the procedure.
      - ▸ Sedate the child, if prescribed.
    - □ Client Education
      - ▸ Provide emotional support.
  - ▪ Evaluation of the growth curve
    - □ Nursing Actions
      - ▸ Accurately obtain and plot height and weight measurements.
      - ▸ Assess height velocity or height over time.
      - ▸ Determine height-to-weight relationship.
      - ▸ Project target height in context of genetic potential.

Patient-Centered Care

- Nursing Care
  - The child's height and weight are measured and marked on a growth chart as part of every visit to the primary care provider.
    - The height of a child is more affected than weight. Bone age usually matches height age.
    - Measure children who are younger than 3 years of age at least every 6 months and children older than 3 years of age every year.
  - Assess and monitor effectiveness of GH replacement. GH is supplied by recombinant DNA technology.
  - Administer other hormone replacements (thyroid hormone) if prescribed.
  - Provide support to the child and family regarding psychosocial concerns (altered body image, depression). Reassure the child and family that there are no cognitive delays or deficits.
  - Stress the importance of maintaining realistic expectations based on the child's age and abilities.
- Medications
  - Somatropin
    - Used as a human growth hormone that is a replacement for deficiency in growth hormones
    - Nursing Considerations
      - Administer the medication via subcutaneous injections.
      - Use cautiously in children who are receiving insulin.
- Teamwork and Collaboration
  - Consult with an endocrinologist.
  - Psychological counseling may be indicated to help the child and family cope during this period of time.
- Care After Discharge
  - Nursing Actions
    - Inform the child and parents that there should not be any significant side effects when GH replacement therapy is used in appropriate doses for GH deficiency.
    - Inform the child and parents that GH will assist with muscle growth and help improve self-esteem.

  - Client Education
    - Teach the child and parents how to administer medication by subcutaneous injection for home use.
    - Instruct the child and parents that GH should be administered 6 to 7 days a week.
    - Inform the child and parents that GH usually is continued until bone maturation takes place. Radiologic evidence of epiphyseal closure is a criterion for ending therapy. This may be 16 years of age or older for boys and 14 years of age or older for girls.
    - Encourage the child and family to seek evaluation during early adulthood. Children with GH deficiency in childhood should be evaluated in early adulthood to determine the need for continued replacement therapy.

Complications

- GH deficiency without hormone replacement may result in disruption of vertical growth, delayed epiphyseal closure, retarded bone age, delayed sexual development, and premature aging later in life.

APPLICATION EXERCISES

1. A nurse is caring for a child who has short stature. Which of the following diagnostic tests should be completed to confirm growth hormone (GH) deficiency? (Select all that apply.)

_____ A. CT scan of the head

_____ B. Bone age scan

_____ C. GH stimulation test

_____ D. Serum IGF-1

_____ E. DNA testing

2. A parent of a school-age child with GH deficiency asks the nurse how long his son will need to take injections for his growth delay. Which of the following is an appropriate response by the nurse?

A. "Injections are usually continued until age 10 for girls and age 12 for boys."

B. "Injections continue until your child reaches the fifth percentile on the growth chart."

C. "Injections should be continued until there is evidence of epiphyseal closure."

D. "The injections will need to be administered throughout your child's entire life."

3. A nurse is assessing a child with short stature. Which of the following findings would indicate a growth hormone deficiency?

A. Proportional height to weight

B. Height proportionally greater than weight

C. Weight proportionally greater than height

D. BMI greater than height/weight ratio

4. A nurse is teaching the parent of a child who has a growth hormone deficiency. Which of the following are complications of untreated growth hormone deficiency? (Select all that apply.)

_____ A. Delayed sexual development

_____ B. Premature aging

_____ C. Advanced bone age

_____ D. Short stature

_____ E. Increased epiphyseal closure

5. A nurse is preparing to administer somatropin (Genotropin) 0.2 mg/kg/week divided into six doses to a child who weighs 22 kg. Available is somatropin 5 mg/1.5 mL. How many mL should the nurse administer per dose? (Round the answer to the nearest tenth.)

6. A nurse is planning care for a child who is to undergo a growth hormone (GH) stimulation test. Which interventions should the nurse include in the plan of care? Use the ATI Active Learning Template: Nursing Skill to complete this item to include two preprocedure nursing actions and three intraprocedure actions.

APPLICATION EXERCISES KEY

1. A. **CORRECT:** A CT scan of the head is conducted to determine whether there is a structural component to the short stature.

   B. **CORRECT:** A bone age scan is conducted to determine the development of the bones.

   C. **CORRECT:** A GH stimulation test is conducted to confirm diagnosis of GH deficiency.

   D. **CORRECT:** A serum IGF-1 is obtained as a preliminary test to determine GH deficiency.

   E. INCORRECT: DNA testing is not a diagnostic test to determine GH deficiency.

   Ⓝ NCLEX® Connection: Reduction of Risk Potential, Diagnostic Tests

2. A. INCORRECT: Injections are continued until there is evidence of epiphyseal closure; age will be variable among clients.

   B. INCORRECT: Injections are continued until there is evidence of epiphyseal closure; growth will be variable among clients.

   C. **CORRECT:** Injections are continued until there is evidence of epiphyseal closure on radiographic tests.

   D. INCORRECT: Injections are continued until there is evidence of epiphyseal closure; age will be variable among clients.

   Ⓝ NCLEX® Connection: Pharmacological and Parenteral Therapies, Medication Administration

3. A. **CORRECT:** Children who have growth hormone deficiency present with short stature with proportional height and weight.

   B. INCORRECT: Children who have growth hormone deficiency present with short stature with proportional height and weight.

   C. INCORRECT: Children who have growth hormone deficiency present with short stature with proportional height and weight.

   D. INCORRECT: Children who have growth hormone deficiency present with short stature with proportional height and weight.

   Ⓝ NCLEX® Connection: Physiological Adaptations, Pathophysiology

4.   A. **CORRECT:** A complication of untreated growth hormone deficiency includes delayed sexual development.

    B. **CORRECT:** A complication of untreated growth hormone deficiency includes premature aging.

    C. INCORRECT: A complication of untreated growth hormone deficiency includes retarded bone age.

    D. **CORRECT:** A complication of untreated growth hormone deficiency includes short stature.

    E. INCORRECT: A complication of untreated growth hormone deficiency includes delayed epiphyseal closure.

   (N) NCLEX® Connection: Physiological Adaptations, Unexpected Response to Therapies

5.   **0.2** mL

Using Ratio and Proportion

STEP 1: *What is the unit of measurement to calculate?*
mg

STEP 2: *Set up an equation and solve for X.*
mg x kg/week = X
0.2 mg x 22 kg = 4.4 mg

STEP 3: *Round if necessary.*

STEP 4: *Reassess to determine whether the amount makes sense.*
If the prescribed amount is 0.2 mg/kg/week and the client weighs 22 kg, it makes sense to give 4.4 mg/week or 0.7333 mg per dose.

STEP 5: *What is the unit of measurement to calculate?*
mL

STEP 6: *What is the dose available? Dose available = Have.*
5 mg

STEP 7: *Should the nurse convert the units of measurement?*
No

STEP 8: *What is the quantity of the dose available?*
1.5 mL

STEP 9: *Set up an equation and solve for X.*

$$\frac{\text{Have}}{\text{Quantity}} = \frac{\text{Desired}}{\text{X}}$$

$$\frac{5 \text{ mg}}{1.5 \text{ mL}} = \frac{0.7333 \text{ mg}}{\text{X mL}}$$

X = 0.2199

STEP 10: *Round if necessary.*
0.2199 = 0.2

STEP 11: *Reassess to determine whether the amount to give makes sense.*
If there are 5 mg/1.5 mL and the prescribed amount is 0.7333 mg, it makes sense to give 0.2 mL. The nurse should administer somatropin injection 0.2 mL subcutaneous per dose.

Using Desired over Have

STEP 1: *What is the unit of measurement to calculate?*
mg

STEP 2: *Set up an equation and solve for X.*
mg x kg/week = X
0.2 mg x 22 kg = 4.4 mg

STEP 3: *Round if necessary.*

STEP 4: *Reassess to determine whether the amount makes sense.*
If the prescribed amount is 0.2 mg/kg/week and the client weighs 22 kg, it makes sense to give 4.4 mg/week or 0.7333 mg per dose.

STEP 5: *What is the unit of measurement to calculate?*
mL

STEP 6: *What is the dose available? Dose available = Have.*
5 mg

STEP 7: *Should the nurse convert the units of measurement?*
No

STEP 8: *What is the quantity of the dose available?*
1.5 mL

STEP 9: *Set up an equation and solve for X.*

$$\frac{\text{Desired} \times \text{Quantity}}{\text{Have}} = X$$

$$\frac{0.7333 \text{ mg} \times 1.5 \text{ mL}}{5 \text{ mg}} = X \text{ mL}$$

$$0.2199 = X$$

STEP 10: *Round if necessary.*
0.2199 = 0.2

STEP 11: *Reassess to determine whether the amount to give makes sense.*
If there are 5 mg/1.5 mL and the prescribed amount is 0.7333 mg, it makes sense to give 0.2 mL. The nurse should administer somatropin injection 0.2 mL subcutaneous per dose.

Using Dimensional Analysis

STEP 1: *What is the unit of measurement to calculate?*
mg

STEP 2: *Set up an equation and solve for X.*
mg x kg/week = X
0.2 mg x 22 kg = 4.4 mg

STEP 3: *Round if necessary.*

STEP 4: *Reassess to determine whether the amount makes sense.*
If the prescribed amount is 0.2 mg/kg/week and the client weighs 22 kg, it makes sense to give 4.4 mg/week or 0.7333 mg per dose.

STEP 5: *What is the unit of measurement to calculate?*
mL

STEP 6: *What is the dose available? Dose available = Have.*
5 mg

STEP 7: *Should the nurse convert the units of measurement?*
No

STEP 8: *What is the quantity of the dose available?*
1.5 mL

STEP 9: *Set up an equation and solve for X.*

$$X = \frac{\text{Quantity}}{\text{Have}} \times \frac{\text{Conversion (Have)}}{\text{Conversion (Desired)}} \times \text{Desired}$$

$$X \text{ mL} = \frac{1.5 \text{ mL}}{5 \text{ mg}} \times \frac{0.7333 \text{ mg}}{}$$

$$X = 0.2199$$

STEP 10: *Round if necessary.*
0.2199 = 0.2

STEP 11: *Reassess to determine whether the amount to give makes sense.*
If there are 5 mg/1.5 mL and the prescribed amount is 0.7333 mg, it makes sense to give 0.2 mL. The nurse should administer somatropin injection 0.2 mL subcutaneous per dose.

(N) NCLEX® Connection: Pharmacological and Parenteral Therapies, Dosage Calculation

6. *Using the ATI Active Learning Template: Nursing Skill*
   - Preprocedure
     ○ Nothing to eat or drink 10 to 12 hr prior to procedure.
     ○ Limit activity 10 to 12 hr prior to procedure.
   - Intraprocedure
     ○ Draw baseline blood sample between 0600 and 0800.
     ○ Administer medication that triggers the release of GH (arginine or GH-releasing hormone).
     ○ Obtain blood sample every 30 min during a 3-hr period following medication administration.

(N) NCLEX® Connection: Reduction of Risk Potential, Diagnostic Tests

UNIT 2   Nursing Care of Children with System Disorders

SECTION: IMMUNE AND INFECTIOUS DISORDERS

› Immunizations
› Communicable Diseases
› Acute Otitis Media
› HIV/AIDS

NCLEX® CONNECTIONS

When reviewing the chapters in this unit, keep in mind the relevant sections of the NCLEX® outline, in particular:

Client Needs: Safety and Infection Control	Client Needs: Health Promotion and Maintenance	Client Needs: Physiological Adaptation

› Relevant topics/tasks include
 	
» Standard Precautions/ Transmission-Based Precautions/Surgical Asepsis
 	
  › Understand communicable diseases and the modes of organism transmission.
 	
  › Apply principles of infection control.
 	
  › Utilize appropriate precautions for immunocompromised clients.
	› Relevant topics/tasks include
	
	» Health Promotion/Disease Prevention
	
	  › Provide information about health promotion and maintenance recommendations.
		› Relevant topics/tasks include
		
		» Alterations in Body Systems
		
		  › Identify signs, symptoms and incubation periods of infectious diseases.
		
		» Pathophysiology
		
		  › Identify pathophysiology related to an acute or chronic condition.
		
		» Unexpected Response to Therapies
		
		  › Recognize signs and symptoms of complications and intervene appropriately when providing client care.

UNIT 2   **NURSING CARE OF CHILDREN WITH SYSTEM DISORDERS**
          SECTION: IMMUNE AND INFECTIOUS DISORDERS

CHAPTER 35   Immunizations

Overview

- Administration of a vaccine stimulates the immune system to produce anitbodies against that specific disease.
- Vaccines have the same anitgen as the disease, but it is either killed or weakened, therefore not strong enough to cause the disease.
- Antibodies will disappear after they have destroyed the infection/antigen. But memory cells are formed to protect from future exposures to that same infection. This is called immunity.
- The Advisory Committee on Immunization Practices (ICIP) makes recommendations and creates guidelines regarding immunizations.
- The most up-to-date information can be found at the Centers for Disease Control and Prevention website (www.cdc.gov).

Childhood Immunizations

CHILDHOOD IMMUNIZATIONS			
MINIMUM AGE	NUMBER OF DOSES	SCHEDULE	CONSIDERATIONS
Hepatitis B (HepB)			
Birth	3	Birth 1 to 2 months 6 to 18 months	› Minimum of 4 weeks between doses 1 and 2. › Minimum of 8 weeks between doses 2 and 3. › Final dose no earlier than 24 weeks and at least 16 weeks after first dose.
Rotavirus (RV)			
6 weeks	2	2 months 4 months	› Maximum age for the first dose is 14 weeks, 6 days. › Maximum age for the last dose is 8 months. › Series should not be initiated for children older than 15 weeks.
Diphtheria, tetanus, pertussis (DTaP)			
6 weeks	4	2 months 4 months 6 months 15 to 18 months 4 to 6 years 11 to 12 years Booster every 10 years	› Minimum of 6 months between doses 3 and 4. › Booster can be either Tdap or Td.

CHILDHOOD IMMUNIZATIONS

MINIMUM AGE	NUMBER OF DOSES	SCHEDULE	CONSIDERATIONS
Haemophilus influenzae type b (Hib)			
6 weeks	3	2 months 4 months 12 to 15 months	
Pneumococcal (PCV)			
6 weeks	4	2 months 4 months 6 months 12 to 15 months	
Inactivated poliovirus (IPV)			
6 weeks	4	2 months 4 months 6 to 18 months 4 to 6 years	› Final dose should be administered after 4 years and at least 6 months from the previous dose.
Influenza (TIV)			
6 weeks	Yearly	Yearly	› Must be 2 years or older to receive live vaccine (LAIV). › Children who have medical conditions that predispose them to influenza should not receive the live vaccine. › Administer starting with availability, usually October.
Measles, mumps, rubella (MMR)			
12 months	2	12 to 15 months 4 to 6 years	› MMR should be given to children ages 6 months through 11 months if traveling internationally. However, these children still need the scheduled MMR immunizations.
Varicella (VAR)			
12 months	2	12 to 15 months 4 to 6 years	
Hepatitis A (HepA)			
12 months	2	12 months to 2 years 6 to 18 months following	› Administer the final dose 6 to 18 months after the first.
Meningococcal (MCV4)			
9 months	1	11 to 12 years	› Can be given earlier for high-risk groups. › If vaccine given prior to 16 years, a booster is recommended.
Human papillomavirus			
9 years	3	11 to 12 years	› Administer second dose 1-2 months after first dose. › Administer third dose 6 months after first dose.

• For children who have missed scheduled immunizations, use the "catch-up" schedule.

Purpose

- Decrease or eliminate certain infectious diseases in society.
- Prevent infectious diseases and their complications.

Complications/Contraindications/Precautions

- An anaphylactic reaction to a vaccine is a contraindication for receiving further doses of that vaccine.
- An anaphylactic reaction to a vaccine is a contraindication for using other vaccines containing that substance.
- Contraindications to all immunizations include severe allergies to any component of a vaccine.
- Moderate or severe illnesses with or without fever are contraindications to receiving immunizations. With acute febrile illness, immunization is deferred until symptoms resolve. The common cold and other minor illnesses are not contraindications.
- Contraindications to immunizations require health care providers to analyze data and weigh the risks that come with vaccinating or not vaccinating.

IMMUNIZATION SIDE EFFECTS AND CONTRAINDICATIONS	
SIDE EFFECTS	**CONTRAINDICATIONS**
DTaP	
› Local reaction at the injection site › Fever and irritability › Crying that cannot be consoled and lasts up to 3 hr › Seizures › Rare – acute encephalopathy	› An occurrence of encephalopathy 7 days after the administration of the vaccine › An occurrence of seizures within 3 days of the immunization › A history of uncontrollable, inconsolable crying after a prior immunization (may have lasted more than 3 hr and occurred within 48 hr of immunization)
Hib	
› Mild local reactions and a low-grade fever › Rare – temperature greater than 38.5° C (101.3° F), vomiting, and crying	
RV	
› Irritability › Mild, temporary diarrhea or vomiting	› Intussusception › Immunocompromised
IPV	
› Local reaction at injection site	› Allergy to neomycin (Mycifradin) and/or streptomycin and polymyxin B › Pregnancy
MMR	
› Local reactions (rash; fever; swollen glands in cheeks, neck, and under the jaw) › Possibility of joint pain lasting for days to weeks › Risk for anaphylaxis and thrombocytopenia	› Pregnancy › Allergy to gelatin and neomycin › History of thrombocytopenia or thrombocytopenic purpura › Immunosuppression (with HIV infection or from medication administration) › Recent transfusion with blood products or immunoglobulins

IMMUNIZATION SIDE EFFECTS AND CONTRAINDICATIONS	
SIDE EFFECTS	**CONTRAINDICATIONS**
Varicella vaccine	
› Varicella-like rash that is local or generalized (vesicles on the body) › Seizure	› Pregnancy › Cancers of blood and lymphatic system › Allergy to gelatin neomycin › Corticosteriods › Immunosuppression (with HIV or from medication administration)
PCV	
› Mild local reactions	
HepA	
› Local reaction at the injection site › Headache › Loss of appetite › Tiredness	
HepB	
› Local reaction at the injection site › Temperature of 37.7° C (99.9° F) or higher	› Allergy to baker's yeast
Influenza vaccine; TIV: Influenza (inactivated) vaccine; LAIV: Influenza (live) vaccine (nasal)	
› TIV – mild local reaction, and fever › LAIV – headache, cough, and fever › Rare – risk for Guillain-Barré syndrome	› Hypersensitivity to eggs › LAIV › Younger than 2 years old › Immunosuppression › Chronic disease
Meningococcal Conjugate vaccine (MCV4)	
› Mild local reaction › Rare – risk for allergic response	› History of Guillain-Barré syndrome
HPV2 and HPV4	
› Mild local reaction and fever › Fainting (shortly after receiving the immunization) › Headache	› Pregnancy › Hypersensitivity to yeast

Nursing Administration

- Infants and Children
  - Obtain parental consent for children.
  - Note the date, route, and site of immunization on the child's immunization record at the time of immunization.
  - Give intramuscular immunizations in the vastus lateralis or ventrogluteal muscle in infants and young children, and into the deltoid muscle for older children and adolescents.
  - Give subcutaneous injections in the outer aspect of the upper arm or anterolateral thigh.
  - Use an appropriately sized needle for the route, site, age, and amount of medication.
  - Use strategies to minimize discomfort.
  - Provide for distraction.
  - Encourage the parents to use comforting measures during the procedure (cuddling, pacifiers) and after the procedure (application of cool compresses to injection site, gentle movement of the involved extremity).
  - Provide praise afterward.
  - Apply a colorful bandage, if appropriate.
  - Have emergency medications and equipment on standby in case the child experiences an allergic response, such as anaphylaxis (rare).
  - Follow storage and reconstitution directions. If reconstituted, use within 30 min.
  - Provide written vaccine information sheets and review the content with parents or clients.
  - Instruct the parents and child to observe for complications and to notify the provider if side effects occur.
  - Encourage the parents to maintain up-to-date immunizations for the child.
  - Document the administration of the vaccine, including the date, route, and site of immunization; type, manufacturer, lot number, and expiration date of the vaccine; and name, address and signature of the child and/or parent.
  - Instruct the parents to avoid administering aspirin to the child to treat fever or local reaction due to the risk of the development of Reye syndrome
  - Give an infant concentrated oral sucrose solution on a pacifier 2 min prior to, during, and 3 min after injections.
  - Apply a topical anesthetic prior to the injection.
  - Report any adverse reactions to the Vaccine Adverse Event Reporting System.

Nursing Evaluation of Medication Effectiveness

- Depending on therapeutic intent, effectiveness may be evidenced by:
  - Improvement of local reaction to immunization with absence of pain, fever, and swelling at the site of injection
  - Development of immunity

APPLICATION EXERCISES

1. A nurse is preparing to administer immunizations to a 6-month-old infant. Which of the following is an appropriate action for the nurse to take in providing atraumatic care?

    A. Administer 81 mg of aspirin.

    B. Use the Z-track method when injecting.

    C. Ask the parents to leave the room during the injection.

    D. Provide sucrose solution on the pacifier.

2. A nurse is planning to administer immunizations to a 2-month-old infant. Which of the following should the nurse anticipate giving? (Select all that apply.)

    _____ A. Rotavirus (RV)

    _____ B. Diphtheria, tetanus, pertussis (DTaP)

    _____ C. Haemophilus influenzae type b (Hib)

    _____ D. Hepatitis A (HepA)

    _____ E. Pneumococcal (PCV)

    _____ F. Inactivated poliovirus (IPV)

3. A nurse is planning to administer immunizations to a 4-year-old child who has up-to-date immunizations. Which of the following should the nurse anticipate giving? (Select all that apply.)

    _____ A. Inactivated poliovirus (IPV)

    _____ B. Haemophilus influenzae type b (Hib)

    _____ C. Measles, mumps, rubella (MMR)

    _____ D. Varicella (VAR)

    _____ E. Hepatitis B (HepB)

    _____ F. Diphtheria, tetanus, pertussis (DTaP)

4. A nurse is preparing to administer varicella vaccine to an adolescent. Which of the following questions should the nurse ask to determine whether there is a contraindication to administering the vaccine?

    A. "Do you have an allergy to eggs?"

    B. "Have you ever had encephalopathy following immunizations?"

    C. "Are you currently taking corticosteroid medication?"

    D. "Do you have a hypersensitivity to yeast?"

5. A nurse is caring for a toddler in a clinic. Which of the following is an appropriate action for the nurse to take? (See the chart below for additional client information.)

DEMOGRAPHICS	IMMUNIZATION RECORD	NURSE'S NOTES
› 15 months old › Female	› HepB: 1 month, 2 months, 12 months › Rotavirus: 2 months, 4 months, 6 months › DTaP: 2 months, 4 months, 6 months › Hib: 2 months, 4 months, 12 months › IPV: 2 months, 4 months, 6 months › MMR: 12 months › Varicella: 12 months › HepA: 12 months	› Temperature: 38.4° C (101.1° F) › Sore throat › Family history of seizures

    A. Administer diphtheria, tetanus, pertussis (DTaP) vaccine.

    B. Administer haemophilus influenzae type b (Hib) vaccine.

    C. Administer immunizations when febrile.

    D. Administer hepatitis A (HepA) vaccine.

6. A nurse is preparing to work in an immunization clinic. Use the ATI Active Learning Template: Basic Concept to complete this item to include the following: Related Concept: List all immunizations given during childhood. Underlying Principles: List the recommended ages of each immunization.

APPLICATION EXERCISES KEY

1. A. INCORRECT: Aspirin is contraindicated in children because of the risk of Reye's syndrome. Therefore, this is not an appropriate action for the nurse to take.

    B. INCORRECT: Using the Z-track method is not recommended with immunizations. Therefore, this is not an appropriate action for the nurse to take.

    C. INCORRECT: Separating the parents from the infant can produce anxiety in the infant. Therefore, this is not an appropriate action for the nurse to take.

    D. **CORRECT:** Allowing an infant to suck on a pacifier with sucrose solution can decrease pain with immunizations and is an appropriate action for the nurse to take in providing atraumatic care.

    (N) NCLEX® Connection: Basic Care and Comfort, Non-Pharmacological Comfort Interventions

2. A. **CORRECT:** Two doses of rotavirus vaccine are given during childhood starting at 2 months of age.

    B. **CORRECT:** Six doses of diphtheria, tetanus, pertussis vaccine are given during childhood starting at 2 months of age.

    C. **CORRECT:** Three doses of haemophilus influenzae type b vaccine are given during childhood starting at 2 months of age.

    D. INCORRECT: Two doses of hepatitis A vaccine are given during childhood starting at 12 months of age.

    E. **CORRECT:** Four doses of pneumococcal vaccine are given during childhood starting at 2 months of age.

    F. INCORRECT: Four doses of inactivated poliovirus vaccine are given during childhood starting at 2 months of age.

    (N) NCLEX® Connection: Health Promotion and Maintenance, Health Promotion/Disease Prevention

3. A. **CORRECT:** Four doses of inactivated poliovirus vaccine are given during childhood with a dose given at 4 years of age.

    B. INCORRECT: Three doses of haemophilus influenzae type b vaccine are given during childhood scheduled at 2, 4, and 12 months of age.

    C. **CORRECT:** Two doses of measles, mumps, and rubella vaccine are given during childhood with a dose given at 4 years of age.

    D. **CORRECT:** Two doses of varicella vaccine are given during childhood with a dose given at 4 years of age.

    E. INCORRECT: Three doses of hepatitis B vaccine are given during childhood scheduled at birth, 2, and 6 to 18 months of age.

    F. **CORRECT:** Six doses of diphtheria, tetanus, pertussis vaccine are given during childhood with a dose given at 4 years of age.

    (N) NCLEX® Connection: Pharmacological and Parenteral Therapies, Adverse Effects/ Contraindications/Side Effects/Interactions

4.   A. INCORRECT: Influenza vaccine is contraindicated in clients who have an allergy to eggs.

   B. INCORRECT: DTaP vaccine is contraindicated in clients who have a history of encephalopathy following immunizations.

   C. **CORRECT:** Varicella vaccine is contraindicated in clients who are currently taking corticosteroid medications.

   D. INCORRECT: HepB vaccine is contraindicated in clients who have a hypersensitivity to yeast.

   Ⓝ NCLEX® Connection: Health Promotion and Maintenance, Health Promotion/Disease Prevention

5.   A. **CORRECT:** Five diphtheria, tetanus, pertussis (DTaP) immunizations are given during early childhood, with one at 15 months of age.

   B. INCORRECT: Three haemophilus influenzae type b immunizations are given during childhood.

   C. INCORRECT: Temperature of 38.4° C (101.1° F) is a contraindication to administering immunizations. Immunizations with moderate to severe illness should be deferred.

   D. INCORRECT: Two hepatitis A immunizations are given during childhood, with the second one 6 to 18 months after the first.

   Ⓝ NCLEX® Connection: Health Promotion and Maintenance, Health Promotion/Disease Prevention

6.   *Using the ATI Active Learning Template: Basic Concept*

- Hepatitis B (HepB)
  - Birth
  - 1 to 2 months
  - 6 to 18 months
- Rotavirus (RV)
  - 2 months
  - 4 months
- Diphtheria, tetanus, pertussis (DTaP)
  - 2 months
  - 4 months
  - 6 months
  - 15 to 18 months
  - 4 to 6 years
  - 11 to 12 years
  - Booster every 10 years

- Haemophilus influenzae type b4 (Hib)
  - 2 months
  - 4 months
  - 12 to 15 months
- Pneumococcal (PCV)
  - 2 months
  - 4 months
  - 6 months
  - 12 to 15 months
- Inactivated poliovirus (IPV)
  - 2 months
  - 4 months
  - 6 to 18 months
  - 4 to 6 years

- Measles, mumps, rubella (MMR)
  - 12 to 15 months
  - 4 to 6 years
- Varicella (VAR)
  - 12 to 15 months
  - 4 to 6 years
- Hepatitis A (HepA)
  - 12 months to 2 years
  - 6 to 18 months following
- Meningococcal (MCV4)
  - 11 to 12 years
- Influenza (TIV)
  - Yearly
- Human papillomavirus
  - 11 to 12 years (3 doses)

   Ⓝ NCLEX® Connection: Health Promotion and Maintenance, Health Promotion/Disease Prevention

chapter 36

Overview

- Communicable diseases are easily spread through airborne, droplet, or direct contact transmission.
- Most communicable disease can be prevented with immunizations.

Health Promotion and Disease Prevention

SPREAD	INCUBATION	COMMUNICABILITY
Conjunctivitis		
› Direct contact (viral and bacterial)	› Depends on the infection	› Viral: Appears secondary to a viral infection; clears on own in 7 to 14 days. › Bacterial: Starts in one eye, spreads to the other, clears with antibiotics. › Allergic: Occurs in people who have other allergic conditions; clears with allergy medications.
Epstein-Barr virus (EBV)/mononucleosis		
› Saliva	› 4 to 6 weeks	› Healthy people can carry EBV in saliva, transmitting the virus for a lifetime. › People who have mononucleosis can transmit for weeks.
Erythema infectiosum (fifth disease)/parvovirus B19		
› Droplet › Blood	› 4 to 14 days, sometimes up to 20 days	› Onset of symptoms before rash appears.
Hand, foot, and mouth disease (HFMD)		
› Direct contact	› 4 to 6 days	› Most contagious during the first week of illness, contagious even when free from symptoms.
Mumps/paramyxovirus		
› Direct contact › Droplet › Surfaces, contaminated objects	› 12 to 25 days	› Immediately before and 5 days after swelling begins.

SPREAD	INCUBATION	COMMUNICABILITY
Pertussis (whooping cough)/Bordetella pertussis		
› Direct contact › Droplet	› 7 to 10 days	› Catarrhal stage through 2 weeks into the paroxysmal stage.
Rubella (German measles)/rubella virus		
› Direct contact › Droplet	› 12 to 23 days	› 7 days before to 5 to 7 days after the rash.
Rubeola (measles)/rubeola virus		
› Direct contact › Droplet › Can survive 2 hr on surfaces	› 7 to 18 days	› 4 days before to 4 days after rash.
Varicella (chickenpox)/ varicella-zoster virus		
› Direct contact › Droplet › From person with shingles	› 10 to 21 days	› 1 to 2 days before lesions appear until all lesions have scabs.

View Images
- › Chickenpox
- › Rubella
- › Mumps

Assessment

- Risk Factors
  - Immunocompromised status
  - Crowded living conditions
  - Poor sanitation
  - Poor nutrition
  - Poor oxygenation and impaired circulation
  - Chronic illness
  - Recent exposure to a known case of a communicable disease
  - Not immunized or up to date on immunizations
- Subjective and Objective Data
  - Conjunctivitis
    - Pink or red color in the whites of the eyes
    - Swelling of the conjunctiva
    - Tearing
    - Yellow-green pus discharge from the eyes
    - Crusting of the eyelids in the morning

- ○ Fifth Disease
  - ▪ Before rash (several days)
    - ▫ Fever, runny nose, headache
  - ▪ Rash (7 to 10 days to several weeks)
    - ▫ Red rash on face (slapped cheek)
    - ▫ Secondary itchy rash may appear on rest of body, especially on the soles of the feet
- ○ Hand, Foot, and Mouth Disease
  - ▪ 1 to 2 days before rash and mouth sores
    - ▫ Fever and sore throat
    - ▫ Malaise and poor appetite
  - ▪ Rash and mouth sores
    - ▫ Painful sores in the mouth, blisters that become ulcers
    - ▫ Skin rash that is flat or raised red spots, usually on the hands and soles of the feet
- ○ Infectious Mononucleosis
  - ▪ Fever
  - ▪ Sore throat
  - ▪ Swollen lymph glands
  - ▪ Increased WBC
  - ▪ Atypical lymphocytes
  - ▪ Splenomegaly
  - ▪ Enlarged liver
- ○ Measles (rubeola)
  - ▪ 3 to 5 days prior to rash
    - ▫ Mild to moderate fever
    - ▫ Cough, runny nose, red eyes, sore throat
  - ▪ Rash
    - ▫ Koplik's spots (tiny white spots) appear in mouth
    - ▫ Red or reddish-brown rash beginning on the face spreading downward
    - ▫ Spike in fever with rash
- ○ Mumps
  - ▪ Painful swollen salivary glands
  - ▪ Fever and muscle aches
  - ▪ Abdominal pain
  - ▪ Fatigue and loss of appetite

- ○ Pertussis (whooping cough)
  - ■ Common cold symptoms (runny nose/congestion, sneezing, mild fever, mild cough)
  - ■ Severe coughing starts in 1 to 2 weeks
    - □ Coughing fits
    - □ Violent and rapid coughing
    - □ Loud "whooping" sound
- ○ Rubella (German measles)
  - ■ Low-grade fever and sore throat
  - ■ Red rash that starts on the face and spreads to the rest of the body, lasting 2 to 3 days.
- ○ Varicella (chickenpox)
  - ■ Symptoms 1 to 2 days prior to rash
    - □ High fever
    - □ Fatigue
    - □ Loss of appetite
    - □ Headache
  - ■ Rash
    - □ Macules start in trunk and face, spreading to rest of the body, progressing to papules.
    - □ Vesicles follow, with crusts forming.
    - □ Scabs appear in approximately 1 week.
- • Laboratory Tests
  - ○ CBC
  - ○ Electrolyte panels
  - ○ Mono spot blood test for infectious mononucleosis

Patient-Centered Care

- • Nursing Care
  - ○ Symptomatic treatment
    - ■ Isolation Precautions
      - □ Airborne/Contact
        - ‣ Varicella
      - □ Droplet
        - ‣ Rubella
        - ‣ Fifth disease
        - ‣ Pertussis
        - ‣ Mumps

- Standard
  - ‣ Mononucleosis
  - ‣ Hand, foot, and mouth disease
  - ‣ Conjunctivitis
- Administer an antipyretic for fever. Do not administer aspirin, due to the risk of Reye syndrome.
- Administer analgesics for pain.
- Provide fluids and nutritious foods the child prefers.
- Skin care
  - Provide calamine lotion for topical relief.
  - Keep the child's skin clean and dry to prevent secondary infection.
  - Keep the child cool, but prevent chilling.
  - Dress the child in lightweight, loose clothing.
  - Give baths in tepid water, possibly with oatmeal.
  - Keep the child's fingernails clean and short.
  - Apply mittens if the child scratches.
  - Teach good oral hygiene. The child may gargle with warm water for a sore throat.
  - Change linens daily.
- Provide quiet diversional activities.
- Promote adequate rest with naps if necessary.
- Keep lights dim if the child develops photophobia.
- Keep the child out of the sun.
- Notify the child's school or day care center of the child's infection. Obtain a plan from the school so that the child can continue working on schoolwork at home.
- Notify the health department of communicable diseases.
- Medications
  - Antihistamine – Diphenhydramine hydrochloride (Benadryl) and hydroxyzine (Atarax)
    - Used to controls pruritus
    - Nursing Considerations
      - Monitor the child's reaction to the medication because some children may become hyperalert with the administration of a medication from this group.
      - Monitor the child for drowsiness.
    - Client Education
      - Educate the family about safety precautions.
  - Antibiotic or antiviral therapy
    - Acyclovir (Zovirax) for high-risk clients who have varicella or mononucleosis
    - Antibiotics for pertussis
    - Antibiotic eye drops for bacterial conjunctivitis

- ◦ NSAIDs or acetaminophen (Tylenol)
  - ▪ Decreases fever
  - ▪ Nursing Considerations
    - ▫ Be alert for allergies.
  - ▪ Client Education
    - ▫ Teach parents the appropriate dosing for acetaminophen.
- • Care After Discharge
  - ◦ Client Education
    - ▪ Good hand hygiene prevents spread of infection.
    - ▪ Encourage adherence with antibiotic or antiviral therapy.
    - ▪ Instruct parents to teach the child to cover her nose and mouth when coughing or sneezing.
    - ▪ Instruct parents to wash the child's bed linens daily in mild detergent.
    - ▪ Teach parents of children who are immunocompromised to seek prompt medical care if symptoms develop.
    - ▪ Encourage adolescents to participate in decision-making.

Complications

- • Fifth Disease
  - ◦ People who have a weakened immune system are at risk for serous complications, anemia, secondary infections
- • Hand, Foot, and Mouth Disease
  - ◦ Viral or aseptic meningitis
- • Mononucleosis
  - ◦ Ruptured spleen
- • Mumps
  - ◦ Orchitis, encephalitis, meningitis, oophoritis, mastitis, deafness
- • Pertussis
  - ◦ Infants and children: pneumonia, convulsions, apnea, encephalopathy, death
  - ◦ Teens and adults: weight loss, loss of bladder control, passing out, rib fractures
- • Rubella
  - ◦ Birth defects (deafness; heart defects; mental, liver, and spleen damage) in fetus of women infected during pregnancy
- • Rubeola
  - ◦ Ear infections, pneumonia, diarrhea, encephalitis, death
- • Varicella
  - ◦ Dehydration, pneumonia, bleeding problems, bacterial infection of the skin, sepsis, toxic shock syndrome, bone or joint infections, death

APPLICATION EXERCISES

1. A nurse is teaching a group of parents about complications of communicable diseases. Which of the following communicable diseases may lead to pneumonia? (Select all that apply.)

_____ A. Rubella (German measles)

_____ B. Rubeola (measles)

_____ C. Pertussis (whooping cough)

_____ D. Varicella (chickenpox)

_____ E. Mumps

2. A nurse is caring for an adolescent client who has mononucleosis. The nurse assesses fever, fatigue, swollen lymph nodes, sore throat, and a sore upper abdomen. Which of the following instructions should the nurse discuss with the adolescent and her parents? (Select all that apply.)

_____ A. Take antibiotics until symptoms subside.

_____ B. Drink plenty of liquids.

_____ C. Avoid participating in strenuous activities.

_____ D. Allow for periods of rest.

_____ E. Take aspirin as needed for fever and discomfort.

_____ F. Gargle with saltwater every 2 to 3 hr.

3. A nurse is teaching the parent of a child who has hand, foot, and mouth disease. Which of the following should be included in the teaching?

A. "Your child can be contagious when the symptoms are gone."

B. "The incubation period is 10 to 21 days."

C. "It is transmitted by droplet."

D. "Once infected, your child will be a lifetime carrier."

4. A nurse is assessing a client who has pertussis. Which of the following are clinical manifestations of pertussis? (Select all that apply.)

_____ A. Runny nose

_____ B. Mild fever

_____ C. Whooping sound cough

_____ D. Swollen salivary glands

_____ E. Red rash

5. A nurse is teaching a group of parents about communicable diseases. Which of the following is the most appropriate method to prevent a communicable disease?

A. Handwashing

B. Avoiding persons with active disease

C. Covering your cough

D. Obtaining immunizations

6. A nurse is planning care for a group of clients who have communicable diseases. Use the ATI Active Learning Template: Basic Concept to complete this item to include the following sections:

A. Related Content: List the communicable diseases that require more than standard isolation precautions during hospitalization.

B. Nursing Interventions: Identify the type of isolation precaution to be implemented with the communicable disease identified above.

APPLICATION EXERCISES KEY

1. A. INCORRECT: Complications of rubella include birth defects (deafness; heart defects; mental, liver, and spleen damage) in the fetus of a woman infected during pregnancy.

    B. **CORRECT:** Complications of rubeola include ear infections, pneumonia, diarrhea, encephalitis, and death.

    C. **CORRECT:** Complications of pertussis include: infants and children – pneumonia, convulsions, apnea, encephalopathy, and death; teens and adults – weight loss, loss of bladder control, passing out, and rib fractures.

    D. **CORRECT:** Complications of varicella include dehydration, pneumonia, bleeding problems, bacterial infection of the skin, sepsis, toxic shock syndrome, bone or joint infections, and death.

    E. INCORRECT: Complications of mumps include orchitis, encephalitis, meningitis, oophoritis, mastitis, and deafness.

     NCLEX® Connection: Safety and Infection Control, Standard Precautions/Transmission-Based Precautions/Surgical Asepsis

2. A. INCORRECT: Antivirals are prescribed to clients who have mononucleosis.

    B. **CORRECT:** Fluids are encouraged to prevent dehydration with illness.

    C. **CORRECT:** The spleen could rupture as a result of injury. Therefore, strenuous activities should be avoided.

    D. **CORRECT:** Fatigue is common in clients who have mononucleosis. Therefore, allowing for periods of rest facilitates healing.

    E. INCORRECT: Acetaminophen (Tylenol) is used to control fever and discomfort.

    F. **CORRECT:** It can soothe discomfort associated with a sore throat.

     NCLEX® Connection: Physiological Adaptations, Alterations in Body Systems

3. A. **CORRECT:** Children are most contagious the first week of illness. However, they can be contagious even when symptoms are gone.

    B. INCORRECT: The incubation period of varicella is 10 to 21 days.

    C. INCORRECT: Varicella, rubella, rubeola, and mumps are examples of communicable diseases transmitted by droplet.

    D. INCORRECT: Healthy people who have EBV can transmit infection for a lifetime.

     NCLEX® Connection: Safety and Infection Control, Standard Precautions/Transmission-Based Precautions/Surgical Asepsis

4.   A. **CORRECT:** A client who has pertussis has coldlike symptoms, including runny nose, congestion, and mild fever.

    B. **CORRECT:** A client who has pertussis has coldlike symptoms, including runny nose, congestion, and mild fever.

    C. **CORRECT:** A client who has pertussis will experience coughing fits and a whooping sound.

    D. INCORRECT: A client who has mumps will have enlarged lymph nodes.

    E. INCORRECT: A client who has measles will have a red rash.

    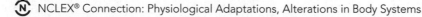 NCLEX® Connection: Physiological Adaptations, Alterations in Body Systems

5.   A. INCORRECT: Handwashing will decrease the spread of infection. However, this is not the best method to prevent communicable disease.

    B. INCORRECT: Avoiding people who have active disease will decrease the spread of infection. However, this is not the best method to prevent communicable disease.

    C. INCORRECT: Covering coughs will decrease the spread of infection. However, this is not the best method to prevent communicable disease.

    D. **CORRECT:** Obtaining immunizations has decreased the rate of communicable diseases and is the best method to prevent further spread of illness.

    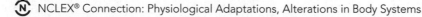 NCLEX® Connection: Safety and Infection Control, Standard Precautions/Transmission-Based Precautions/Surgical Asepsis

6.   *Using ATI Active Learning Template: Basic Concept*

    A. Related Content
       • Varicella
       • Rubella
       • Fifth disease
       • Pertussis
       • Mumps

    B. Nursing Interventions
       • Airborne/contact: varicella
       • Droplet: rubella, fifth disease, pertussis, mumps

    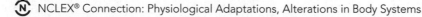 NCLEX® Connection: Safety and Infection Control, Standard Precautions/Transmission-Based Precautions/Surgical Asepsis

chapter 37

Overview

- Acute otitis media (AOM) is an infection of the structures of the middle ear with rapid clinical symptoms of infection.

- Otitis media with effusion (OME) is a collection of fluid in the middle ear but no infection.

- Repeated infections may cause impaired hearing and speech delays.

- Many infections clear spontaneously in a few days.

- The majority of incidences are related to eustachian tube malfunction.

Assessment

- Risk Factors

    ○ The eustachian tubes in children are shorter and more horizontal than those of adults. Otitis media is most common in the first 24 months of life and again when children enter school (ages 5 to 6). Otitis media occurs infrequently after age 7.

    ○ Otitis media is usually triggered by a bacterial infection (Streptococcus pneumoniae, Haemophilus influenzae, Moraxella catarrhalis), a viral infection (respiratory syncytial virus or influenza), allergies, or enlarged adenoids.

    ○ There is a lower incidence of otitis media in infants who are breastfed (possibly due to the presence of immunoglobulin A [IgA] in breast milk), which protects against infection.

    ○ Incidence is higher in the winter months.

    ○ Exposure to large numbers of children (day care).

    ○ Exposure to secondhand smoke.

    ○ Cleft lip and/or cleft palate.

    ○ Down syndrome.

- Subjective Data

    ○ Recent history of upper respiratory infection; acute onset of changes in behavior; frequent crying, irritability, and fussiness; inconsolability; tugging at ear; and reports of ear pain, loss of appetite, nausea, and vomiting.

- Objective Data
  - Physical Assessment Findings
    - AOM
      - Rubbing or pulling on ear
      - Crying
      - Lethargy
      - Bulging yellow or red tympanic membrane
      - Purulent material in middle ear or drainage from external canal
      - Decreased or no tympanic movement with pneumatic otoscopy
      - Lymphadenopathy of the neck and head
      - Temperature (may be as high as 40° C [104° F])
      - Hearing difficulties and speech delays if otitis media becomes a chronic condition
    - OME
      - Feeling of fullness in the ear
      - Orange discoloration of the tympanic membrane with decreased movement
      - Vague findings including rhinitis, cough, and diarrhea
      - Transient hearing loss and balance disturbances
  - Diagnostic Procedures
    - Pneumatic otoscope
      - A pneumatic otoscope is used to visualize the tympanic membrane and middle ear structures. The otoscope also assesses tympanic membrane movement.
      - Nursing Actions
        - ▸ Gently pull the pinna down and back to visualize the tympanic membrane of a child younger than 3 years old. For a child older than 3 years, gently pull the pinna up and back.

Patient-Centered Care

- Nursing Care
  - Provide comfort measures.
    - Administer pain medication as needed.
    - Provide diversional activities.
  - Place child in an upright position.
  - Management of fevers.
- Medications
  - Acetaminophen (Tylenol) or ibuprofen (Advil)
    - Used to provide analgesia and reduce fever
    - Nursing Considerations
      - Obtain a liquid preparation.
      - Use age-appropriate techniques to administer medication.

- ○ Antibiotics
  - ■ Amoxicillin (Amoxil), amoxicillin-culavulate (Augmentin), or azithromycin (Zithromax) PO (10 to 14 days)
  - ■ Ceftriaxone (Rocephin) IM (once)
  - ■ Nursing Considerations
    - □ Wait 72 hr for spontaneous resolution of otitis media before starting antibiotic.
    - □ Administer in high doses orally, usually 80 to 90 mg/kg/day in two divided doses.
    - □ The usual course of treatment orally is 10 to 14 days in children younger than 6 years of age. The course may be shorter for older children.
    - □ IM is used for resistant organisms or for client-specific reasons (difficulty taking oral medications, inability to complete the oral course).
  - ■ Client Education
    - □ Instruct the family that the child should complete the total course of treatment.
    - □ Observe for signs of allergy to the antibiotic, such as rash or difficulty breathing.
  - ○ Benzocaine (Americaine-Otic)
    - ■ Ear drops for topical pain relief
    - ■ Client Education
      - □ Instruct the family how to properly administer ear drops.
      - □ Discourage the use of decongestants or antihistamines.
- • Therapeutic Procedures
  - ○ Myringotomy and placement of tympanoplasty tubes may be indicated for a child who has multiple episodes of otitis media. This procedure may now be performed by laser treatment.
    - ■ This procedure is performed in an outpatient setting with the administration of general anesthesia. It is usually completed in 15 min.
    - ■ A small incision is made in the tympanic membrane, and tiny plastic or metal tubes are placed into the eardrum to equalize pressure and minimize effusion.
    - ■ Recovery takes place in a PACU, and discharge usually occurs within 1 hr.
    - ■ Postoperative pain is not common and, if present, will be mild.
    - ■ The tubes come out spontaneously (usually in 6 to 12 months).
    - ■ Client Education
      - □ Limit the child's activities for a few days following surgery.
      - □ Instruct parents to notify the provider when tubes come out. This usually does not require replacement of tubes.
- • Surgical Interventions
  - ○ Instruct the family to avoid getting water into the child's ears while the tubes are in place. The effectiveness of earplugs is not conclusive. Advise the parents to follow the health care provider's instructions.

- Care After Discharge
  - Client Education
    - Inform the client/parents about comfort measures.
    - Encourage the parents to feed the child in an upright position when bottle or breastfeeding.
    - If drainage is present, clean the external ear with sterile cotton swabs. Apply antibiotic ointment.
    - Teach the parents to avoid exposure of child to risk factors if possible (secondhand smoke, exposure to individuals with viral/bacterial respiratory infections).
    - Stress the importance of seeking medical care at initial signs and symptoms of infections (change in child's behavior, tugging on ear).
    - Encourage the parents to keep the child's immunizations up to date.
- Client Outcomes
  - The child will be free of infection.

Complications

- Hearing loss and/or speech delays
  - Nursing Actions
    - Assess and monitor for deficits.
    - Refer the child for audiology testing if needed.
  - Client Education
    - Speech therapy may be necessary.

APPLICATION EXERCISES

1. A nurse is caring for a toddler who has acute otitis media. Which of the following is the priority action for the nurse to take?

    A. Provide emotional support to the family.

    B. Educate the family on care of the child.

    C. Prevent clinical complications.

    D. Administer analgesics.

2. A nurse is caring for a 2-year-old child who has had three ear infections in the past 5 months. The nurse should know that the child is at risk for developing which of the following as a long-term complication?

    A. Balance difficulties

    B. Prolonged hearing loss

    C. Speech delays

    D. Mastoiditis

3. An infant who has clinical manifestations of acute otitis media (AOM) is brought to an outpatient facility by his parent. The nurse should recognize that which of the following factors places the infant at risk for otitis media? (Select all that apply.)

    _____ A. Breastfeeding without formula supplementation.

    _____ B. Attends day care 4 days per week.

    _____ C. Immunizations are up to date.

    _____ D. History of a cleft palate repair.

    _____ E. Parents smoke cigarettes outside.

4. A nurse is caring for a toddler who has rhinitis, cough, and diarrhea for 2 days. Upon assessment, it is noted that the tympanic membrane has a orange discoloration and decreased movement. Which of the following is an appropriate statement for the nurse to make?

    A. "Your child has an ear infection that requires antibiotics."

    B. "Your child could experience transient hearing loss."

    C. "Your child will need to be on a decongestant until this clears."

    D. "Your child will need to have a myringotomy."

5. A nurse is assessing an infant. Which of the following findings are clinical manifestations of acute otitis media? (Select all that apply.)

_____ A. Decreased pain in the supine position

_____ B. Rolling head side to side

_____ C. Loss of appetite

_____ D. Increased sensitivity to sound

_____ E. Crying

6. A nurse is caring for an infant who has acute otitis media for the first time. Use the ATI Active Learning Template: Systems Disorder to complete this item to include the following:

A. Description of Disorder/Disease Process

B. Nursing Care: Describe two interventions.

C. Medications: List two.

D. Care after Discharge: Describe two teaching points.

E. Potential Complication: Identify one.

APPLICATION EXERCISES KEY

1. A. INCORRECT: Providing emotional support to the family for the families psychological well-being is an important action for the nurse to take. However, it is not the priority action.

   B. INCORRECT: Educating the family on the care of the child to promote recovery from illness is an important action for the nurse to take. However, it is not the priority action.

   C. INCORRECT: Preventing clinical complications by administering antibiotics and monitoring the child's status is an important action for the nurse to take. However, it is not the priority action.

   D. **CORRECT:** The priority action the nurse should take when using Maslow's hierarchy of needs is to meet the toddler's physiological need first. Therefore, administering analgesics to alleviate or decrease physical pain is the priority action for the nurse to take.

    NCLEX® Connection: Pharmacological and Parenteral Therapies, Pharmacological Pain Management

2. A. INCORRECT: Balance difficulties may be present with otitis media. However, it is not a long-term complication.

   B. INCORRECT: Prolonged hearing loss may be present with otitis media. However, it is not a long-term complication.

   C. **CORRECT:** Speech delay is a common complication of otitis media.

   D. INCORRECT: Mastoiditis may be a result of otitis media. However, it is not a long-term complication.

    NCLEX® Connection: Physiological Adaptations, Unexpected Response to Therapies

3. A. INCORRECT: Breastfeeding helps to protect against AOM because breast milk contains secretory immunoglobulin A.

   B. **CORRECT:** Infants who attend day care have an increased risk of OM because of the exposure to multiple people.

   C. INCORRECT: The pneumococcal conjugate vaccine decreases the incidence of OM.

   D. **CORRECT:** Infants born with cleft palate are more prone to AOM because micro-organisms can easily enter the eustachian tubes.

   E. **CORRECT:** Exposure to secondhand smoke increases an infant's risk for AOM.

    NCLEX® Connection: Health Promotion and Maintenance, Health Promotion/Disease Prevention

4. A. INCORRECT: Rhinitis, cough, diarrhea, and an orange discoloration of the tympanic membrane are clinical findings of otitis media with effusion (OME). Therefore, antibiotics are not recommended.

    B. **CORRECT:** Rhinitis, cough, diarrhea, and an orange discoloration of the tympanic membrane are clinical findings of OME. Transient hearing loss is a complication of OME.

    C. INCORRECT: Rhinitis, cough, diarrhea, and an orange discoloration of the tympanic membrane are clinical findings of OME. Therefore, decongestants are not recommended.

    D. INCORRECT: Myringotomy is recommended for clients with chronic OME.

     NCLEX® Connection: Physiological Adaptations, Unexpected Response to Therapies

5. A. INCORRECT: Infants who have acute otitis media will have an increase in pain in the supine position from the fluid and pressure in the ear.

    B. **CORRECT:** Infants who have acute otitis media will roll their head side to side because of the pain and pressure in the ear.

    C. **CORRECT:** Infants who have acute otits media will exhibit a loss of appetite due to the pain and pressure in the ear.

    D. INCORRECT: Infants who have acute otitis media have a decreased sensitivity to sound from the fluid and pressure in the ear.

    E. **CORRECT:** Infants who have acute otitis media will exhibit crying and irritability from the pain.

     NCLEX® Connection: Physiological Adaptations, Pathophysiology

6. *Using the ATI Active Learning Template: Systems Disorder*

    A. Description of Disorder/Disease Process
       • Acute otitis media (AOM) is an infection of the structures of the middle ear with rapid clinical symptoms of infection.

    B. Nursing Care
       • Comfort care with pain medications and distraction.
       • Management of fevers
       • Place child in an upright position

    C. Medications
       • Amoxicillin (Amoxil), amoxicillin-clavulanate (Augmentin) or azithromycin (Zithromax) PO or ceftriaxone (Rocephin) IM
       • Acetaminophen (Tylenol) or ibuprofen (Advil) for pain and fever
       • Benzocaine (Americaine Otic)

    D. Care After Discharge
       • Inform the parents about comfort measures.
       • Encourage the parents to feed the child in an upright position when bottle or breastfeeding.
       • If drainage is present, clean the external ear with sterile cotton swabs. Apply antibiotic ointment.
       • Teach parents to avoid risk factors (secondhand smoke, exposure to individuals with viral/bacterial respiratory infections).
       • Stress the importance of seeking medical care at the onset of signs and symptoms of infections (change in child's behavior, tugging on ear).
       • Eliminate exposure to secondhand smoke.
       • Encourage the parents to keep the child's immunizations up to date.

    E. Potential Complication
       • Hearing loss and/or speech delays

    (N) NCLEX® Connection: Physiological Adaptations, Pathophysiology

chapter 38

Overview

- HIV infection is a viral infection in which the virus infects the T-lymphocytes, causing immune dysfunction. This leads to organ dysfunction and a variety of opportunistic illnesses in a weakened host.

Assessment

- Risk Factors

  - Infants of mothers who are infected with HIV/AIDs can transmit the virus perinatally or by breast milk.

  - Blood products that contain the HIV virus.

  - Sexual abuse.

  - Risky behaviors such as unprotected sexual activity and IV drug use.

  - Sexually transmitted infections.

  - Lack of awareness.

- Objective Data

  - Physical Assessment Findings and Laboratory Tests

    - HIV infection – Birth to 12 years

HIV INFECTION: BIRTH TO 12 YEARS					
	LESS THAN 12 MONTHS		1 TO 5 YEARS		6 TO 12 YEARS
	Cells/mEq/L*	%**	Cells/mEq/L	%	Cells/mEq/L	%
No suppression	1,500 or more	25 or more	1,000 or more	25 or more	500 or more	25 or more
Moderate suppression	750 to 1,499	15 to 24	500 to 999	15 to 24	200 to 499	15 to 24
Severe suppression	less than 750	less than 15	less than 500	less than 15	less than 200	less than 15

*CD4+ T-lymphocyte count = cells/mEq/L
**CD4+ T-lymphocyte percentage of total lymphocytes = %

NOT SYMPTOMATIC

› No signs or symptoms considered to be the result of HIV infection are present, or the child has only one of the conditions listed in the mildly symptomatic section.

MILDLY SYMPTOMATIC

› Two or more of the following conditions are present, but the child has none of the conditions listed in the moderately or severely symptomatic sections.

  » Lymphadenopathy

  » Hepatomegaly

» Splenomegaly

» Recurrent upper respiratory infections, sinusitis, or otitis media

» Dermatitis

» Parotitis

MODERATELY SYMPTOMATIC

› Children with the following conditions are considered moderately symptomatic.

  » Anemia

  » Bacterial meningitis, pneumonia, or sepsis (single episode)

  » Oropharyngeal candidiasis

  » Cardiomyopathy

  » Cytomegalovirus infection, with onset before 1 month of age

  » Recurrent or chronic diarrhea

  » Hepatitis

» Herpes simplex virus (HSV), stomatitis, bronchitis, pneumonitis, or esophagitis

» Herpes zoster

» Nephropathy

» Leiomyosarcoma

» Lymphoid interstitial pneumonia (LIP) or pulmonary lymphoid hyperplasia complex

» Persistent fever (lasting more than 1 month)

» Toxoplasmosis before 1 month of age

» Disseminated varicella

SEVERELY SYMPTOMATIC

› Children with the following conditions are considered severely symptomatic.

  » Multiple serious bacterial infections (meningitis, bone or joint, abscesses of internal organ or body cavity, septicemia, pneumonia)

  » Esophageal or pulmonary candidiasis, (bronchi, trachea, lungs)

  » Cytomegalovirus disease (greater than 1 month of age with site other than liver, spleen, or lymph nodes)

  » HSV stomatitis, bronchitis, pneumonitis, or esophagitis lasting longer than 1 month

  » Kaposi's sarcoma

  » Brain or Burkitt's lymphoma

» Disseminated or extrapulmonary mycobacterium tuberculosis

» Encephalopathy with developmental delays

» Disseminated coccidioidomycosis

» Extrapulmonary cryptococcosis

» Cryptosporidiosis or isosporiasis with diarrhea longer than 1 month

» Disseminated histoplasmosis

» Pneumocystis carinii pneumonia

» Multifocal leukoencephalopathy

» Salmonella septicemia

» Toxoplasmosis of the brain

» Wasting syndrome

*Human Immunodeficiency Virus Infection (HIV) (retrieved from www.cdc.gov). To read more about HIV, go to the website of the Centers for Disease Control and Prevention (www.cdc.gov).

  ▪ HIV infection – 13 to 20 years (See the chapter on *HIV/AIDS* in the *Adult Medical Surgical Nursing Review Module*.)

- ○ Diagnostic Procedures
  - ▪ Laboratory criteria for diagnosis – 18 months or older
    - ☐ Positive result from HIV enzyme-linked immunosorbent assay (ELISA) and Western blot immunoassay.
  - ▪ Laboratory criteria for diagnosis of infants who are less than 18 months of age and were born to infected mothers
    - ☐ Positive result from polymerase chain reaction (PCR) and virus culture.
  - ▪ Classification
    - ☐ Children less than 13 are classified by the following criteria.
      - ▸ N: No signs or symptoms
        - ▹ N1 = no evidence of suppression
        - ▹ N2 = evidence of moderate suppression
        - ▹ N3 = severe suppression
      - ▸ A: Mild signs of symptoms
        - ▹ A1 = no evidence of suppression
        - ▹ A2 = evidence of moderate suppression
        - ▹ A3 = severe suppression
      - ▸ B: Moderate signs or symptoms
        - ▹ B1 = no evidence of suppression
        - ▹ B2 = evidence of moderate suppression
        - ▹ B3 = severe suppression
      - ▸ C: Severe signs or symptoms
        - ▹ C1 = no evidence of suppression
        - ▹ C2 = evidence of moderate suppression
        - ▹ C3 = severe suppression

Patient-Centered Care

- Nursing Care
  - ○ Encourage a balanced diet that is high in calories and protein. Obtain the child's preferred food and beverages. Give nutritional supplements.
  - ○ Administer total parental nutrition (TPN) if prescribed.
  - ○ Provide good oral care and report abnormalities for treatment.
  - ○ Keep the child's skin clean and dry.
  - ○ Provide nonpharmacological methods of pain relief.
  - ○ Assess the child for pain and provide adequate pain management. Use of medications may include nonsteroidal anti-inflammatory drugs (NSAIDs), acetaminophen (Tylenol), opioids, muscle relaxants, and/or a eutectic mixture of local anesthetics (EMLA cream) for numerous diagnostic procedures.

- Protect/prevent infection using standard precautions.
  - Encourage deep breathing and coughing.
  - Maintain good hand hygiene.
  - Teach the child and parents to avoid individuals who have colds/infections/viruses.
  - Encourage immunizations, such as pneumococcal vaccine (PCV) and yearly seasonal influenza vaccine.
  - Monitor for signs of opportunistic infections.
- Administer medications as prescribed for opportunistic infections.

- Medications
  - Antiretroviral medications are given at various stages of the HIV cycle to inhibit reproduction of the virus.
    - Nucleoside reverse transcriptase inhibitors (NRTIs) – zidovudine, didanosine, lamivudine, abacavir
      - Suppress the synthesis of viral DNA
    - Non-nucleoside reverse transcriptase inhibitors (NNRTIs) – delavirdine, efavirenz, nevirapine
      - Bind to the viral DNA causing direct inhibition
    - Nucleotide reverse transcriptase inhibitors such as adefovir.
      - Inhibit viral DNA synthesis
    - Protease inhibitors – indinavir, ritonavir, nelfinavir, amprenavir
      - Inhibit an enzyme needed for the virus to replicate
    - Adjunctive antiretrovirals such as hydroxyurea
      - Suppress DNA replication
    - Nursing considerations
      - Monitor laboratory results (CBC, WBC, liver function tests). Antiretroviral medications can increase alanine aminotransferase (ALT), aspartate aminotransferase (AST), bilirubin, mean corpuscular volume (MCV), high-density lipoproteins (HDLs), total cholesterol, and triglycerides.
    - Client education
      - Educate about the side effects of the medications and ways to decrease the severity of the side effects.
      - Educate about the need to take the medication on a regular schedule and to not miss doses.
  - Antibiotics
    - Trimethoprim-sulfamethoxazole (TMZ-SMZ)
      - Administer to all infants who are born to infected mothers until HIV infection is excluded.
  - IV gamma globulin
    - To prevent recurrent or serious bacterial infections
- Teamwork and Collaboration
  - Social services can help with access to health care and medication acquisition.
  - Dietician can assist with nutritional support and promote good nutrition.

- Care After Discharge
    - Client Education
        - Educate the child and parents about the chronicity of the illness and the need for lifelong medication administration.
        - Instruct the parents when to notify the provider. Signs and symptoms requiring medical care include headache, fever, lethargy, warmth, tenderness, redness at joints, and neck stiffness.
        - Educate the child and parents about transmission of the virus (high-risk behaviors).
        - Identify stressors that may be affecting the family and make appropriate referrals (school/community response to child, finances, access to health care).
        - Instruct the child and parents about safe practice when using needles/syringes and administering medications.

Complications

- Failure to thrive
    - Nursing Actions
        - Obtain a baseline height and weight, and continue to monitor.
        - Promote optimal nutrition. This may require the administration of total parenteral nutrition.
        - Assess growth and development. Monitor for delays.
        - Provide opportunities for normal development (age-appropriate toys, play with children of the same age).
    - Client Education
        - Educate the child and parents about appropriate nutrition and how to meet nutritional needs.
- *Pneumocystis carinii* pneumonia (PCP)
    - Nursing Actions
        - Assess and monitor respiratory status, which includes respiratory rate and effort, oxygen saturation, and breath sounds.
        - Administer appropriate antibiotics.
        - Administer an antipyretic and/or analgesics.
        - Provide adequate hydration and maintain fluid and electrolyte balance.
        - Use postural drainage and chest physiotherapy to mobilize and remove fluid from the lungs.
        - Promote adequate rest.
    - Client Education
        - Educate the child and parents about the infectious process and how to prevent infection.
        - Educate the child and parents about the importance of medication and the need to maintain the medication regimen.

APPLICATION EXERCISES

1. A nurse is teaching a parent of a child who has HIV. Which of the following should be included? (Select all that apply.)

_____ A. Obtain yearly influenza vaccination.

_____ B. Avoid live immunizations.

_____ C. Avoid individuals who have colds.

_____ D. Provide nutritional supplements.

_____ E. Administer aspirin for fever.

2. A nurse is caring for a child who has AIDS. Which of the following isolation precautions should the nurse implement?

A. Contact

B. Airborne

C. Droplet

D. Standard

3. A nurse is admitting a child who has HIV. Which of the following are clinical manifestations of a child who is mildly symptomatic? (Select all that apply.)

_____ A. Herpes zoster

_____ B. Anemia

_____ C. Dermatitis

_____ D. Hepatomegaly

_____ E. Lymphadenopathy

4. A nurse is teaching a group of adolescents about HIV/AIDS. Which of the following should be included in the teaching?

A. "You can contract HIV through casual kissing."

B. "You can contract HIV by sharing eating utensils."

C. "The incubation period can be months to years."

D. "Medications inhibit transmission of the virus."

5. A nurse is admitting a child who has HIV. Which of the following are clinical manifestations of a child who is severly symptomatic? (Select all that apply.)

_____ A. Kaposi's sarcoma

_____ B. Hepatitis

_____ C. Wasting syndrome

_____ D. Pulmonary candidiasis

_____ E. Cardiomyopathy

6. A nurse is teaching a parent of a child who has AIDS. Use the ATI Active Learning Template: Systems Disorder to complete this item. List two complications of AIDS and include four nursing actions for each.

APPLICATION EXERCISES KEY

1. A. **CORRECT:** Obtaining a yearly influenza vaccination is recommended to protect the child from opportunistic infections.

    B. **CORRECT:** Live vaccines should not be given to children who are immunocompromised.

    C. **CORRECT:** Avoiding individuals who have colds will assist in protecting the child from opportunistic infections.

    D. **CORRECT:** Nutritional supplements are recommended to promote improved nutrition of the child who has HIV.

    E. INCORRECT: Acetaminophen should be administered to a child who has a fever.

     NCLEX® Connection: Physiological Adaptations, Illness Management

2. A. INCORRECT: Contact isolation precautions are used to protect transmission of disease that is skin-to-skin or direct contact.

    B. INCORRECT: Airborne isolation precautions are used to protect transmission of disease that is small-particles droplets.

    C. INCORRECT: Droplet isolation precautions are used to protect transmission of disease that is large-particles droplets.

    D. **CORRECT:** Standard isolation precautions are used to protect transmission of disease that is bloodborne or present in a body substance.

     NCLEX® Connection: Safety and Infection Control, Standard Precautions/Transmission-Based Precautions/Surgical Asepsis

3. A. INCORRECT: Herpes zoster is a clinical manifestation of a child who is moderately symptomatic.

    B. INCORRECT: Anemia is a clinical manifestation of a child who is moderately symptomatic.

    C. **CORRECT:** Dermatitis is a clinical manifestation of a child who is mildly symptomatic.

    D. **CORRECT:** Hepatomegaly is a clinical manifestation of a child who is mildly symptomatic.

    E. **CORRECT:** Lymphadenopathy is a clinical manifestation of a child who is mildly symptomatic.

     NCLEX® Connection: Physiological Adaptations, Alterations in Body Systems

4. A. INCORRECT: HIV is transmitted via blood, semen, vaginal secretions, and breast milk. There is no evidence that casual contact spreads the virus.

    B. INCORRECT: HIV is transmitted via blood, semen, vaginal secretions, and breast milk. There is no evidence that casual contact spreads the virus.

    C. **CORRECT:** The incubation period can be months to years depending on the individual, how HIV was acquired, and interventions.

    D. INCORRECT: Medications suppress the progression of the virus.

     NCLEX® Connection: Safety and Infection Control, Standard Precautions/Transmission-Based Precautions/Surgical Asepsis

5. A. **CORRECT:** Kaposi's sarcoma is a clinical manifestation of a child who is severely symptomatic.

    B. INCORRECT: Hepatitis is a clinical manifestation of a child who is moderately symptomatic.

    C. **CORRECT:** Wasting syndrome is a clinical manifestation of a child who is severely symptomatic.

    D. **CORRECT:** Pulmonary candidiasis is a clinical manifestation of a child who is severely symptomatic.

    E. INCORRECT: Cardiomyopathy is a clinical manifestation of a child who is moderately symptomatic.

    NCLEX® Connection: Physiological Adaptations, Alterations in Body Systems

6. *Using the ATI Active Learning Template: Systems Disorder*
    - Failure to thrive
      ○ Nursing Actions
        - Obtain a baseline height and weight, and continue to monitor.
        - Promote optimal nutrition. This may require the administration of total parenteral nutrition.
        - Assess growth and development. Monitor for delays.
        - Provide opportunities for normal development (age-appropriate toys, play with children of the same age).
        - Educate the child and parents about appropriate nutrition and how to meet nutritional needs.
    - *Pneumocystis carinii* pneumonia (PCP)
      ○ Nursing Actions
        - Assess and monitor respiratory status, which includes respiratory rate and effort, oxygen saturation, and breath sounds.
        - Administer appropriate antibiotics.
        - Administer an antipyretic and/or analgesics.
        - Provide adequate hydration and maintain fluid and electrolyte balance.
        - Use postural drainage and chest physiotherapy to mobilize and remove fluid from the lungs.
        - Promote adequate rest.
        - Educate the child and parents about the infectious process and how to prevent infection.
        - Educate the child and parents about the importance of medication and the need to maintain the medication regimen.

    NCLEX® Connection: Physiological Adaptations, Unexpected Response to Therapies

UNIT 2   Nursing Care of Children with System Disorders

SECTION: NEOPLASTIC DISORDERS

› Organ Neoplasms
› Blood Neoplasms
› Bone and Soft Tissue Cancers

NCLEX® CONNECTIONS

When reviewing the chapters in this unit, keep in mind the relevant sections of the NCLEX® outline, in particular:

Client Needs: Basic Care and Comfort	Client Needs: Pharmacological and Parenteral Therapies	Client Needs: Reduction of Risk Potential
› Relevant topics/tasks include: » Mobility/Immobility › Perform a skin assessment and implement measures to maintain skin integrity and prevent skin breakdown. » Nonpharmacological Comfort Interventions › Assess the client's need for palliative care. » Nutrition and Oral Hydration › Manage the client who has an alteration in nutritional intake.	› Relevant topics/tasks include: » Adverse Effects/ Contraindications/Side Effects/Interactions › Assess client for actual or potential side effects and adverse effects of medications. » Expected Actions/Outcomes › Evaluate client response to medication. » Pharmacological Pain Management › Administer and document pharmacological pain management appropriate for client age and diagnoses.	› Relevant topics/tasks include: » Diagnostic Tests › Monitor the results of diagnostic testing and intervene as needed. » Potential for Complications of Diagnostic Tests/ Treatments/Procedures › Monitor the client for signs of bleeding. » Therapeutic Procedures › Provide preoperative care.

UNIT 2   NURSING CARE OF CHILDREN WITH SYSTEM DISORDERS
SECTION: NEOPLASTIC DISORDERS

CHAPTER 39   Organ Neoplasms

Overview

- Refer to the AMS review module for organ neoplasms that both adults and children can acquire, such as lymphoma, brain tumor, and liver and testicular cancer.
- Wilms' tumor (nephroblastoma) is a malignancy that occurs in the kidneys or abdomen.
  - The tumor is usually unilateral, with 10% of cases affecting both kidneys.
  - Diagnosis typically occurs at an age younger than 5, with the majority of cases being diagnosed at about age 3.
  - Metastasis is rare.
- Neuroblastoma is a malignancy that occurs in the adrenal gland, sympathetic chain of the retroperitoneal area, head, neck, pelvis, or chest.
  - Usually manifested during the toddler years, with 95% of cases prior to age 10.
  - Half of all cases have metastasized before diagnosis.
- Treatment varies with each child and can be any combination of surgery, chemotherapy, and radiation.

Assessment

- Risk Factors
  - There are no known risk factors for Wilms' tumor or neuroblastoma.
- Subjective and Objective Data
  - Wilms' Tumor
    - Firm, nontender abdominal swelling or mass
    - Fatigue, malaise, weight loss
    - Fever
    - Hematuria
    - Hypertension
    - Signs and symptoms of metastasis include dyspnea, cough, and shortness of breath.
  - Neuroblastoma
    - Symptoms depend upon the location and stage of disease.
    - Half of children who have neuroblastoma have few symptoms.
    - Signs and symptoms of metastasis include an ill appearance, periorbital ecchymoses, proptosis, bone pain, and irritability.

- ○ Laboratory Tests
  - ■ Wilms' Tumor
    - □ BUN, creatinine
    - □ CBC
    - □ Urinalysis
  - ■ Neuroblastoma
    - □ CBC and coagulation studies
    - □ Urine catecholamines (vanillylmandelic acid, homovanillic acid, dopamine, and norepinephrine)
- ○ Diagnostic Procedures
  - ■ Wilms' Tumor
    - □ Abdominal ultrasonography
    - □ Abdominal and chest computed tomography (CT) scan
    - □ Inferior venacavogram (rule out involvement with the vena cava)
    - □ Bone marrow aspiration (rule out metastasis)
  - ■ Neuroblastoma
    - □ Skeletal survey
    - □ Skull, neck, chest, abdominal, and bone CT scans
    - □ Bone marrow aspiration (rule out metastasis)
    - □ Metaiodobenzylguanidine (MIBG) scan (determine bone, bone marrow and soft tissue involvement)
    - □ Biopsy of tumor
  - ■ Nursing Actions
    - □ Assess the child for allergies to dye or shellfish.
    - □ Assist the child to remain still during the procedure.
    - □ Instruct the child to drink oral contrast if prescribed.
    - □ Sedate the child if prescribed.
  - ■ Client Education

    - □ Provide emotional support.

Patient-Centered Care

- • Nursing Care
  - ○ If Wilms' tumor is suspected, do not palpate the abdomen.
  - ○ Assess the child and family's coping and support.
  - ○ Assess for developmental delays related to illness.
  - ○ Assess physical growth (height and weight).
  - ○ Provide education and support to the child and family regarding diagnostic testing, treatment plan, ongoing therapy, and prognosis.

- ○ Monitor for signs of infection.
- ○ Administer antibiotics as prescribed for infection.
- ○ Keep the child's skin clean, dry, and lubricated.
- ○ Provide oral hygiene and keep the child's lips lubricated.
- ○ Provide age-appropriate diversional activities.
- ○ Provide support to the child and family.
  - Avoid false reassurance.
  - Listen to the child's concerns.
  - Allow time for the child and family to discuss feelings regarding loss and to grieve.
- Teamwork and Collaboration
  - ○ Social services may be of assistance with access to medications and durable medical equipment if needed.
  - ○ A nutritionist may be consulted for development of a diet plan.
- Therapeutic Procedures
  - ○ Treatment for Wilms' tumor
    - Surgical removal of the tumor and kidney soon after diagnosis
    - Preoperative chemotherapy or radiation if both kidneys are involved to decrease the size of the tumors and potentially preserve one kidney.
    - Postoperative radiation and/or chemotherapy for children with large tumors, metastasis, reoccurrence, and residual disease
  - ○ Treatment for neuroblastoma
    - Surgical removal of the tumor
    - Chemotherapy and/or radiation used for metastasis and residual disease
  - ○ Chemotherapy
    - Wilms' Tumor
      - □ Dactinomycin (Cosmegen) and vincristine (Vincasar PFS)
      - □ For tumors at more advanced stages, those with unfavorable histology, or tumors that recur after treatment, other drugs such as doxorubicin hydrochloride (Adriamycin), cyclophosphamide (Cytoxan), etoposide (Etopophos), irinotecan (Camptosar), and carboplatin may be used.
    - Neuroblastoma
      - □ Various combination of agents are used: cyclophosphamide, doxorubicin, cisplatin, etoposide, vincristine, ifosfamide, and carboplatin
    - The child may have a long-term central venous access device or a peripherally inserted central catheter (PICC) in place.
    - Nursing Actions
      - □ Handle the chemotherapeutic agents carefully.
      - □ Medicate the child with an antiemetic prior to administration.
      - □ Allow the child several food choices. Allow the child to choose favorite foods.
      - □ Observe the mouth for mucosal ulcerations.
      - □ Offer cool fluids to prevent dehydration and soothe sore mucous membranes.

- Client Education
  - Educate the child and family about the side effects of chemotherapy (mouth sores, loss of appetite, nausea and vomiting, hair loss, diarrhea or constipation, increased risk of infection, easy bruising or bleeding, and fatigue).
  - Educate the child and family about the importance of immunizations and follow-up appointments.
  - Educate the child and family about good infection control practices.
- Radiation
  - Radiation is dose-calculated and usually delivered in divided treatments over several weeks.
  - Radiation affects rapidly growing cells in the body. Therefore, cells that normally have a fast turnover may be affected in addition to cancer cells.
  - Nursing Actions
    - Take care when radiation is in use. Wear lead aprons.
  - Client Education
    - Educate the child and family about the procedure and provide support.
    - Instruct the child and family not to wash off marks on skin that outline the targeted areas.
    - Teach the child and family to wash the marked areas with lukewarm water, use hands instead of a washcloth, pat dry, and take care not to remove the markings. Avoid using hot or cold water.
    - Teach the child and family to avoid the use of soaps, creams, lotions, and/or powders unless they are prescribed.
    - Encourage wearing loose cotton clothing.
    - Remind the child and family to keep the areas protected from the sun by wearing a hat and long-sleeved shirts.
    - Instruct the family to seek medical care for blisters, weeping, and red/tender skin.
- Surgical Interventions
  - Tumor debulking
    - Nursing Actions
      - Preoperative
        - Avoid palpation of Wilms' tumor.
      - Postoperative
        - Monitor gastrointestinal activity (bowel sounds, bowel movements, distention, nausea, vomiting).
        - Provide pain relief.
        - Monitor vital signs and assess for any signs and symptoms of infection.
        - Encourage pulmonary hygiene.
    - Client Education
      - Provide preoperative teaching to the child and family that includes length of surgery, where the child will recover, and what equipment will be in place (nasogastric tube, IV line, indwelling urinary catheter).

Complications

- Metastasis
- Kidney failure
- Pancytopenia
  - Bone marrow depression resulting in anemia, neutropenia, and/or thrombocytopenia
  - Nursing Actions
    - Monitor vital signs and report them to the health care provider. Report a temperature greater than 37.8° C (100° F).
    - Monitor for signs of infection (lung congestion; redness, swelling, and pain around IV sites) and lesions in the mouth, and monitor the client's wound site and immunization status.
    - Administer antimicrobial, antiviral, and antifungal medications as prescribed.
    - Protect the child from sources of possible infection.
      - Use good hand hygiene.
      - Encourage the child and family to use good hand hygiene.
    - Encourage the child to avoid crowds while undergoing chemotherapy.
    - Instruct the child to avoid fresh fruits and vegetables.
    - Avoid invasive procedures (injections, rectal temperatures, catheters). Apply pressure to puncture sites for 5 min.
    - Monitor for signs of bleeding.
    - Avoid aspirin/NSAIDs.
    - Administer filgrastim (Neupogen), a granulocyte colony-stimulating factor that stimulates WBC production, subcutaneously daily.
    - Monitor the child for headache, fever, and mild to moderate bone pain.
    - Administer epoetin alfa (Procrit) subcutaneously two to three times per week as prescribed to stimulate RBC formation.
    - Monitor blood pressure.
    - Administer oprelvekin (Interleukin-11, Neumega) subcutaneously daily as prescribed to stimulate platelet formation.
    - Encourage the use of a soft toothbrush.
    - Use gentle handling and positioning to protect from injury.
    - Organize care to provide for rest. Schedule rest periods.

  - Client Education
    - Educate the child and family about infection control procedures at home.
    - Provide support.

- Anorexia, nausea, vomiting
  - These are side effects of chemotherapy and radiation therapy.
  - Nursing Actions
    - Avoid strong odors. Provide a pleasant atmosphere for meals.
    - Suggest and assist in selecting foods/fluids.
    - Provide small, frequent meals.
    - Administer antiemetics as prescribed, usually before meals.
- Alteration in bowel elimination
  - Diarrhea is a result of radiation to the abdominal area. Some chemotherapeutic agents may cause constipation. If mobility and nutrition decrease, the child is more likely to develop constipation.
  - Nursing Actions
    - Provide meticulous skin care.
    - Provide a nutritious diet.
    - Determine if certain foods or drinks (high-fiber, lactose-rich) worsen the child's condition.
    - Monitor intake and output and daily weight.
- Mucositis and dry mouth
  - Nursing Actions
    - Provide a soft toothbrush and/or swabs.
    - Lubricate the child's lips.
    - Give soft, nonacidic foods. A puréed or liquid diet may be required.
    - Provide analgesics.

  - Client Education
    - Encourage the parents and child to visit a dentist before therapy.
    - Encourage the use of mouth washes, such as 1 tsp salt mixed with 1 pint water or 1 tsp baking soda mixed with 1 quart water.
- Alopecia
  - Occurs with chemotherapy and radiation of the head and/or neck
  - Nursing Actions
    - Assess the child's feelings.
    - Discuss cutting long hair.
    - Use gentle shampoos. Gently brush the child's hair.
    - Avoid blow dryers and curling irons.
    - Suggest wearing a cotton hat or scarf.
  - Client Education
    - Discuss the use of a wig, turbans, or hats.
    - Instruct the child and family to avoid blow dryers and curling irons.

APPLICATION EXERCISES

1. A nurse is teaching the parent of a child who has a neuroblastoma. Which of the following statements should the nurse include in the teaching? (Select all that apply.)

_____ A. "Half of the children who have neuroblastoma have metastatic disease."

_____ B. "Your child will need a bone marrow biopsy."

_____ C. "Your child will be paralyzed because of this tumor."

_____ D. "Most children are diagnosed around age 12."

_____ E. "Your child will need surgery for resection of the tumor."

2. A nurse is caring for a toddler who has a Wilms' tumor. Which of the following should be included in the plan of care?

A. Abdominal palpation to identify the size of the tumor

B. Preparation for surgery

C. Teaching about dialysis

D. Obtaining 24-hr urine specimen

3. A nurse is teaching the parent of a child who has a Wilms' tumor. Which of the following statements should the nurse include in the teaching? (Select all that apply.)

_____ A. "Your child will need to have chemotherapy for 12 months."

_____ B. "Wilms' tumors are typically genetic in nature."

_____ C. "Surgery is done usually within 48 hours of diagnosis."

_____ D. "Palpating the tumor could cause spread of the cancer."

_____ E. "Further treatments will start immediately after surgery.

4. A nurse is caring for a child who is postoperative following surgical removal of a Wilms' tumor. Which of the following assessments is an indication to continue NPO status?

A. Abdominal girth 1 cm larger than yesterday

B. Report of pain at the operative site

C. Absent bowel sounds

D. Passing of flatus every 30 min

5. A nurse is assessing a child who has neuroblastoma of the adrenal gland. Which of the following are clinical manifestations of metastasis from the primary site? (Select all that apply.)

_____ A. Weight gain

_____ B. Bone pain

_____ C. Periorbital ecchymoses

_____ D. Proptosis

_____ E. Ill appearance

6. A nurse is caring for a child who has an organ neoplasm. Use the ATI Active Learning Template: Systems Disorder to complete this item to include the following:

A. Nursing Care: Describe seven actions.

B. Teamwork and Collaboration: Identify two potential referrals.

APPLICATION EXERCISES KEY

1. A. **CORRECT:** Half of the children who have neuroblastoma have metastatic disease. Therefore, this should be included in the teaching.

    B. **CORRECT:** Diagnostic testing for neuroblastoma includes a bone marrow biopsy. Therefore, this should be included in the teaching.

    C. INCORRECT: Physical effects are dependant on the size and location of the tumor. Therefore, this should not be included in the teaching.

    D. INCORRECT: The majority of cases occur before the age of 10, with a median age of 23 months. Therefore, this should not be included in the teaching.

    E. **CORRECT:** Resection of the tumor is the treatment of choice. Therefore, this should be included in the teaching.

     NCLEX® Connection: Reduction of Risk Potential, Therapeutic Procedures

2. A. INCORRECT: Pressure applied to the abdomen could rupture the encapsulated tumor. Therefore, palpating the abdomen should not be included in the plan of care.

    B. **CORRECT:** Removal of the tumor occurs within 24 to 48 hr of admission. Therefore, preparation for surgery should be included in the plan of care.

    C. INCORRECT: Wilms' tumor is usually unilateral. Therefore, teaching about dialysis should not be included in the plan of care.

    D. INCORRECT: A urine specimen is usually obtained for diagnostic evaluation of Wilms' tumor. Therefore, obtaining a 24-hr urine specimen should not be included in the plan of care.

     NCLEX® Connection: Reduction of Risk Potential, Therapeutic Procedures

3. A. INCORRECT: Chemotherapy treatment is dependant on the stage of the tumor. Therefore, this should not be included in the teaching.

    B. INCORRECT: About 2% of Wilms' tumors have a familial origin. Therefore, this should not be included in the teaching.

    C. **CORRECT:** Prompt removal of the tumor is best practice for treatment of Wilms' tumor. Therefore, this should be included in the teaching.

    D. **CORRECT:** Palpating the tumor could cause rupture of the encapsulated tumor. Therefore, this should be included in the teaching.

    E. **CORRECT:** Chemotherapy and/or radiation are started immediately after surgery. Therefore, this should be included in the teaching.

     NCLEX® Connection: Physiological Adaptations, Illness Management

4.　A. INCORRECT: An abdominal girth increase of 1 cm could indicate edema. However, it is not an indication to continue with NPO status.

　　B. INCORRECT: Report of pain at the operative site is an expected postoperative finding and is not an indication to continue with NPO status.

　　C. **CORRECT:** Absent bowel sounds is an indication that gastrointestinal motility is absent and a reason to continue with NPO status.

　　D. INCORRECT: Passing flatus is an indication that gastrointestinal motility has resumed and is an indication to advance the diet.

　　 NCLEX® Connection: Reduction of Risk Potential, Potential for Alterations in Body Systems

5.　A. INCORRECT: A child who has metastatic neuroblastoma would have weight loss rather than weight gain.

　　B. **CORRECT:** A child who has metastatic neuroblastoma will report bone pain.

　　C. **CORRECT:** A child who has metastatic neuroblastoma will have periorbital ecchymoses.

　　D. **CORRECT:** A child who has metastatic neuroblastoma will have proptosis.

　　E. **CORRECT:** A child who has metastatic neuroblastoma will have an ill appearance.

　　 NCLEX® Connection: Physiological Adaptations, Unexpected Response to Therapies

6.　*Using ATI Active Learning Template: Systems Disorder*

　　A. Nursing Care

　　　• If Wilms' tumor is suspected, do not palpate the abdomen.

　　　• Assess the child and family's coping and support.

　　　• Assess for developmental delays related to illness.

　　　• Assess physical growth (height and weight).

　　　• Provide education and support to the child and family regarding diagnostic testing, treatment plan, ongoing therapy, and prognosis.

　　　• Monitor for signs of infection.

　　　• Administer antibiotics as prescribed for infection.

　　　• Keep the child's skin clean, dry, and lubricated.

　　　• Provide oral hygiene, and keep the child's lips lubricated.

　　　• Provide age-appropriate diversional activities.

　　　• Provide support to the child and family.

　　B. Teamwork and Collaboration

　　　• Social services

　　　• Nutritionist

　　 NCLEX® Connection: Physiological Adaptations, Pathophysiology

Overview

- Leukemia is the term for a group of malignancies that affect the bone marrow and lymphatic system.
- Leukemia is classified by the type of WBCs that becomes neoplastic and is commonly divided into two groups: acute lymphoid leukemia (ALL) and acute myelogenous or nonlymphoid leukemia (AML/ANLL).
- Leukemia causes an increase in the production of immature WBCs, which leads to infiltration of organs and tissues.
  - Bone marrow infiltration causes crowding of cells that would normally produce RBCs, platelets, and mature WBCs.
    - Deficient RBCs cause anemia.
    - Deficient mature WBCs (neutropenia) increase the risk for infection.
    - Deficient platelets (thrombocytopenia) cause bleeding and bruising.
  - Infiltration of spleen, liver, and lymph nodes leads to tissue fibrosis.
  - Infiltration of the CNS causes increased intracranial pressure.
  - Other tissues may also be infiltrated (testes, prostate, ovaries, gastrointestinal tract).

Assessment

- Risk Factors
  - Leukemia is the most common cancer of childhood.
  - Leukemia is more common in boys and Caucasians.
  - The peak onset is between 2 and 5 years of age.
  - There is a family history of leukemia.
  - Children with trisomy 21 (Down syndrome) have a greater risk of developing leukemia.
- Subjective Data
  - History and physical assessment findings may reveal vague reports (anorexia, headache, fatigue).
- Objective Data
  - Physical Assessment Findings
    - Early manifestations
      - Low-grade fever
      - Pallor
      - Increased bruising and petechiae
      - Listlessness

- Enlarged liver, lymph nodes, and joints
- Abdominal, leg, and joint pain
- Constipation
- Headache
- Vomiting and anorexia
- Unsteady gait
  - Late manifestations
    - Pain
    - Hematuria
    - Ulcerations in the mouth
    - Enlarged kidneys and testicles
    - Signs of increased intracranial pressure
  - Laboratory Tests
    - Complete blood counts
      - Anemia (low blood counts)
      - Thrombocytopenia (low platelets)
      - Neutropenia (low neutrophils)
      - Leukemic blasts (immature WBCs)
  - Diagnostic Procedures
    - Bone marrow aspiration or biopsy analysis
      - Bone marrow aspiration or biopsy is the most definitive diagnostic procedure. If leukemia is present, the specimen will show prolific quantities of immature leukemic blast cells and protein markers indicating a specific type of leukemia.
      - Nursing Actions
        - ▶ Assist the provider with the procedure.
        - ▶ Topical anesthetic, such as a eutectic mixture of local anesthetics (EMLA), may be applied over the biopsy area 45 min to 1 hr prior to the procedure.
        - ▶ Unconscious sedation is induced using a general anesthetic, such as propofol (Diprivan).
        - ▶ Positioning depends on the access site to be used (posterior or anterior iliac crest is most common; tibia can be used in infants because it is easier to access and hold the infant).
        - ▶ A specimen is obtained by the provider.
        - ▶ Postprocedure
          - ▷ Apply pressure to the site for 5 to 10 min, then apply a pressure dressing.
          - ▷ Assess vital signs frequently.
          - ▷ Monitor for signs of bleeding and infection for 24 hr.
      - Client Education
        - ▶ Educate the child and parents about the procedure and postprocedure care.

- Cerebrospinal fluid (CSF) analysis
  - CSF, obtained by lumbar puncture, is assessed to determine CNS involvement.
  - Nursing Actions
    - Have the child empty his bladder.
    - Assist the provider with the procedure.
    - A topical anesthetic (EMLA cream) may be applied over the biopsy area 45 min to 1 hr prior to the procedure.
    - Place the child in the side-lying position with the head flexed and knees drawn up toward the chest, and assist in maintaining the position. Distraction may need to be used.
    - The child may be sedated with fentanyl (Sublimaze) and midazolam (Versed).
    - The provider will clean the skin and inject a local anesthetic.
    - The provider will take pressure readings and collect three to five test tubes of CSF.
    - Pressure and an elastic bandage will be applied to the puncture site after the needle is removed.
    - Label specimens appropriately, and deliver them to the laboratory.
    - Monitor the site for bleeding, hematoma, or infection.
  - Client Education
    - Instruct the child to remain in bed for 4 to 8 hr in a flat position to prevent leakage and a resulting spinal headache. This may not be possible for an infant, toddler, or preschooler.
- Liver and Kidney Function Studies
  - These studies are used for baseline functioning before chemotherapy.
  - Nursing Actions
    - Draw the appropriate amount of serum.
  - Client Education
    - Educate the child and parents about the length of time to receive results.

Patient-Centered Care

- Nursing Care
  - Provide emotional support to the child and parents.
  - Encourage peer contact if appropriate.
  - Assess pain using an age-appropriate pain scale.
  - Use pharmacological and nonpharmacological interventions to provide around-the-clock pain management.

- Medications
  - Chemotherapy
    - The agents to be used depend on the type of leukemia, age, and whether leukemic cells are found in the cerebrospinal fluid.
    - Chemotherapy is administered in four phases to treat leukemia.
      - Induction therapy – To achieve complete remission or less than 5% of leukemic cells in the bone marrow
      - CNS prophylactic therapy – To prevent invasion of the CNS by leukemic cells
      - Intensification therapy (consolidation) – To destroy any remaining leukemic cells followed by a delayed intensification to prevent any resistant leukemic cells from emerging
      - Maintenance therapy – To sustain the remission phase
    - Nursing Considerations
      - Control nausea and vomiting with antiemetics prior to treatment.
      - Manage side effects of treatment.

CHEMOTHERAPY SIDE EFFECTS AND NURSING INTERVETIONS	
SIDE EFFECT	NURSING INTERVENTIONS
Mucosal ulceration	› Provide frequent oral care.
	› Inspect the child's mouth for ulceration and hemorrhage.
	› Use a soft-bristled toothbrush or a soft, disposable toothbrush for oral care.
	› Lubricate lips with lip balm to prevent cracking.
	› Offer foods that are soft and bland.
	› Assist the child to use mouthwashes (such as 1 tsp salt mixed with 1 pint of water or 1 tsp baking soda mixed with 1 qt of water) frequently.
	› Apply local anesthetics (hydrocortisone dental paste [Orabase], antiseptic mouth rinse [UlcerEase]), aluminum and magnesium hydroxide (Maalox) to mucosa to minimize pain.
	› Use agents (mouthwashes, lozenges) that are effective against fungal and bacterial infections (chlorhexidine gluconate [Peridex]).
	› Avoid viscous lidocaine (causes risk of aspiration from depressed gag reflex), hydrogen peroxide (delays healing), milk of magnesia (dries mucous membranes), and lemon glycerin swabs (causes tooth decay and erosion of tissue).
Skin breakdown	› Inspect skin daily.
	› Assess rectal mucosa for fissures.
	› Avoid rectal temperatures.
	› Provide sitz baths as needed.
	› Reposition frequently.
	› Use a pressure reduction system.

CHEMOTHERAPY SIDE EFFECTS AND NURSING INTERVETIONS	
SIDE EFFECT	**NURSING INTERVENTIONS**

Neuropathy	› Constipation
	  » Encourage a diet high in fiber.
	  » Administer stool softeners and laxatives as needed.
	  » Encourage fluids.
	› Foot drop
	  » Use a footboard in bed.
	  » Weakness and numbness of extremities
	  » Assist with ambulation.
	› Jaw pain
	  » Provide a soft diet.

Loss of appetite	› Monitor fluid intake and hydration status. › Provide small, frequent, well-balanced meals. › Involve the child in meal planning. › Administer enteral nutrition if needed. › Weigh the child daily. › Monitor electrolyte values. › Administer chemotherapy early in the day.
Hemorrhage cystitis	› Encourage fluids. › Encourage frequent voiding. › Administer chemotherapy early in the morning to promote adequate fluid intake and voiding. › Administer mesna (Mesnex) to provide protection to the bladder.
Alopecia	› Prepare the child and parents in advance for hair loss. › Encourage the use of a cotton hat or scarf, or a wig if the child is self-conscious about hair loss.

- Client Education
  - Instruct the parents that the use of steroid treatment may cause moon face.
  - Instruct the parents that the child may experience mood changes.
  - Teach the parents to recognize signs of infection, skin breakdown, and nutritional deficiency.
  - Encourage the child and parents to maintain good hygiene.
  - Teach the child and parents to avoid individuals who have infectious diseases.
  - Instruct the child and parents how to administer medications and provide nutritional support at home.
  - Instruct the parents in the proper use of vascular access devices.
  - Instruct the child and parents about bleeding precautions and the management of active bleeding.

- Teamwork and Collaboration
  - Provide information regarding support services for the child and parents.
- Therapeutic Procedures
  - Hematopoietic stem cell transplant (HCST)
    - HCST may be indicated for children who have AML during the first remission and for children who have ALL after a second remission.
    - Allogeneic transplant: The blood-forming stem cells generally are donated by another person.
    - Nursing Actions
      - Coordinate administration of high-dose chemotherapy and possible full-body radiation.
      - Administer donor stem cells via IV infusion.
      - Implement protective isolation.
        - A private, positive-pressure room
        - At least 12 air exchanges/hr
        - HEPA filtration for incoming air
        - Respirator mask, gloves, and gowns
        - No dried or fresh flowers, and no potted plants
    - Client Education
      - The child is at an increased risk for infection and bleeding until the transfused stem cells grow.
  - Radiation therapy to the brain
    - Nursing Actions
      - Assist with positioning.
      - Provide support to the child and parents.
      - Manage side effects.
    - Client Education
      - Educate the child and parents regarding side effects (fatigue, infection).
      - Encourage adequate rest and a healthy diet.

Complications

- Infection
  - Infection can be a complication of myelosuppression.
  - Nursing Actions
    - Provide the child with a private room. The room should be designed to allow for adequate air flow to reduce airborne pathogens.
    - Restrict visitors and health personnel who have active illnesses.
    - Adhere to strict hand hygiene.

- Assess potential sites of infections (oral ulcer, open cut), and monitor temperature.
- Administer antibiotics as prescribed.
- Monitor the child's absolute neutrophil count (ANC).
  - Calculation of the ANC
    - Determine the total percent of neutrophils (the "polys" or "segs" plus the "bands").
    - Convert the percentage of neutrophils to a decimal.
    - Multiply the total WBC count by the percentage of neutrophils to equal the ANC.
- Encourage adequate protein and caloric intake.
  - Client Education
    - Educate about infection control practices.
    - Educate the child and parents about signs and symptoms of infection and when to call the provider.
    - Avoid live vaccines while the immune system is depressed.
- Hemorrhage
  - Bleeding (thrombocytopenia) can be a complication of myelosuppression.
  - Nursing Actions
    - Monitor for signs of bleeding (petechiae, ecchymoses, hematuria, bleeding gums, hematemesis, tarry stools).
    - Avoid unnecessary skin punctures, and use surgical aseptic technique when performed. Apply pressure for 5 min to stop bleeding.
    - Treat a nosebleed with cold and pressure.
    - Administer platelets as ordered.
    - Avoid obtaining temperatures rectally.

  - Client Education
    - Encourage/provide meticulous oral care to prevent gingival bleeding. Use a soft toothbrush, and avoid astringent mouthwashes.
    - Teach the parents measures for controlling epistaxis.
    - Teach the parents and child to avoid activities that may lead to injury or bleeding.
- Anemia
  - Anemia can be a complication of myelosuppression.
  - Nursing Actions
    - Administer blood transfusions as prescribed.
    - Allow for frequent rest periods.
    - Administer oxygen therapy.
    - Administer IV fluid replacement.

  - Client Education
    - Educate the child and parents about foods high in iron.

APPLICATION EXERCISES

1. A nurse is assessing a child who has leukemia. Which of the following are early clinical manifestations of leukemia? (Select all that apply.)

_____ A. Hematuria

_____ B. Anorexia

_____ C. Petechiae

_____ D. Ulcerations in the mouth

_____ E. Unsteady gait

2. A nurse is caring for a child who has thrombocytopenia. Which of the following are appropriate actions for the nurse to take? (Select all that apply.)

_____ A. Monitor for signs of bleeding.

_____ B. Administer routine immunizations.

_____ C. Obtain rectal temperatures.

_____ D. Avoid peripheral venipunctures.

_____ E. Limit visitors.

3. A nurse is caring for a child who is receiving chemotherapy. Which of the following are clinical manifestations of neuropathy? (Select all that apply.)

_____ A. Constipation

_____ B. Skin breakdown

_____ C. Foot drop

_____ D. Jaw pain

_____ E. Hemorrhage cystitis

4. A nurse is caring for a child who has oral mucositis. Which of the following is an appropriate action for the nurse to take? (Select all that apply.)

_____ A. Swab the mucosa with lemon glycerine swabs.

_____ B. Apply viscous lidocaine.

_____ C. Offer soft foods.

_____ D. Use a soft, disposable toothbrush for oral care.

_____ E. Encourage gargling with a warm saline mouthwash.

5. A nurse is planning care for an infant who is has been prescribed a lumbar puncture. Which of the following is an appropriate action for the nurse to take?

    A. Cleanse the thoracic area of the infant's back with an antiseptic solution.

    B. Apply a eutectic mixture of local anesthetics (EMLA) cream just before the procedure begins.

    C. Restrain the infant during the procedure to prevent movement.

    D. Position the infant with his head extended and chin raised.

6. A nurse is preparing to assist with a lumbar puncture. Use the ATI Active Learning Template: Diagnostic Procedure to complete this item to include the following sections:

    A. Description of the procedure.

    B. Nursing Actions: Describe six.

    C. Potential Complications: Identify two.

APPLICATION EXERCISES KEY

1. A. INCORRECT: Hematuria is a late clinical manifestation of leukemia.

    B. **CORRECT:** Anorexia is an early clinical manifestation of leukemia.

    C. **CORRECT:** Petechiae is an early clinical manifestation of leukemia.

    D. INCORRECT: Ulcerations in the mouth are a late clinical manifestation of leukemia.

    E. **CORRECT:** Unsteady gait is an early clinical manifestation of leukemia.

    Ⓝ NCLEX® Connection: Physiological Adaptations, Pathophysiology

2. A. **CORRECT:** The child who has thrombocytopenia is at risk for hemorrhage. Therefore, monitoring for signs of bleeding is an appropriate action for the nurse to take.

    B. INCORRECT: The child who has thrombocytopenia is at risk for bleeding, and skin punctures should be avoided. Therefore, administering routine immunizations is not an appropriate action for the nurse to take.

    C. INCORRECT: The child who has thrombocytopenia is at risk for bleeding, and obtaining a rectal temperature could cause tissue injury. Therefore, this is not an appropriate action for the nurse to take.

    D. **CORRECT:** The child who has thrombocytopenia is at risk for bleeding. Therefore, avoiding venipunctures is an appropriate action for the nurse to take.

    E. INCORRECT: The child who has thrombocytopenia is at risk for bleeding. Limiting visitors protects the child from infection. Therefore, it is not an appropriate action to prevent bleeding.

    Ⓝ NCLEX® Connection: Physiological Adaptations, Unexpected Response to Therapies

3. A. **CORRECT:** Constipation is a clinical manifestation of neuropathy.

    B. INCORRECT: Skin breakdown is an adverse effect of chemotherapy.

    C. **CORRECT:** Foot drop is a clinical manifestation of neuropathy.

    D. **CORRECT:** Jaw pain is a clinical manifestation of neuropathy.

    E. INCORRECT: Hemorrhage cystitis is an adverse effect of chemotherapy.

    Ⓝ NCLEX® Connection: Reduction of Risk Potential, System Specific Assessments

4. A. INCORRECT: Lemon glycerine swabs may cause tooth decay and erosion of the tissues. They should not be used.

    B. INCORRECT: Viscous lidocaine can depress the gag reflex and cause aspiration. It should not be used.

    C. **CORRECT:** Offering soft foods decreases the amount of chewing needed and possible irritation. This is an appropriate action for the nurse to take.

    D. **CORRECT:** A soft toothbrush allows for adequate cleaning of the mouth and decreases irritation. It is an appropriate action for the nurse to take.

    E. **CORRECT:** A warm saline mouthwash is effective in soothing mucositis. It is an appropriate action for the nurse to take.

     NCLEX® Connection: Physiological Adaptations, Alterations in Body Systems

5. A. INCORRECT: The lumbar area of the infant's back should be cleansed prior to the procedure.

    B. INCORRECT: EMLA cream should be applied 60 min prior to the procedure.

    C. **CORRECT:** Restraining the infant during the procedure to prevent movement will decrease the potential for injury. It is an appropriate action for the nurse to take.

    D. INCORRECT: The infant should be positioned with his neck flexed and chin to the chest.

     NCLEX® Connection: Reduction of Risk Potential, Diagnostic Tests

6. *Using the ATI Active Learning Template: Diagnostic Procedure*
    A. Description of the procedure

      • CSF is obtained to determine whether there is CNS involvement.

    B. Nursing Actions

      • Have the child empty his bladder.

      • Apply a topical anesthetic 45 to 60 min before the procedure.

      • Administer fentanyl (Sublimaze) and midazolam (Versed) if prescribed.

      • Position the child in a side-lying position with the head flexed and knees drawn up toward the chest.

      • Use distraction techniques if needed.

      • Assist with the procedure.

      • Apply pressure and an elastic bandage to the site after the needle is withdrawn.

      • Label the specimens, and deliver them to the laboratory.

      • Monitor for hematoma, bleeding, and infection.

      • Keep the bed flat.

      • Instruct the child to remain in bed.

    C. Potential Complications

      • Spinal headache

      • Hematoma

      • Infection

      • Bleeding

     NCLEX® Connection: Reduction of Risk Potential, Diagnostic Tests

chapter 41

Overview

- Malignant tumors in bone may originate from all tissues involved in bone growth, including osteoid matrix, blood vessels, and cartilage.

  - Osteosarcoma usually occurs in the metaphysis of long bones, most often in the femur. Treatment frequently includes amputation or limb salvage procedure of the affected extremity as well as chemotherapy.

  - Ewing's sarcoma (a primitive neuroectodermal tumor [PNET]) occurs in the shafts of long bones and of trunk bones. Treatment includes surgical biopsy, intensive radiation therapy to tumor site, and chemotherapy, but not amputation.

  - Prognosis depends on how quickly the disease is diagnosed and whether metastasis has occurred.

- Soft tissue malignancies arise from undifferentiated cells in the soft tissues (muscles, tendons), in connective or fibrous tissue, or in blood or lymph vessels. These malignancies can begin in any area of the body.

  - Rhabdomyosarcoma originates in skeletal muscle in any part of the body, but it most commonly occurs in the head and neck, with the orbit of the eye frequently affected. Treatment consists of surgical biopsy, local radiation therapy, and chemotherapy, rather than radical surgical procedures.

- Children who undergo irradiation for malignancies in or near the pelvic area may experience sterilization and/or secondary cancers.

Assessment

- Risk Factors

  - Osteosarcoma peaks at age 15 during growth spurts and is more common in boys.

  - Ewing's sarcoma occurs prior to 30 years of age and is more common in Caucasians.

  - Rhabdomyosarcoma occurs in children of all ages (but more commonly in children younger than 5 years of age) and is more common in Caucasians.

- Subjective and Objective Data

BONE CANCERS	
Subjective Data	› Nonspecific bone pain that is often mistaken for an injury or growing pains › Temporary relief of pain when extremity is flexed
Objective Data	› Weakness, swelling, or decreased movement of the extremity › Palpable lymph nodes near the tumor › Anemia, generalized infection, or unexplained weight loss › Limpness or inability to hold a heavy object
RHABDOMYOSARCOMA	
Subjective Data	› May cause pain in local areas related to compression by the tumor (sore throat may occur with tumor of the nasopharynx) › Possible absence of pain in some parts of the body, such as in the retroperitoneal area, until the tumor begins to obstruct organs
Objective Data	› Based on affected area » CNS – headaches, diplopia, vomiting » Orbit – unilateral proptosis, ecchymosis of conjunctiva, strabismus » Nasopharynx – stuffy nose, pain, nasal obstruction, epistaxis, palpable neck nodes, visible mass (late) » Paranasal sinuses – nasal obstruction, pain, discharge, sinusitis, swelling » Middle ear – chronic otitis media, pain, sanguinopurulent discharge, facial paralysis » Retroperitoneal area – usually no symptoms, abdominal mass, pain, intestinal or genitourinary obstruction » Perineum – visible superficial mass, bowel or bladder obstruction » Extremity – pain, palpable fixed mass, lymph node enlargement

- Laboratory Tests
  - Complete blood count (CBC) and other common tests can help rule out infection, iron deficiency anemia, and other possible causes of findings.
- Diagnostic Procedures
  - Bone Cancers
    - X-rays, CT scans, or magnetic resonance imaging (MRI) of the primary site
    - Bone marrow biopsy
    - CT of the chest and bone scans to evaluate metastasis.
  - Rhabdomyosarcoma
    - CT scans or MRI of the primary site
    - Biopsy of tumor is possible
    - CT of the chest, bone scans, bone marrow biopsy, and lumbar puncture to evaluate metastasis

Patient-Centered Care

- Nursing Care
  - Be honest when answering questions and when giving information about the disease and treatment.
  - Allow the child time, usually several days, to prepare emotionally for surgery and chemotherapy.
  - Avoid overwhelming the child with information.
- Medications
  - Chemotherapy
    - Osteosarcoma
      - Various agents used singly or in combination before and/or after surgery
      - High-dose methotrexate with citrovorum factor rescue, doxorubicin, cisplatin, ifosfamide, and etoposide
    - Ewing's sarcoma
      - Vincristine, doxorubicin, and cyclophosphamide alternating with ifosfamide and etoposide
    - Rhabdomyosarcoma
      - Vincristine, actinomycin D, cyclophosphamide, ifosfamide, topotecan, irinotecan, and doxorubicin for about 1 year
    - Nursing Considerations
      - Control nausea and vomiting with antiemetics prior to treatment.
      - Manage side effects of treatment.
    - Client Education
      - Teach the family to recognize signs of infection, skin breakdown, and nutritional deficiency.
      - Encourage the child and family to maintain good hygiene.
      - Instruct the family in the proper use of vascular access devices.
      - Instruct the child and family about bleeding precautions and management of active bleeding.
  - Amitriptyline (Elavil)
    - A tricyclic antidepressant (TCA) for use with neuropathic pain or phantom pain in adolescents who have amputated limbs.
    - Nursing Considerations
      - Monitor the child for drowsiness, orthostatic hypotension, anticholinergic effects, seizures, mania, and cardiac dysfunction.
    - Client Education
      - Teach the child and family how to manage side effects.
      - Caution the child and parents about taking only the prescribed dosage to prevent toxic reactions.

- Teamwork and Collaboration
  - Older children and adolescents may benefit from attending a support group for children who have cancer and/or amputations.
  - Initiate a referral for mental health counseling to assist the child to resume normal activities.
  - Initiate physical and occupational therapy referrals to start while in the hospital and to continue after discharge.
- Therapeutic Procedures
  - Localized radiation therapy
    - Radiation therapy may be used in combination with chemotherapy and surgery.
    - Nursing Actions
      - Assist the child with positioning.
      - Monitor for side effects.
    - Client Education
      - Educate the child and family regarding the course of therapy.
- Surgical Interventions
  - Surgical biopsy for any of the bone or soft tissue cancers
    - Tumor is biopsied under anesthesia to determine presence and/or tissue type of cancer.
    - Nursing Actions
      - Provide routine pre- and postoperative care.
      - Provide for adequate pain relief.
      - Monitor wound for signs of infection.
      - Actions vary with extent and area of surgery, but nursing actions should include pre- and postprocedure assessment, including vital signs, medication for pain, and wound care as necessary.
    - Client Education
      - Educate the child and family regarding postoperative care.
  - Limb salvage procedure for bone cancers
    - It involves a preoperative course of chemotherapy to shrink the tumor and then total bone and joint replacement after the tumor and affected bone are removed.
    - Nursing Actions
      - Administer preoperative chemotherapy.
      - Assist with managing side effects.
      - Provide routine postoperative care.
      - Provide adequate pain relief.
    - Client Education
      - Educate the child and family regarding postoperative care.
      - Teach the child and family about any expected effects of preoperative chemotherapy, such as hair loss.

- ○ Limb amputation for bone cancer
    - ▪ The child may receive chemotherapy both preoperatively and postoperatively.
    - ▪ Nursing Actions
        - □ Provide routine pre- and postoperative care.
        - □ Provide emotional support.
        - □ Care for the stump as prescribed.
        - □ Assess for the presence of phantom limb pain postoperatively, and medicate appropriately.
    - ▪ Client Education
        - □ Prepare the child for fitting of a temporary prosthesis, which may occur immediately after surgery.
        - □ Encourage cooperation with postoperative physical therapy.
        - □ Work with the child and family to plan for issues such as appropriate clothing to wear with prosthesis.
        - □ Role-play issues that the child will need to deal with after discharge, such as talking to strangers who ask about the prosthesis.
        - □ Assist the family to recognize that the child's emotions, such as anger, are normal grief reactions after amputation, chemotherapy, and other treatments.
- • Care After Discharge
    - ○ Client Education
        - ▪ Educate the child and family regarding the importance of follow-up care.
    - ○ Community Services
        - ▪ Initiate appropriate referrals to assist the child to resume normal activities (school attendance, physical activities).

Complications

- • Skin desquamation (either dry or moist) with permanent hyperpigmentation and possible damage to underlying structures
    - ○ Nursing Actions
        - ▪ Assess the site frequently for infection.
        - ▪ Assess for damage to underlying structures (nerves, blood vessels) by assessing circulation and movement.
    - ○ Client Education
        - ▪ Teach the parents methods to prevent additional irritation to the site (use loose-fitting clothing, prevent exposure to sunlight or extremes of temperature).
        - ▪ Teach adolescents about risks of sterilization if indicated.
        - ▪ Explain the importance of continuing follow-up examinations.

- Myelosuppression
  - Elimination of normal blood cells along with cancer cells is a risk with treatment by most chemotherapeutic agents. This may cause infection (reduced leukocytes), hemorrhage (reduced thrombocytes), and anemia (reduced red blood cells).
  - Nursing Actions
    - Evaluate laboratory data and assess for symptoms of complications.
      - Infection – elevated WBC and fever
      - Hemorrhage – blood in urine or stool, bruising, and petechiae
      - Anemia – fatigue and decreased hemoglobin/hematocrit
    - Prevent infection
      - Provide a private room when hospitalized.
      - Restrict staff/visitors who have infections.
      - Promote frequent hand hygiene by staff/visitors.
      - Avoid all live-virus vaccines during periods of immunosuppression.
      - Ensure that siblings are up to date on vaccinations.
      - Provide a diet adequate in proteins and calories.
    - Prevent hemorrhage or injury from bleeding.
      - Use a strict aseptic technique for all invasive procedures.
      - Use gentle technique when providing mouth care.
      - Clean the perineal area carefully to prevent trauma, and avoid obtaining temperatures rectally.
      - Infuse platelets as prescribed.
    - Prevent anemia or injury from anemia.
      - Provide rest periods as needed.
      - Infuse packed red blood cells as prescribed.
  - Client Education
    - Teach family members strategies to recognize complications at home and to prevent damage from infection, hemorrhage, or bleeding.

APPLICATION EXERCISES

1. A nurse is caring for a child following an above-the-knee left-leg amputation. Which of the following is an appropriate action for the nurse to take?

    A. Avoid discussing the amputation.

    B. Administer aspirin for phantom pain.

    C. Prepare the child for a prosthesis fitting.

    D. Maintain the affected limb in the dependent position.

2. A nurse is caring for an adolescent who has been diagnosed with osteosarcoma. Which of the following actions should the nurse take?

    A. Ensure that the adolescent has a referral for a psychiatrist visit.

    B. Prepare a teaching plan to educate the adolescent in detail about what he should know regarding his diagnosis and treatment.

    C. Spend time with the adolescent to answer any questions he may have.

    D. Perform a mental status examination to assess the adolescent's thought patterns.

3. A nurse is teaching a parent of a child who is receiving chemotherapy for bone cancer. Which of the following should be included in the teaching? (Select all that apply.)

    _____ A. Signs of infection

    _____ B. Bleeding precautions

    _____ C. Hand hygiene

    _____ D. Home schooling

    _____ E. Nutritional requirements

4. A nurse is assessing a child who has rhabdomyosarcoma of the nasopharynx. Which of the following are clinical manifestations of this disorder? (Select all that apply.)

    _____ A. Enlarged neck lymph nodes

    _____ B. Pain

    _____ C. Vomiting

    _____ D. Epistaxis

    _____ E. Diplopia

5. A nurse is assessing a child who has rhabdomyosarcoma of an extremity. Which of the following are clinical manifestations of this condition? (Select all that apply.)

_____ A. Pain

_____ B. Discoloration of the skin

_____ C. Lymph node enlargement

_____ D. Moveable mass

_____ E. Palpable mass

6. A nurse is teaching a parent of a child who has bone cancer and is receiving chemotherapy about myelosuppression. Use the ATI Active Learning Template: Systems Disorder to complete this item to include the following:

A. Nursing Actions: Describe two actions related to each of the following areas.
- Evaluating laboratory data to assess for complications
- Preventing infection
- Preventing hemorrhage or injury from bleeding
- Preventing anemia or injury from anemia

APPLICATION EXERCISES KEY

1. A. INCORRECT: The loss of a limb entails a grieving process. Therefore, avoiding discussion of the amputation is not an appropriate action for the nurse to take.

    B. INCORRECT: Amitriptyline (Elavil) should be given for phantom pain because aspirin should be avoided in children.

    C. **CORRECT:** Temporary prostheses are fitted soon after surgery. Therefore, preparing the child for a prosthesis is an appropriate action for the nurse to take.

    D. INCORRECT: The affected limb should be elevated after surgery to decrease swelling.

    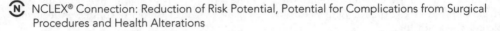 NCLEX® Connection: Reduction of Risk Potential, Potential for Complications from Surgical Procedures and Health Alterations

2. A. INCORRECT: A psychiatrist referral is not indicated at the time of diagnosis. Therefore, this is not an appropriate action for the nurse to take.

    B. INCORRECT: A detailed teaching plan is not indicated at the time of diagnosis. Therefore, this is not an appropriate action for the nurse to take.

    C. **CORRECT:** The nurse should be available to answer the client's questions and to listen as he talks about his feelings.

    D. INCORRECT: Performing a mental status examination is not indicated at the time of diagnosis. Therefore, this is not an appropriate action for the nurse to take.

    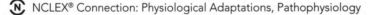 NCLEX® Connection: Physiological Adaptations, Pathophysiology

3. A. **CORRECT:** Chemotherapy destroys healthy WBCs, which increases the risk of infection. Therefore, signs of infection should be included in the teaching.

    B. **CORRECT:** Chemotherapy destroys healthy platelets, which increases the risk of bleeding. Therefore, bleeding precautions should be included in the teaching.

    C. **CORRECT:** Chemotherapy destroys healthy WBCs, which increases the risk of infection. Therefore, hand hygiene should be included in the teaching.

    D. INCORRECT: Children who are receiving chemotherapy can continue to attend school following recommendations of the provider. Therefore, home schooling should not be included in the teaching.

    E. **CORRECT:** Chemotherapy destroys healthy blood cells. Therefore, nutritional requirements should be included in the teaching.

    NCLEX® Connection: Psychosocial Integrity, Therapeutic Communication

4. A. **CORRECT:** Palpable neck lymph nodes is a clinical manifestation of rhabdomyosarcoma of the nasopharynx.

    B. **CORRECT:** Pain is a clinical manifestation of rhabdomyosarcoma of the nasopharynx.

    C. INCORRECT: Vomiting is a clinical manifestation of rhabdomyosarcoma of the central nervous system.

    D. **CORRECT:** Epistaxis is a clinical manifestation of rhabdomyosarcoma of the nasopharynx.

    E. INCORRECT: Diplopia is a clinical manifestation of rhabdomyosarcoma of the central nervous system.

    (N) NCLEX® Connection: Physiological Adaptations, Alterations in Body Systems

5. A. **CORRECT:** Pain is a clinical manifestation of rhabdomyosarcoma of an extremity.

    B. INCORRECT: Rhabdomyosarcoma is a soft tissue cancer. Therefore, discoloration of the skin is not a clinical manifestation.

    C. **CORRECT:** Lymph node enlargement is a clinical manifestation of rhabdomyosarcoma of an extremity.

    D. INCORRECT: Fixed mass is a clinical manifestation of rhabdomyosarcoma of an extremity.

    E. **CORRECT:** Palpable mass is a clinical manifestation of rhabdomyosarcoma of an extremity.

    (N) NCLEX® Connection: Physiological Adaptations, Pathophysiology

6. Using the ATI Active Learning Template: Systems Disorder
    A. Nursing Actions
    - Evaluating laboratory data to assess for complications
      - Infection – elevated WBC and fever
      - Hemorrhage – blood in urine or stool, bruising, and petechiae
      - Anemia – fatigue and decreased hemoglobin/hematocrit
    - Preventing infection
      - Provide a private room when hospitalized.
      - Restrict staff/visitors who have infections.
      - Promote frequent hand hygiene by staff/visitors.
      - Avoid all live-virus vaccines during periods of immunosuppression.
      - Ensure that siblings are up to date on vaccinations.
      - Provide a diet adequate in proteins and calories.
    - Preventing hemorrhage or injury from bleeding
      - Use a strict aseptic technique for all invasive procedures.
      - Use gentle technique when providing mouth care.
      - Clean the perineal area carefully to prevent trauma, and avoid obtaining temperatures rectally.
      - Infuse platelets as prescribed.
    - Preventing anemia or injury from anemia
      - Provide rest periods as needed.
      - Infuse packed red blood cells as prescribed.

    (N) NCLEX® Connection: Physiological Adaptations, Pathophysiology

UNIT 3   Nursing Care of Children with Special Needs

CHAPTERS

› Pediatric Emergencies
› Psychosocial Issues of Infants, Children, and Adolescents

NCLEX® CONNECTIONS

When reviewing the chapters in this unit, keep in mind the relevant sections of the NCLEX® outline, in particular:

Client Needs: Health Promotion and Maintenance	Client Needs: Psychosocial Integrity	Client Needs: Physiological Adaptation
› Relevant topics/tasks include: » Developmental Stages and Transitions › Compare the client's development to expected age/developmental stage and report any deviations. » High-Risk Behaviors › Perform health history/health and risk assessment. » Health Promotion/Disease Prevention › Assist the client in maintaining an optimum level of health.	› Relevant topics/tasks include: » Abuse/Neglect › Identify risk factors for domestic, child, elder abuse/neglect, and sexual abuse. » Family Dynamics › Assess parental techniques related to discipline.	› Relevant topics/tasks include: » Medical Emergencies › Apply knowledge of nursing procedures and psychomotor skills when caring for a client experiencing a medical emergency.

chapter 42

Overview

- In caring for children, nurses often deal with emergent care situations that require rapid assessment and intervention and offer opportunities for parent and community education.

  ○ Respiratory emergencies

  ○ Drowning

  ○ Apparent life-threatening event

  ○ Sudden infant death syndrome (SIDS)

  ○ Poisoning

RESPIRATORY EMERGENCIES

Overview

- Respiratory insufficiency

  ○ Increased work of breathing with mostly adequate gas exchange or hypoxia with acidosis

- Respiratory failure

  ○ Inability to maintain adequate oxygenation of the blood

- Apnea

  ○ The cessation of respirations for more than 20 seconds

  ○ May be associated with hypoxemia or bradycardia

  ○ Can be central or obstructive

- Respiratory arrest

  ○ The complete cessation of respirations

- Airway obstruction

  ○ May be due to aspiration of a foreign body

Assessment

- Risk Factors
  - Toddlers
  - Primary inefficient gas exchange due to cerebral trauma, brain tumor, overdose, asphyxia, or CNS infection
  - Obstructive lung disease caused by aspiration, infection, tumor, anaphylaxis, laryngospasm, or asthma
  - Restrictive lung disease resulting from cystic fibrosis, pneumonia, or respiratory distress syndrome
- Subjective Data
  - History of illnesses (chronic or acute)
  - History of events leading to respiratory emergency
  - Allergies
- Objective Data
  - Early signs of respiratory distress
    - Restlessness
    - Tachypnea
    - Tachycardia
    - Diaphoresis
    - Nasal flaring
    - Retractions
    - Grunting
    - Dyspnea
    - Wheezing
  - Advanced hypoxia
    - Bradypnea
    - Bradycardia
    - Peripheral or central cyanosis
    - Stupor
    - Coma
  - Signs of choking
    - Universal choking sign (clutching neck with hands)
    - Inability to speak
    - Weak, ineffective cough
    - High-pitched sounds or no sound
    - Dyspnea
    - Cyanosis
- Laboratory Tests – arterial blood gases (ABGs)
- Diagnostic Procedures – chest x-rays

Patient-Centered Care

- Nursing Care
    - ○ Follow the American Heart Association (AHA) guidelines for CPR for respiratory and cardiac arrest.
    - ○ Follow the facility's protocol for activating the rapid response team.
    - ○ Use current basic life support (BLS) and advanced cardiac life support (ACLS) guidelines for neonates (NALS) and for pediatric clients (PALS).
    - ○ Obstructed Airway
        - ▪ Follow the American Heart Association (AHA) guidelines for a choking child.
        - ▪ Infants – Use a combination of back blows and chest thrusts.
        - ▪ Children and adolescents – Use abdominal thrusts.
        - ▪ Remove any visual obstruction or large debris from the mouth, but do not perform blind finger sweep.
        - ▪ Place the recovered child (one who resumes breathing) into the recovery position (side-lying position with legs bent at knees for stability).
    - ○ Position to maintain patent airway. Monitor respiratory status. Monitor vital signs.
    - ○ Administer oxygen as prescribed.
    - ○ Suction as needed.
    - ○ Prepare for intubation if needed.
    - ○ Use a calm approach with the child and family.
    - ○ Administer medications, IV fluids, and emergency medications as prescribed.
    - ○ Keep the family informed of the child's status.
    - ○ Client Education
        - ▪ Teach the family clinical manifestations of respiratory distress.
        - ▪ Encourage the family to learn CPR.
        - ▪ Teach the family about strategies to prevent respiratory emergencies, such as recognizing choking hazards for toddlers.

DROWNING

Overview

- Asphyxiation while child is submerged in fluid may occur in any standing body of water that is at least 1 inch deep (bathtub, toilet, bucket, pool, pond, lake).
- Submersion injury (near-drowning) incidents are those in which children have survived for 24 hr after being submerged in fluid.
- Families should be taught preventive measures.

Assessment

- Risk Factors
  - Children over 12 months of age
  - Swimming (may be overconfident or lack ability)
  - Inadequate supervision or unattended in bathtub, pools
  - Not wearing life jackets when in water
  - Diving
  - Child abuse
- Subjective Data
  - History of event including location and time of submersion
  - Type and temperature of the fluid
- Objective Data
  - Respiratory assessment (see respiratory emergencies)
  - Body temperature (hypothermia)
  - Bruising, spinal cord injury, or other physical injuries
- Laboratory Tests – ABGs
- Diagnostic Procedures – chest x-rays

Patient-Centered Care

- Nursing Care (based on degree of cerebral insult)
  - Administer oxygen, may need mechanical ventilation.
  - Monitor vital signs.
  - Administer medications, IV fluids, and emergency medications as prescribed.
  - Provide chest physiotherapy.
  - Monitor for complications that can occur 24 hr after incident (cerebral edema, respiratory distress).
  - Use a calm approach with the child and family.
  - Keep the family informed of the child's status.
  - Client Education
    - Encourage parents of toddlers to lock toilet seats when their child is at home.
    - Instruct parents to not leave the child unattended in the bathtub.
    - Inform parents to not leave the child unattended in a swimming pool, even if the child can swim.
    - Instruct parents to make sure private pools are fenced with locked gates to prevent children from wandering into the pool area.
    - Encourage parents to provide life jackets when boating.

APPARENT LIFE-THREATENING EVENT

Overview

- Sudden event where the infant exhibits apnea, change in color, change in muscle tone, and choking

Assessment

- Risk Factors
  - Gastroesophageal reflux
  - Respiratory infections
  - Seizure
  - Urinary tract infection (UTI)
- Subjective data
  - Description of the event by the observer
  - CPR efforts provided
  - Maternal history
  - Family history of seizures
- Objective data
  - Event
    - Apnea may or may not be present during event.
    - Change in color: pallor, redness, cyanosis.
    - Change in muscle tone: hypotonia.
    - Choking, gagging, coughing.
  - Head-to-toe assessment
- Laboratory Tests
  - Blood cultures – bacterial or viral infection
  - Urine culture – UTI
  - CBC
  - Serum glucose
  - Electrolytes
- Diagnostic Procedures
  - ECG (long QT syndrome or dysrhythmias)
  - EEG (epilepsy)
  - pH study (reflux)
  - MRI (hemorrhage or cerebral abnormalities/injuries)
  - Sleep study (sleep apnea)

Patient-Centered Care

- Nursing Care
  - Prepare infant and family for testing
  - Monitor infant for recurrent events
  - Encourage the family to learn CPR
  - Client teaching – use of an apnea monitor, if prescribed

SUDDEN INFANT DEATH SYNDROME (SIDS)

Overview

- SIDS is the sudden, unpredictable death of an infant without an identified cause, even after investigation and autopsy.
- Preventive measures should be taught to families.

Assessment

- Risk Factors
  - Maternal smoking during pregnancy
  - Secondhand smoke
  - Cosleeping with parent or adult
  - Nonstandard bed (sofa, soft bedding, water beds, pillows)
  - Prone or side-lying sleeping
  - Low birth weight
  - Prematurity
  - Twin or multiple birth
  - Low Apgar scores
  - Viral illness
  - Family history of SIDS
  - Poverty
- Subjective data
  - History of events prior to discover of infant
  - History of illnesses
  - Pregnancy and birth history
  - Presence of risk factors

Patient-Centered Care

- Nursing Care
  - Teach the family how to reduce the risks of SIDS.
    - Place infant on back for sleep.
    - Avoid exposure to tobacco smoke.
    - Prevent overheating.
    - Use a firm, tight-fitting mattress in the infant's crib.
    - Remove pillows, quilts, and sheepskins from the crib during sleep.
    - Ensure that the infant's head is kept uncovered during sleep.
    - Offer pacifier at naps and night.
    - Encourage breastfeeding.
    - Avoid cosleeping.
    - Maintain immunizations up to date.
  - Provide support.
  - Allow the infant's family an opportunity to express feelings.
  - Plan a home health visit to follow a death.
  - Refer to support groups, counseling, or community groups.

POISONING

Overview

- Ingestion of or exposure to toxic substances.
- Preventive measures should be taught to families.

Assessment

- Risk Factors
  - Children younger than 6 years of age
  - Improperly stored medications, household chemicals, and hazardous substances
  - Exposure to plants, cosmetics, and heavy metals, which are potential sources of toxic substances
  - Lead ingestion from lead-based paint, soil contamination
- Subjective data
  - Information regarding poisonous agent
    - Name and location
    - Amount ingested
    - Time of ingestion

- Objective data
  - Physical response will depend on specific poison
    - Acetaminophen (Tylenol)
      - 2 to 4 hr after ingestion – nausea, vomiting, sweating, and pallor
      - 24 to 36 hr after ingestion – improvement in the child's condition
      - 36 hr to 7 days or longer (hepatic stage) – pain in upper right quadrant, confusion, stupor, jaundice, and coagulation disturbances
      - Final stage – death or gradual recovery
    - Acetylsalicylic acid (aspirin)
      - Acute poisoning – nausea, vomiting, disorientation, diaphoresis, tachypnea, tinnitus, oliguria, lightheadedness, and seizures
      - Chronic poisoning – subtle version of acute manifestations, bleeding tendencies, dehydration, and seizures more severe than acute poisoning
    - Supplemental iron
      - Initial period (30 min to 6 hr after ingestion) – vomiting, hematemesis, diarrhea, gastric pain, and bloody stools
      - Latency period (2 to 12 hr after ingestion) – improvement of condition
      - Systemic toxicity period (4 to 24 hr after ingestion) – metabolic acidosis, hyperglycemia, bleeding, fever, shock, and possible death
      - Hepatic injury period (48 to 96 hr after ingestion) – seizures or coma
    - Hydrocarbons (gasoline, kerosene, lighter fluid, paint thinner, turpentine)
      - Gagging, choking, coughing, nausea, and vomiting
      - Lethargy, weakness, tachypnea, cyanosis, grunting, and retractions
    - Corrosives (household cleaners, batteries, denture cleaners, bleach)
      - Pain and burning in mouth, throat, and stomach
      - Edematous lips, tongue, and pharynx with white mucous membranes
      - Violent vomiting with hemoptysis
      - Drooling
      - Anxiety
      - Shock
    - Lead
      - Low-dose exposure – easily distracted, impulsive, hyperactive, hearing impairment, and mild intellectual difficulty
      - High-dose exposure – cognitive delays varying in severity, blindness, paralysis, coma, seizures, and death
      - Other manifestations – kidney impairment, impaired calcium function, and anemia

- Laboratory Tests
  - Serum lead
  - CBC with differential
  - ABGs
  - Serum iron
  - Serum acetaminophen
  - Liver function tests
  - Blood alcohol and toxicology screening

Patient-Centered Care

- Nursing Care
  - Depends on the poison ingested – monitor for ongoing changes.
  - Terminate exposure.
  - Provide cardiorespiratory support as needed.
  - Notify local or regional poison control center.
  - Administer IV fluids as prescribed.
  - Provide for cardiac monitoring.
  - Monitor vital signs and oxygen saturation.
  - Monitor I&O.
  - Administer antidote if indicated.
  - Assist with gastric decontamination if indicated.
    - Activated charcoal
    - Gastric lavage
    - Increasing bowel motility
    - Syrup of ipecac is contraindicated for routine poison control treatment
  - Keep the family informed of the child's condition.

INTERVENTIONS FOR SPECIFIC SUBSTANCES	
SUBSTANCE	INTERVENTION
Acetaminophen (Tylenol)	› N-acetylcysteine (Mucomyst) given orally
Acetylsalicylic acid (Aspirin)	› Activated charcoal › Gastric lavage › Sodium bicarbonate › Oxygen and ventilation › Vitamin K › Hemodialysis for severe cases

INTERVENTIONS FOR SPECIFIC SUBSTANCES	
SUBSTANCE	INTERVENTION
Supplemental iron	› Emesis or lavage › Chelation therapy using deferoxamine mesylate (Desferal)
Hydrocarbons (gasoline, kerosene, lighter fluid, paint thinner, turpentine)	› Do not induce vomiting › Intubation with cuffed endotracheal tube prior to any gastric decontamination › Treatment of chemical pneumonia
Corrosives (household cleaners, batteries, denture cleaners, bleach)	› Airway maintenance › NPO › No attempt to neutralize acid (corrosive) › Do not induce vomiting › Analgesics for pain
Lead	› Chelation therapy using calcium EDTA (calcium disodium versenate)

- ○ Client Education
  - Poison prevention
    - □ Keep toxic agents out of reach of children.
    - □ Lock cabinets containing potentially harmful substances.
    - □ Do not take medication in front of children.
    - □ Discard unused medications.
    - □ When giving a child medication, do not tell them it is candy.
    - □ Use nonmercury thermometers.
    - □ Eliminate lead-based paint in the environment.
    - □ Encourage hand hygiene prior to eating.
    - □ Do not store food in lead-based containers.

Complications

- Cognitive Impairments
  - ○ Varies with degree of anoxic insult or lead levels in the blood.
  - ○ Provide prevention measures to families.
  - ○ Routine screening for lead levels at 1, 2, and 3 years of age.
  - ○ Provide case management for children who have elevated lead levels.
  - ○ Make appropriate referrals (community nurse, teacher, early intervention).

APPLICATION EXERCISES

1. A nurse is caring for a child who has respiratory distress. Which of the following are early clinical manifestations? (Select all that apply.)

_____ A. Bradypnea

_____ B. Peripheral cyanosis

_____ C. Tachycardia

_____ D. Diaphoresis

_____ E. Restlessness

2. A nurse is preparing to admit an infant who experienced an apparent life-threatening event. Which of the following prescriptions by the provider should the nurse anticipate? (Select all that apply.)

_____ A. EEG

_____ B. ECG

_____ C. Urine culture

_____ D. Arterial blood gases

_____ E. Blood culture

3. A nurse is teaching a parent about acetaminophen (Tylenol) poisoning. Which of the following statements by the nurse should be included in the teaching?

A. "Nausea begins 24 hours after ingestion."

B. "Pallor can appear as early as 2 hours after ingestion."

C. "Jaundice will appear in 12 hours if your child is toxic."

D. "Children can have 4 grams of acetaminophen per day."

4. A nurse is caring for a child who has swallowed paint thinner. The child is lethargic, gagging, and cyanotic. Which of the following is an appropriate action for the nurse to take?

A. Induce vomiting with syrup of ipecac.

B. Insert a nasogastric tube and administer activated charcoal.

C. Prepare for intubation with a cuffed endotracheal tube.

D. Administer chelation therapy using deferoxamine mesylate.

5. A nurse in the emergency department is assisting with the admission of a child who experienced an obstructed airway in which the parent performed CPR. Which of the following statements by the parent requires clarification?

      A. "I pushed on my son's abdomen."

      B. "I tilted my son's head back while lifting his chin."

      C. "I listened for sounds of breathing by my son."

      D. "I used my finger to check my son's mouth."

6. A nurse is teaching a group of parents about prevention of sudden infant death syndrome (SIDS). What should be included in the teaching? Use the ATI Active Learning Template: Basic Concept to identify methods to reduce the risk of SIDS.

APPLICATION EXERCISES KEY

1. A. INCORRECT: Bradypnea is an advanced clinical manifestation of hypoxia.

    B. INCORRECT: Cyanosis is an advanced clinical manifestation of hypoxia.

    C. **CORRECT:** Tachycardia is an early clinical manifestation of respiratory distress.

    D. **CORRECT:** Diaphoresis is an early clinical manifestation of respiratory distress.

    E. **CORRECT:** Restlessness is an early clinical manifestation of respiratory distress.

     NCLEX® Connection: Physiological Adaptations, Medical Emergencies

2. A. **CORRECT:** EEG is performed to assess for epilepsy.

    B. **CORRECT:** ECG is performed to assess for long QT syndrome or dysrhythmias.

    C. INCORRECT: A urine specimen is obtain for a culture to assess for a UTI.

    D. INCORRECT: ABGs are not routinely performed for an infant who experienced an apparent life-threatening event.

    E. **CORRECT:** A blood culture is obtained to assess for bacterial or viral infections.

     NCLEX® Connection: Physiological Adaptations, Medical Emergencies

3. A. INCORRECT: Nausea is a clinical manifestation that begins 2 to 4 hr after ingestion.

    B. **CORRECT:** Pallor is a clinical manifestation that starts 2 to 4 hr after ingestion.

    C. INCORRECT: Jaundice will appear in 36 hr to 7 days.

    D. INCORRECT: The maximum dose of acetaminophen in children 2 to 5 years of age is 720 mg/day. In children 6 to 12 years of age, it is 2.6 g/day.

     NCLEX® Connection: Pharmacological and Parenteral Therapies, Adverse Effects/Contraindications/ Side Effects/Interactions

4. A. INCORRECT: Inducing vomiting with syrup of ipecac is contraindicated as a poison control measure.

    B. INCORRECT: Activated charcoal is indicated for acetylsalicylic acid poisoning.

    C. **CORRECT:** Treatment for poisoning with hydrocarbons includes intubation to protect the airway before proceeding with gastric decontamination.

    D. INCORRECT: Chelation therapy is indicated for lead poisoning.

    Ⓝ NCLEX® Connection: Physiological Adaptations, Medical Emergencies

5. A. INCORRECT: Abdominal thrusts are performed to open an obstructed airway in a child as part of CPR.

    B. INCORRECT: The head-tilt, chin-lift method during CPR is used to open an obstructed airway.

    C. INCORRECT: Checking for chest motion and listening for normal breath sounds are steps in evaluating airway clearance when performing CPR.

    D. **CORRECT:** Finger sweeps to check for an impaired airway are not performed as part of CPR.

    Ⓝ NCLEX® Connection: Physiological Adaptations, Medical Emergencies

6. *Using the ATI Active Learning Template: Basic Concept*
    - Methods to reduce the risks of SIDS
      ○ Place infant on back for sleep.
      ○ Avoid exposure to tobacco smoke.
      ○ Prevent overheating.
      ○ Use a firm, tight-fitting mattress in the infant's crib.
      ○ Remove pillows, quilts, and sheepskins from the crib during sleep.
      ○ Ensure that the infant's head is kept uncovered during sleep.
      ○ Offer pacifier at naps and night.
      ○ Encourage breastfeeding.
      ○ Avoid cosleeping.
      ○ Maintain immunizations up to date.

    Ⓝ NCLEX® Connection: Safety and Infection Control, Accident/Error/Injury Prevention

chapter 43

Overview

- Depression
- Posttraumatic stress disorder (PTSD)
- Attention-deficit/hyperactivity disorder (ADHD)
- Autism spectrum disorder
- Cognitive impairment
- Failure to thrive (FTT)
- Maltreatment of infants and children

DEPRESSION

Overview

- Difficult to detect because children have limitations in expressing their feelings.
- Findings must be present for 1 year to diagnose major depressive disorder in children and adolescents.

Assessment

- Risk Factors
  - Family history
  - Traumatic event
- Subjective and Objective Data
  - Sad facial expressions
  - Tendency to remain alone
  - Withdrawn from family, friends, and activities
  - Fatigue
  - Tearful/crying
  - Ill feeling
  - Weight loss or gain
  - Alterations in sleep
  - Lack of interest in school, drop in performance in school
  - Statements regards low self-esteem
  - Hopelessness
  - Suicidal ideations

Patient-Centered Care

- Nursing Care
  - Plan care that is individualized.
  - Obtain health history.
  - Assess for substance use.
  - Assess for actual or potential risk to self (including a suicide plan, the lethality of that plan, and the means to carry out the plan).
  - Assist with coping strategies.
  - Encourage peer group discussions, mentoring, and counseling.
- Medications
  - Tricyclic antidepressants (TCAs) or selective serotonin reuptake inhibitors (SSRIs)
    - Trazodone (Oleptro), sertraline (Zoloft), paroxetine (Paxil), bupropion (Wellbutrin)
    - Nursing Care
      - Monitor for adverse effects.
      - Monitor for suicidal ideations.
    - Client teaching
      - Teach the client and family about adverse effects.
      - Teach the client and family when to expect therapeutic effectiveness.
      - Teach the client and family not to abruptly discontinue the medication.

Complications

- Suicide

POSTTRAUMATIC STRESS DISORDER (PTSD)

Overview

- Develops following a traumatic event

Assessment

- Risk Factors
  - Potential genetic predisposition
  - Traumatic incident
  - Repeated trauma
  - Psychiatric disorder

- Subjective and Objective Data
  - Initial response
    - Lasting a few minutes to 2 hr
    - Increased stress hormones (fight or flight)
  - Second phase
    - Lasting approximately 2 weeks
    - Period of calm (feeling of numbness, denial)
  - Third phase
    - Extends over 2 to 3 months
    - Client gets worse instead of better.
    - Depression, phobias, anxiety, conversion reactions, repetitive movements, flashbacks

Patient-Centered Care

- Nursing Care
  - Refer to psychotherapy services.
  - Monitor for behavior changes/behavior problems.
  - Monitor school work.
  - Assist the family and client with coping strategies.
  - Allow family and client to express their feelings.
- Medications
  - Selective norepinephrine reuptake inhibitor may be used on an individual basis.

ATTENTION-DEFICIT/HYPERACTIVITY DISORDER (ADHD)

Overview

- Inattentiveness, hyperactivity, and impulsiveness
- A child must meet diagnostic criteria to be diagnosed with ADHD.
  - Symptoms are present between the ages of 4 and 18 years.
  - Manifestations are present in more than one setting.
  - Evidence of social or academic impairment.
  - Six or more findings from a category (inattention or hyperactivity-impulsive).

Assessment

- Risk Factors
  - May be a familial tendency
- Subjective and Objective Data
  - Inattention
    - Fails to pay close attention to detail or makes careless mistakes
    - Difficulty sustaining attention
    - Does not seem to listen
    - Fails to follow through on instructions
    - Difficulty organizing activities
    - Avoids or dislikes activities that require mental effort for a period of time
    - Losses things
    - Easily distracted
    - Forgetful
  - Hyperactivity
    - Fidgety
    - Fails to remain seated
    - Inappropriate running
    - Difficulty engaging in quiet play
    - Seems to be busy all the time
    - Talks excessively
  - Impulsivity
    - Blurts out response before question is asked
    - Difficulty waiting turns
    - Interrupts often

Patient-Centered Care

- Nursing Care/Client Teaching
  - Use a calm, firm, respectful approach with the child.
  - Use modeling to demonstrate acceptable behavior.
  - Obtain the child's attention before giving directions. Provide short and clear explanations.
  - Set clear limits on unacceptable behaviors and be consistent.
  - Plan physical activities through which the child can use energy and obtain success.
  - Focus on the family and child's strengths, not just the problems.
  - Support the parents' efforts to remain hopeful.

- ○ Provide a safe environment for the child and others.
- ○ Provide the child with specific positive feedback when expectations are met.
- ○ Identify issues that result in power struggles.
- ○ Assist the child in developing effective coping mechanisms.
- ○ Encourage the child to participate in a form of group, individual, or family therapy.
- ○ Assist the family with behavioral strategies.
  - ▪ Positive reinforcement
  - ▪ Rewards for good behavior
  - ▪ Age-appropriate consequences
- ○ Assist family with modification of the environment to help the child become successful.
  - ▪ Structured environment
  - ▪ Charts to assist with organization
  - ▪ Decreasing stimuli in the environment
  - ▪ Consistent study area
  - ▪ Model positive behaviors
- ○ Assist with appropriate classroom placement in the school.
  - ▪ Allow more time for testing.
  - ▪ Place in classroom that has order and consistent rules.
  - ▪ Offer verbal instruction combined with visual cues.
  - ▪ Plan academic subjects in the morning.
  - ▪ Include regular breaks.
  - ▪ Provide for small classroom settings or work groups.
- • Medications
  - ○ Methylphenidate (Ritalin) or dextroamphetamine (Dexedrine)
    - ▪ Psychostimulant, which increases dopamine and norepinephrine levels
    - ▪ Nursing Considerations/Client Teaching
      - □ Gradually increase dose to reach therapeutic results.
      - □ Give 30 min before meal.
      - □ Give last dose of the day prior to 1800 to prevent insomnia.
      - □ Monitor for adverse effects.
  - ○ Atomoxetine (Strattera)
    - ▪ Selective norepinephrine reuptake inhibitor
    - ▪ Nursing Considerations/Client Teaching
      - □ Gradual increase in dose to reach therapeutic results.
      - □ Monitor for adverse effects (suicidal ideations).

AUTISM SPECTRUM DISORDER

Overview

- Complex neurodevelopmental disorders with spectrum of behaviors affecting an individual's ability to communicate and interact with others.

Assessment

- Risk Factors
  - Possible genetic component
- Subjective and Objective Data
  - Delays in at least one of the following: social interaction, social communication, imaginative play prior to the age of 3 years
  - Distress when routines are changed
  - Unusual attachments to objects
  - Cannot start or continue conversation
  - Uses gestures instead of words
  - Delayed language development
  - Unable to adjust gaze to look at something else
  - Does not refer to self correctly
  - Withdrawn
  - Lack of empathy
  - Spends time alone rather than play with others
  - Avoids eye contact
  - Withdraw from physical contact
  - Heightened or lowered senses
  - Does not imitate actions of others
  - Minimal pretend play
  - Short attention span
  - Intense temper tantrums
  - Shows aggression
  - Exhibits repetitive movements

Patient-Centered Care

- Nursing Care/Client Teaching
  - ○ Assist with screening assessment tools.
  - ○ Refer to early intervention, physical therapy, occupational therapy, and speech and language therapy.
  - ○ Assist with behavior modification program.
    - Promote positive reinforcement.
    - Increase social awareness.
    - Teach verbal communication.
    - Decrease unacceptable behaviors.
    - Set realistic goals.
    - Structure opportunities for small successes.
    - Set clear rules.
  - ○ Decrease environmental stimulation.
  - ○ Assist with nutritional needs.
  - ○ Introduce the child to new situations slowly.
  - ○ Monitor for behavior changes.
  - ○ Encourage age appropriate play.
  - ○ Communicate at an age-appropriate level.
  - ○ Provide support to the family.
  - ○ Encourage support groups.
- Medications
  - ○ Used on an individual basis to control aggression, anxiety, hyperactivity, irritability, mood swings, compulsions and attention problems.

COGNITIVE IMPAIRMENT

Overview

- Mental difficulty or deficiency

Assessment

- Risk Factors
  - ○ Infections (congenital rubella, syphilis)
  - ○ Fetal alcohol syndrome
  - ○ Chronic lead ingestion
  - ○ Trauma to the brain
  - ○ Preexisting disease (Down syndrome, psychiatric disorders, microcephaly, hydrocephaly, metabolic disorders)

- Subjective and Objective Data
  - Can range from mild to severe
  - Delayed developmental milestones
  - Early clinical manifestations
    - Abnormal eye contact
    - Feeding difficulties
    - Language difficulties
    - Gross motor delays
    - Decrease alertness
    - Unresponsive to contact

Patient-Centered Care

- Nursing Care/Client Teaching
  - Determine the child's deficiency.
  - Care and teaching should be individualized to the client's needs.
  - Make appropriate referrals such as early intervention program, social work, speech therapy, physical therapy, and occupational therapy.
  - Add visual cues with verbal instruction.
  - Give one-step instructions.
  - Assist the family in teaching the child self-cares.
  - Assist the family in promoting development.
  - Encourage play.
  - Assist the family with appropriate activities and toys.
  - Assist with communication skills.
  - Encourage social activities.

FAILURE TO THRIVE (FTT)

Overview

- Inadequate growth resulting from the inability to obtain or use calories required for growth. It is usually described in an infant or child who falls below the fifth percentile for weight (and possibly for height) or who has persistent weight loss.
  - Inadequate caloric intake
  - Inadequate absorption
  - Increased metabolism
  - Defective utilization

Assessment

- Risk Factor
  - Organic causes: cerebral palsy, chronic renal failure, congenital heart disease, hyperthyroidism, cystic fibrosis, celiac disease, hepatic disease, Down syndrome, prematurity, and gastroesophageal reflux
  - Parental neglect, lack of parental knowledge, or a disturbed maternal-child attachment
  - Poverty
  - Health or childrearing beliefs
  - Family stress
  - Feeding resistance
  - Insufficient breast milk
- Subjective and Objective Data
  - Less than the fifth percentile on the growth chart for weight
  - Malnourished appearance
  - No fear of strangers
  - Minimal smiling
  - Decreased activity level
  - Withdrawal behavior
  - Developmental delays
  - Feeding disorder
  - Wide-eyed gaze
  - Stiff or flaccid body

Patient-Centered Care

- Nursing Care
  - Obtain a nutritional history.
  - Observe parent-child interactions.
  - Obtain accurate baseline height and weight. Observe for low weight, malnourished appearance, and signs of dehydration.
  - Weigh the child daily without clothing or a diaper.
  - Maintain I&O and calorie counts as prescribed.
  - Teach parents to recognize and respond to the infant's cues of hunger.
  - Establish a routine for eating that encourages usual times, duration, and setting.
  - Reinforce proper positioning, latching on, and timing for mothers who are breastfeeding.
  - Provide 24 kcal/oz formula as prescribed.
  - Provide high-calorie milk supplements for children.
  - Administer multivitamin supplements including zinc and iron.

- ○ Teach parents how to mix formula properly and provide step by step written instructions.
- ○ Limit juice to 4 oz/day.
- ○ Provide developmental stimulation.
- ○ Encourage parents to:
  - Maintain eye contact and face-to-face posture during feedings.
  - Talk to the infant while feeding.
  - Burp the infant frequently.
  - Keep the environment quiet and avoid distractions.
  - Be persistent, remaining calm during 10 to 15 min of food refusal.
  - Introduce new foods slowly.
  - Never force the infant to eat.

Complications

- Extreme malnourishment
  - ○ Nursing Care – Prepare the client and the parents for tube feedings or IV therapy.

MALTREATMENT OF INFANTS AND CHILDREN

Overview

- Maltreatment of infants and children is attributed to a variety of predisposing factors, which include parental, child, and environmental characteristics. Child maltreatment can occur across all economic and educational backgrounds and racial/ethnic/religious groups.
  - ○ Maltreatment of children is made up of several specific types of behaviors.
    - Physical – causing pain or harm to a child (shaken baby syndrome [due to violent shaking of infants], fractures, Munchausen syndrome by proxy)
    - Sexual – occurring when sexual contact takes place without consent, whether or not the victim is able to give consent (includes any sexual behavior toward a minor and dating violence among adolescents)
    - Emotional – humiliating, threatening, or intimidating a child (includes behavior that minimizes an individual's feelings of self-worth)
    - Neglect – includes failure to provide:
      - □ Physical care (feeding, clothing, shelter, medical or dental care, safety, education)
      - □ Emotional care and/or stimulation to foster normal development (nurturing, affection, attention)

Assessment

- Warning signs of abuse
  - Physical evidence of abuse
  - History of injury incompatible with the findings
  - Vague explanation of injury
  - Other injuries are discovered that are not related to the original client concern
  - Delay in seeking care
  - Multiple fractures at different stages of healing
  - Bruising in a nonmobile client
  - Caregivers/client report conflicting histories
  - Statement of possible abuse from a caregiver or client
- Parental characteristics
  - Younger parents
  - Single parents
  - Socially isolated
  - Low-income situation
  - Lack of lower education level
  - Low self-esteem
  - Lack of knowledge of parenting
  - Substance use disorder
  - History of having been abused
- Characteristics of the child
  - Child 1 year old or younger is at greater risk due to the need for constant attention and increased demands of caregiving.
  - Infants and children who are unwanted, hyperactive, or physically or mentally disabled are at risk due to their increased demands and need for constant attention.
  - Premature infants are at risk due to the possible failure of parent-child bonding at birth.
- Environmental characteristics
  - Chronic stress
  - Divorce, alcohol use disorder, drug addiction, poverty, unemployment, inadequate housing, and crowded living conditions
- Subjective and Objective Data
  - Inconsistencies between the parent/caregiver's report and the child's injuries
  - Inconsistency between nature of injury and developmental level of the child
  - Repeated injuries requiring emergency treatment
  - Inappropriate responses from the parents or child

- ○ Physical neglect
  - ▪ Failure to thrive, malnutrition
  - ▪ Lack of hygiene
  - ▪ Frequent injuries
  - ▪ Delay in seeking health care
  - ▪ Dull affect
  - ▪ School absences
  - ▪ Self-stimulating behaviors
- ○ Physical abuse
  - ▪ Bruises, welts in various stages of healing
  - ▪ Burns
  - ▪ Fractures
  - ▪ Lacerations
  - ▪ Fear of parents
  - ▪ Lack of emotional response/reaction
  - ▪ Superficial relationships
  - ▪ Withdrawal
  - ▪ Aggression
- ○ Emotional neglect and abuse
  - ▪ Failure to thrive
  - ▪ Eating disorder
  - ▪ Enuresis
  - ▪ Sleep disturbances
  - ▪ Self-stimulating behaviors
  - ▪ Withdrawal
  - ▪ Lack of social smile (infant)
  - ▪ Extreme behaviors
  - ▪ Delayed development
  - ▪ Attempts suicide
- ○ Sexual abuse
  - ▪ Bruises, lacerations, bleeding of genitalia, anus, or mouth
  - ▪ Sexually transmitted infection
  - ▪ Difficulty walking or standing
  - ▪ UTI
  - ▪ Regressive behavior
  - ▪ Withdrawn
  - ▪ Personality changes

- Shaken baby syndrome – Shaking can cause intracranial hemorrhage.
    - Manifestations
        - Vomiting, poor feeding and listlessness
        - Respiratory distress
        - Bulging fontanels
        - Retinal hemorrhages
        - Seizures
        - Posturing
        - Alterations in LOC
        - Apnea
        - Bradycardia
    - If bruising is present in an infant before 6 months of age, it should be deemed as suspicious by the nurse.
- Laboratory Tests
    - CBC, urinalysis, and other tests that assess for sexually transmitted infections or bleeding
- Diagnostic Procedures – depend upon the assessment findings and noted findings or injuries.
    - Radiograph
    - CT scan or magnetic resonance imaging scan (MRI)

Patient-Centered Care

- Nursing Care
    - Identify abuse as soon as possible
    - Assess for unusual bruising on the abdomen, back, and/or buttocks.
    - Assess the mechanism of injury, which may not be congruent with the physical appearance of the injury. Many bruises at different stages of healing may indicate ongoing beatings.
    - Observe for bruises or welts in the shape of a belt buckle or other objects.
    - Observe for burns that appear glove- or stocking-like on hands or feet, which may indicate forced immersion into boiling water. Small, round burns may be caused by lit cigarettes.
    - Note fractures with unusual features, such as forearm spiral fractures, which could be caused by twisting the extremity forcefully. The presence of multiple fractures is suspicious.
    - Check the child for head injuries. Assess the child's level of consciousness, making sure to note equal and reactive pupils. Also, monitor the child for nausea/vomiting.
    - The nursing priority is to have the child removed from the abusive situation.
    - Mandatory reporting is required of all health care providers, including suspected or actual cases of child abuse. There are civil and criminal penalties for not reporting.
    - Clearly and objectively document information obtained in the interview and during the physical assessment.

- ○ Photograph and detail all visible injuries.

- ○ Conduct the interview with the client and parents individually.

- ○ Be direct, honest, and professional.

- ○ Use language the child understands.

- ○ Be understanding and attentive.

- ○ Client circumstances are case-sensitive, and referrals are made to always keep the client safe. When applicable, explain the process if a referral is made to child or adult protective services.

- ○ Assess safety and reduce danger for the victim.

- ○ Use open-ended questions that require a descriptive response. These questions are less threatening and elicit more relevant information.

- ○ Provide support for the child and parents.

- ○ Demonstrate behaviors for child-rearing with the parents and child.

- ○ Provide consistent care to the child.

- ○ Avoid asking the child probing questions.

- ○ Promote self-esteem.

- ○ Assist with alleviating feelings of shame and guilt.

- ○ Assist the child with grieving the loss of parents, if indicated.

- ○ Discharge can begin once legal determination of placement has been decided.

- • Teamwork and Collaboration – Initiate appropriate referrals for social services.

APPLICATION EXERCISES

1. A nurse is teaching a group of parents about infants who have failure to thrive. Which of the following characteristics should be included in the teaching?

    A. They have been neglected.

    B. They come from an impoverished environment.

    C. They manifest colicky behaviors.

    D. They exhibit developmental delays.

2. A nurse is providing instruction to the teacher of a child who has attention-deficit/hyperactivity disorder (ADHD). Which of the following classroom strategies should be included in the teaching? (Select all that apply.)

_____ A. Eliminate testing.

_____ B. Allow for regular breaks.

_____ C. Combine verbal instruction with visual cues.

_____ D. Establish consistent classroom rules.

_____ E. Decrease stimuli in the environment.

3. A nurse is teaching a parent about posttraumatic stress disorder (PTSD). Which of the following should be included in the teaching? (Select all that apply.)

_____ A. Children who have PTSD require psychotherapy.

_____ B. A clinical manifestation of PTSD is phobias.

_____ C. Depression is seen within 1 day after the incident.

_____ D. PTSD develops following a traumatic event.

_____ E. There are six stages of PTSD.

4. A nurse is providing teaching to the parent of a child who has attention-deficit/hyperactivity disorder. The nurse should include which of the following as a characteristic of impulsivity?

    A. Loses things

    B. Frequently interrupts

    C. Is easily distracted

    D. Talks excessively

5. A nurse is caring for a child who has depression. Which of the following findings are associated with this diagnosis? (Select all that apply.)

_____ A. Prefers being with peers

_____ B. Weight loss

_____ C. Report of low self-esteem

_____ D. Sleeping more than usual

_____ E. Hyperactivity

6. A nurse is teaching a group of parents about shaken baby syndrome. What clinical manifestations should be included in this presentation? Use the ATI Active Learning Template: Basic Concept to complete this item to include describing at least seven clinical manifestations.

APPLICATION EXERCISES KEY

1. A. INCORRECT: Failure to thrive could be caused by neglect, but there are other risk factors that can cause failure to thrive.

    B. INCORRECT: Poverty could be a risk factor for failure to thrive, but not all clients who have failure to thrive are from impoverished environments.

    C. INCORRECT: Infants who have failure to thrive exhibit a withdrawn behavior.

    D. **CORRECT:** Infants who have failure to thrive exhibit developmental delays as a result of decreased nutritional intake needed for brain development.

    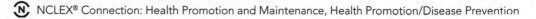 NCLEX® Connection: Health Promotion and Maintenance, Health Promotion/Disease Prevention

2. A. INCORRECT: Allowing for added time when testing may assist the client who has ADHD to be successful.

    B. **CORRECT:** Allowing for regular breaks will assist the client who has ADHD to focus on the required tasks.

    C. **CORRECT:** Combining verbal instruction with visual cues will assist the client who has ADHD with learning information.

    D. **CORRECT:** Providing consistent classroom rules will assist the client who has ADHD to become successful.

    E. **CORRECT:** Stimuli in the environment distract the client who has ADHD, so they should be decreased.

    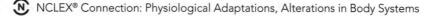 NCLEX® Connection: Physiological Adaptations, Alterations in Body Systems

3. A. **CORRECT:** Children who have PTSD should be referred to psychotherapy to assist with resolution of the traumatic event.

    B. **CORRECT:** The child who is experiencing PTSD often has new phobias that can be related to the traumatic event.

    C. INCORRECT: Depression is a clinical manifestation that is seen approximately 2 weeks following the incident.

    D. **CORRECT:** PTSD develops following a traumatic event such as assault, serious injury, or a life-threatening episode.

    E. INCORRECT: PTSD has three stages: the initial response, second, and third phase.

    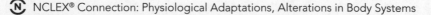 NCLEX® Connection: Physiological Adaptations, Alterations in Body Systems

4.   A. INCORRECT: Losing things is a characteristic of inattention.

     B. **CORRECT:** Frequently interrupting is a characteristic of impulsivity.

     C. INCORRECT: Being easily distracted is a characteristic of inattention.

     D. INCORRECT: Talking excessively is a characteristic of hyperactivity.

     Ⓝ NCLEX® Connection: Physiological Adaptations, Illness Management

5.   A. INCORRECT: A preference for being alone is a finding associated with depression.

     B. **CORRECT:** Weight loss or gain are findings associated with depression.

     C. **CORRECT:** Low self-esteem is a finding associated with depression.

     D. **CORRECT:** Sleeping more than usual is a finding associated with depression.

     E. INCORRECT: Fatigue is a finding associated with depression.

     Ⓝ NCLEX® Connection: Physiological Adaptations, Illness Management

6.   *Using the ATI Active Learning Template: Basic Concept*
     • Clinical Manifestations
       ○ Vomiting, poor feeding, and listlessness
       ○ Respiratory distress
       ○ Bulging fontanels
       ○ Retinal hemorrhages
       ○ Seizures
       ○ Posturing
       ○ Alterations in LOC
       ○ Apnea
       ○ Bradycardia

     Ⓝ NCLEX® Connection: Physiological Adaptations, Pathophysiology

REFERENCES

Dudek, S. G. (2010). *Nutrition essentials for nursing practice* (6th ed.). Philadelphia: Lippincott Williams & Wilkins.

Grodner, M., Roth, S. L., & Walkingshaw, B. C. (2012). *Nutrition foundations and clinical applications of nutrition: A nursing approach* (5th ed.). St. Louis, MO: Mosby.

Hockenberry, M. J., & Winkelstein M. L. (2013). *Wong's essentials of pediatric nursing* (9th ed.). St. Louis, MO: Mosby.

Lowdermilk, D. L., Perry, S. E., Cahsion, M. C., & Aldean, K. R. (2012). *Maternity & women's health care* (10th ed.). St. Louis, MO: Mosby.

Lehne, R. A. (2013). *Pharmacology for nursing care* (8th ed.). St. Louis: Saunders.

Perry, S. E., Hockenberry, M. J., Lowdermilk, D. L., & Wilson, D. (2010). *Maternal child nursing care* (4th ed.). St. Louis, MO: Mosby Elsevier.

Pillitteri, A. (2010). *Maternal and child health nursing: Care of the childbearing and childrearing family* (6th ed.). Philadelphia: Lippincott Williams & Wilkins.

Wilson, B. A., Shannon, M. T., & Shields, K. M. (2013). *Pearson nurse's drug guide 2013*. Upper Saddle River, NJ: Prentice Hall.

Varcarolis, E. M., Carson, V. B., & Shoemaker, N. C. (2010). *Foundations of psychiatric mental health nursing: A clinical approach* (6th ed.). St. Louis, MO: Saunders.

APPENDIX	ACTIVE LEARNING TEMPLATES
TEMPLATE	Basic Concept

CONTENT_____ REVIEW MODULE CHAPTER _____

TOPIC DESCRIPTOR_____

Related Content
(e.g. delegation, levels of prevention, advance directives)

Underlying Principles

Nursing Interventions
› Who?
› When?
› Why?
› How?

Appendix

CONTENT _____ REVIEW MODULE CHAPTER _____

TOPIC DESCRIPTOR _____

DESCRIPTION OF PROCEDURE:

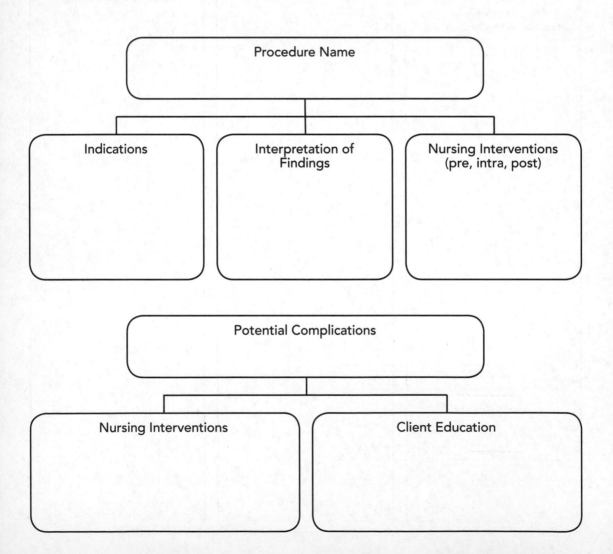

APPENDIX   ACTIVE LEARNING TEMPLATES

TEMPLATE   System Disorder

CONTENT_____ REVIEW MODULE CHAPTER _____

TOPIC DESCRIPTOR_____

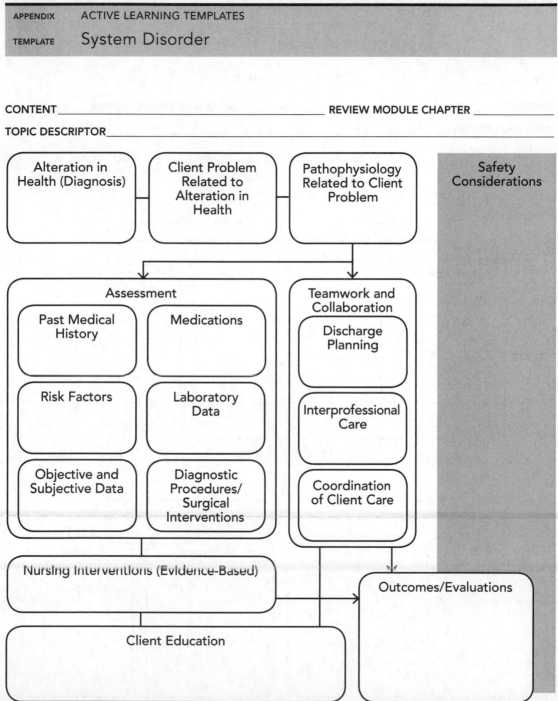

Appendix

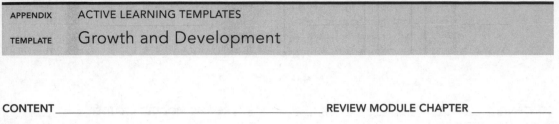

APPENDIX   ACTIVE LEARNING TEMPLATES

TEMPLATE   Growth and Development

CONTENT _____ REVIEW MODULE CHAPTER _____

TOPIC DESCRIPTOR _____

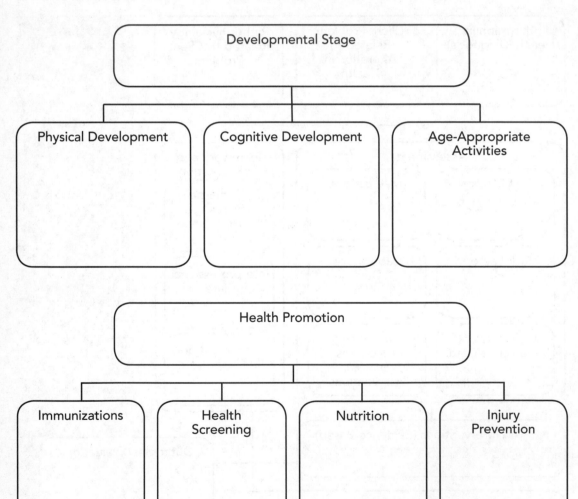

Developmental Stage

Physical Development

Cognitive Development

Age-Appropriate Activities

Health Promotion

Immunizations

Health Screening

Nutrition

Injury Prevention

APPENDIX ACTIVE LEARNING TEMPLATES

TEMPLATE Medication

CONTENT _____ REVIEW MODULE CHAPTER _____

TOPIC DESCRIPTOR_____

MEDICATION _____

EXPECTED PHARMACOLOGICAL ACTION:

Therapeutic Uses

Adverse Effects

Nursing Interventions

Contraindications

Client Education

Medication/Food Interactions

Medication Administration

Evaluation of Medication Effectiveness

Appendix

CONTENT_____ REVIEW MODULE CHAPTER _____

TOPIC DESCRIPTOR_____

DESCRIPTION OF SKILL:

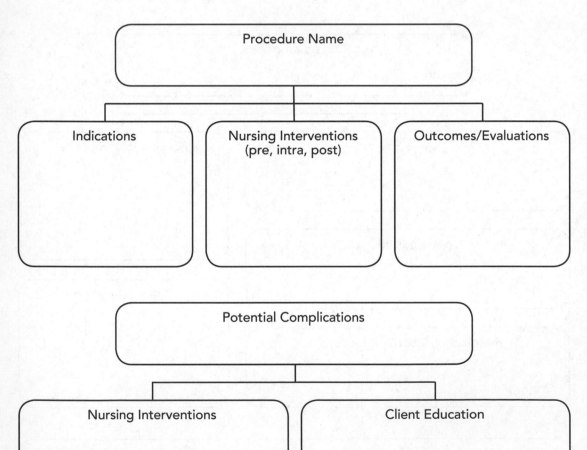

Appendix

CONTENT_____ REVIEW MODULE CHAPTER _____

TOPIC DESCRIPTOR_____

DESCRIPTION OF PROCEDURE:

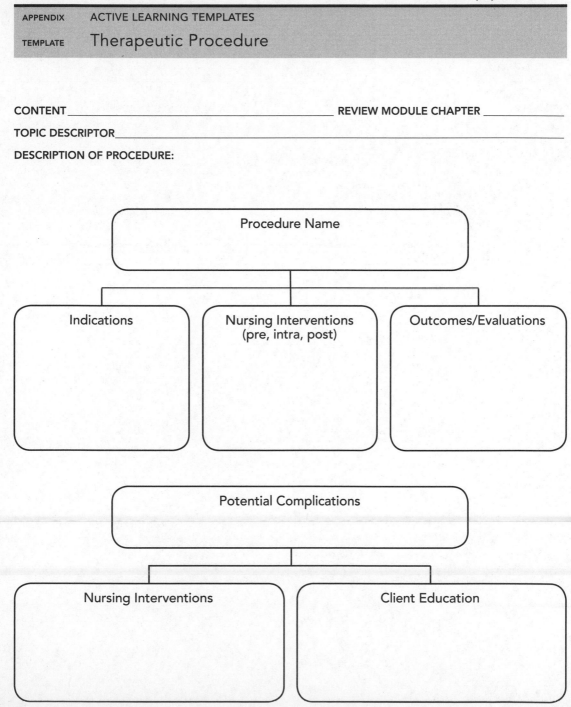

Procedure Name

Indications

Nursing Interventions
(pre, intra, post)

Outcomes/Evaluations

Potential Complications

Nursing Interventions

Client Education